50 Landmark Papers

every

Intensivist Should Know

- 50 Landmark Papers every Spine Surgeon Should Know, Vaccaro, Fisher & Wilson, 9781498768306
- 50 Landmark Papers every Trauma Surgeon Should Know, Cohn & Feinstein, 9781138506299
- 50 Landmark Papers every Acute Surgeon Should Know, Cohn & Rhee, 9781138624443
- 50 Landmark Papers every Vascular & Endovascular Surgeon Should Know, Jimenez & Wilson, 9781138334380
- 50 Landmark Papers every Oral & Maxillofacial Surgeon Should Know, McLeod & Brennan, 9780367210526

Available from www.routledge.com

50 LANDMARK PAPERS

every Intensivist Should Know

EDITED BY

Stephen M. Cohn, MD

Professor of Surgery
Hackensack Meridian School of Medicine
Nutley, New Jersey, USA

Alan Lisbon, MD

Executive Vice Chair, Emeritus
Anesthesia, Critical Care, and Pain Medicine
Beth Israel Deaconess Medical Center
Associate Professor of Anaesthesia
Harvard Medical School
Boston, Massachusetts, USA

Stephen Heard, MD

Professor Emeritus of Anesthesiology and Surgery
Department of Anesthesiology and Perioperative Medicine
UMass Memorial Medical Center, University of Massachusetts Medical School
Worcester, Massachusetts, USA

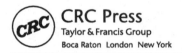

CRC Press
Taylor & Francis Group
Boca Raton London New York

CRC Press is an imprint of the
Taylor & Francis Group, an **informa** business

First edition published 2022
by CRC Press
6000 Broken Sound Parkway NW, Suite 300, Boca Raton, FL 33487-2742

and by CRC Press
2 Park Square, Milton Park, Abingdon, Oxon, OX14 4RN

© 2022 Taylor & Francis Group, LLC
CRC Press is an imprint of Taylor & Francis Group, LLC

Library of Congress Cataloging-in-Publication Data

Names: Cohn, Stephen M., editor. | Lisbon, Alan, editor. | Heard, Stephen, editor.
Title: 50 landmark papers every intensivist should know / edited by Stephen M. Cohn, Alan Lisbon, Stephen Heard.
Other titles: Fifty landmark papers every intensivist should know
Description: Boca Raton : CRC Press, 2021. | Includes bibliographical references and index.
Identifiers: LCCN 2021009259 (print) | LCCN 2021009260 (ebook) | ISBN 9780367486549 (hardback) | ISBN 9780367462413 (paperback) | ISBN 9781003042136 (ebook)
Subjects: MESH: Critical Care | Intensive Care Units | Review
Classification: LCC RC86.8 (print) | LCC RC86.8 (ebook) | NLM WX 218 | DDC 616.02/8--dc23
LC record available at https://lccn.loc.gov/2021009259
LC ebook record available at https://lccn.loc.gov/2021009260

ISBN: 9780367486549 (hbk)
ISBN: 9780367462413 (pbk)
ISBN: 9781003042136 (ebk)

DOI: 10.1201/9781003042136

Typeset in Times
by KnowledgeWorks Global Ltd.

Contents

Section Two   Cardiac

Section Three   Renal

    THERAPY   73
    Review by Kenneth Ralto and Matthew J. Trainor

    **Continuous Venovenous Haemodiafiltration Versus
    Intermittent Haemodialysis for Acute Renal Failure in Patients
    with Multiple-Organ Dysfunction Syndrome: A Multicenter
    Randomised Trial**

    Vinsonneau C et al., *Lancet.* 2006;368(9533):379–385

    Commentary by Christophe Vinsonneau

14 COLLOID VERSUS CRYSTALLOIDS   79
    Review by Peter Rhee and Stephen Heard

    **A Comparison of Albumin and Saline for Fluid Resuscitation in
    the Intensive Care Unit**

    Finfer S et al., *N Engl J Med.* 2004;350(22):2247–2256

    Commentary by Matthew J. Dolich

Section Four   Gastrointestinal

Section Five   Infection

Section Six   Endocrine

Section Seven   Neurological Conditions

Section Eight   Hematology

Section Nine   Trauma

Contributors

Suresh Agarwal
Duke University Hospital
Durham, North Carolina

Abdul Alarhayem
Cleveland Clinic Foundation
Cleveland, Ohio

Hasan B. Alam
University of Michigan Medical School
Ann Arbor, Michigan

Rae M. Allain
Beth Israel Deaconess Medical Center
Boston, Massachusetts

Umar F. Bhatti
University of Michigan Medical School
Ann Arbor, Michigan

John K. Bini
Wilford Hall Medical Center
Dayton, Ohio

Steven Blau
HMH Hackensack University Medical Center
Hackensack, New Jersey

Daniel J. Bonville
University of Houston College of
    Medicine
Houston, Texas

Somnath Bose
Beth Israel Deaconess Medical Center
Boston, Massachusetts

Brian Brisebois
UMass Chan Medical School
Worcester, Massachusetts

Eileen M. Bulger
University of Washington Medicine
Seattle, Washington

Robert J. Canelli
Boston University School of Medicine
Boston, Massachusetts

Raphael A. Carandang
University of Massachusetts Medical School
Worcester, Massachusetts

Jeffrey L. Carson
Robert Wood Johnson University Hospital
New Brunswick, New Jersey

Michael P. Casaer
University Hospitals and Catholic
    University Leuven
Leuven, Belgium

Jessica Cassavaugh
Beth Israel Deaconess Medical Center
Boston, Massachusetts

Philip Chan
Beth Israel Deaconess Medical Center
Boston, Massachusetts

Jean Chastre
Université Pierre et Marie Curie
Paris, France

Michael L. Cheatham
Orlando Regional Medical Center
Orlando, Florida

Randall M. Chesnut
University of Washington School of
    Medicine
Seattle, Washington

Morgan Crigger
The University of Arizona
Phoenix, Arizona

Martin A. Croce
University of Tennessee Health Science Center
Memphis, Tennessee

Bruce Crookes
Medical University South Carolina
Charleston, South Carolina

Saraswati Dayal
HMH Hackensack University Medical Center
Hackensack, New Jersey

Tara DiNitto
Grand Strand Surgical Care
Myrtle Beach, South Carolina

Matthew J. Dolich
University of California, Irvine
Irvine, California

Kevin Dushay
Warren Alpert Medical School of Brown
    University
Providence, Rhode Island

Akpofure Peter Ekeh
Wright State University
Miami, Florida

Richard T. Ellison III
University of Massachusetts Medical School
Worcester, Massachusetts

Eric D. Endean
University of Kentucky College of Medicine
Lexington, Kentucky

Ara J. Feinstein
University of Arizona
Phoenix, Arizona

Dina M. Filiberto
University of Tennessee Health Science Center
Memphis, Tennessee

Andrew L.A. Garton
Weill Cornell Medical College
New York, New York

Enrique Ginzburg
University of Miami Health System
Miami, Florida

E. Wilson Grandin
Beth Israel Deaconess Medical
    Center
Boston, Massachusetts

Michael Gropper
University of California, San Francisco
San Francisco, California

Jan Gunst
University Hospitals and Catholic
    University Leuven
Leuven, Belgium

Morad Hameed
The University of British Columbia
Vancouver, Canada

Dominic A. Harris
Beth Israel Deaconess Medical Center
Boston, Massachusetts

Samuel Isaac Hawkins
HMH Hackensack University Medical
    Center
Hackensack, New Jersey

Stephen Heard
University of Massachusetts Medical
    School
Worcester, Massachusetts

Paul C. Hébert
University of Montreal
Montreal, Quebec, Canada

Nicholas S. Hill
Tufts University School of Medicine
Boston, Massachusetts

Melanie P. Hoenig
Harvard Medical School
Boston, Massachusetts

Robert C. Hyzy
University of Michigan School of Medicine
Ann Arbor, Michigan

Kenji Inaba
Keck School of Medicine of USC
Los Angeles, California

Sandeep Jubbal
University of Massachusetts Medical School
Worcester, Massachusetts

Kunal Karamchandani
UT Southwestern Medical Center
Dallas, Texas

Riyad C. Karmy-Jones
PeaceHealth Medical Group – Vancouver
Vancouver, Canada

Sanjeev Kaul
HMH Hackensack University Medical Center
Hackensack, New Jersey

Josbert Keller
Leiden University Medical Center
Leiden, Belgium

Natasha Keric
Banner University Medical Center
Phoenix, AZ

Jared A. Knopman
Weill Cornell Medical College
New York, NY

Jennifer Kodela
University of Massachusetts Medical School
Worcester, Massachusetts

Scott Kopec
University of Massachusetts Medical School
Worcester, Massachusetts

Jason Kovacevic
UMass Memorial Medical Center
Worcester, Massachusetts

Megan Lynn Krajewski
Beth Israel Deaconess Medical Center
Boston, Massachusetts

John P. Kress
The University of Chicago
Chicago, Illinois

Anand Kumar
University of Manitoba
Winnipeg, Canada

Catherine Kuza
Keck School of Medicine of USC
Los Angeles, California

John G. Laffey
National University of Ireland
Galway, Ireland

Claire Larson Isbell
Baylor Scott and White Hospital
Temple, Texas

James Y. W. Lau
The Chinese University of Hong Kong
Central Ave, Hong Kong

Craig M. Lilly
University of Massachusetts Medical School
Worcester, Massachusetts

Sungho Lim
Cleveland Clinic Foundation
Cleveland, Ohio

Edward Lineen
University of Miami Health System
Miami, Florida

Peter P. Lopez
Henry Ford Health System
Detroit, Michigan

Jennifer Lynde
Wright State University
Miami, Florida

Hesham H. Malik
University of Massachusetts Medical School
Worcester, Massachusetts

Theofilos P. Matheos
University of Massachusetts Medical
    School
Worcester, Massachusetts

Jason Matos
Beth Israel Deaconess Medical Center
Boston, Massachusetts

Addison K. May
Atrium Health
Charlotte, North Carolina

Barbara Mayer
Stanford Health Care
Stanford, California

Joyce McIntyre
University of Massachusetts Medical
    School
Worcester, Massachusetts

Ronny Munoz-Acuna
Beth Israel Deaconess Medical Center
Boston, Massachusetts

Venkatesh A. Murugan
University of Massachusetts Medical
    School
Worcester, Massachusetts

John Muscedere
Faculty of Health Sciences at Queen's
    University
Kingston, Ontario, Canada

Michael F. Musso
Reading Hospital
Reading, Pennsylvania

Els van Nood
Erasmus Medical Center
Rotterdam, the Netherlands

Brian O'Gara
Beth Israel Deaconess Medical Center
Boston, Massachusetts

Adrian W. Ong
Reading Hospital, Tower Health System
Reading, Pennsylvania

Bruck Or
University of Massachusetts Medical School
Worcester, Massachusetts

Ameeka Pannu
Beth Israel Deaconess Medical Center
Boston, Massachusetts

Manish S. Patel
Robert Wood Johnson University Hospital
New Brunswick, New Jersey

Akhil Patel
Cooper University Medical School of
    Rowan University
Camden, New Jersey

Andrew B. Peitzman
University of Pittsburgh
Pittsburgh, Pennsylvania

Javier Martin Perez
HMH Hackensack University Medical
    Center
Hackensack, New Jersey

Juan M. Perez Velazquez
University of Massachusetts Medical
    School
Worcester, Massachusetts

Duane S. Pinto
Beth Israel Deaconess Medical Center
Boston, Massachusetts

Kenneth Ralto
University of Massachusetts Medical
    School
Worcester, Massachusetts

Emily M. Ramasra
Day Kimball Medical Group
Dayville, Connecticut

Todd E. Rasmussen
Uniformed Services University of the
    Health Sciences
Bethesda, Maryland

Peter Rhee
Westchester Medical Center
Valhalla, New York

Emanuel P. Rivers
Henry Ford Hospital
Detroit, Michigan

Ian Roberts
London School of Hygiene and Tropical
    Medicine
London, United Kingdom

Karen Safcsak
Orlando Regional Medical Center
Orlando, Florida

Hjalmar C. van Santvoort
St Antonius Hospital Nieuwegein and
    University Medical Center
Utrecht, the Netherlands

Stephanie A. Savage
University of Wisconsin School of
    Medicine and Public Health
Madison, Wisconsin

Mark D. Sawyer
Mayo Clinic Health System
Rochester, Minnesota

Robert Sawyer
Western Michigan University Homer
    Stryker School of Medicine
Kalamazoo, Michigan

Magdy Selim
Beth Israel Deaconess Medical Center
Boston, Massachusetts

Paulette Seymour-Route
University of Massachusetts Medical School
Worcester, Massachusetts

Jyoti Sharma
HMH Hackensack University Medical
    Center
Hackensack, New Jersey

Shahla Siddiqui
Beth Israel Deaconess Medical Center
Boston, Massachusetts

Vasiliy Sim
Memorial Hospital
Jacksonville, Florida

Mervyn Singer
University College London
London, United Kingdom

Nicholas A. Smyrnios
University of Massachusetts Medical
    School
Worcester, Massachusetts

Emily E. Switzer
Keck School of Medicine of USC
Los Angeles, California

Gavin Tansley
The University of British Columbia
Vancouver, Canada

Ajith J. Thomas
Beth Israel Deaconess Medical Center
Boston, Massachusetts

Allison J. Tompeck
Banner University Medical Center
Phoenix, Arizona

Ulises Torres Cordero
University of Massachusetts Medical
    School
Worcester, Massachusetts

Matthew J. Trainor
University of Massachusetts Medical
    School
Worcester, Massachusetts

Greet Van den Berghe
University Hospitals and Catholic
    University Leuven
Leuven, Belgium

Ana M. Velez-Rosborough
University of Miami Health System
Miami, Florida

Christophe Vinsonneau
Hopital de Bethune
Bethune, France

Daniel Walsh
Beth Israel Deaconess Medical Center
Boston, Massachusetts

Brooks Willar
Beth Israel Deaconess Medical Center
Boston, Massachusetts

Jeffrey H. William
Beth Israel Deaconess Medical Center
Boston, Massachusetts

Paul J. Young
Wellington Regional Hospital
Wellington South, New Zealand

Peter J. Zimetbaum
Beth Israel Deaconess Medical Center
Boston, Massachusetts

CHAPTER 1

Diagnosis and Epidemiology of ARDS

Review by Nicholas S. Hill

Acute respiratory distress syndrome (ARDS) is a disease of modern technology. Without oxygen supplementation and mechanical ventilation as well as modern diagnostic technology, patients with incipient respiratory failure cannot survive long enough to show more than the initial features of ARDS let alone have the diagnosis made. It is not an accident that Ashbaugh and Petty described the syndrome during the 1960s as ICUs and blood gas machines were becoming available, and they also launching their academic careers.

ARDS clearly antedated its description. Mendelsohn's syndrome was an example, described during the late 1940s in women who developed often lethal severe hypoxic respiratory failure after gastric aspiration that occurred as they were being intubated during labor, a common practice at that time. The reports of Da Nang Lung on massive trauma victims during the Vietnam War was another.

The dozen patients described by Ashbaugh and Petty in their *Lancet* 1967 report exemplified the typical findings of the syndrome: acute onset of severe dyspnea, cyanosis, and bilateral patchy infiltrates on chest x-ray. Patients responded poorly to oxygen supplementation unless given positive end-expiratory pressure (PEEP), and lung compliance was low. Pathology revealed diffuse alveolar damage and hyaline membranes. Some patients seemed to respond to corticosteroids, but mortality was still very high at 75%.

In the years since the syndrome was described, the epidemiology of ARDS has been very controversial with estimates of incidence varying from 3.5/100,000/yr on one of the Canary Islands to 58.7/100,000/yr for the Seattle area. On average, the incidence in the US has been much higher than in Europe, sometimes by an order of magnitude. Possible reasons for these disparities are manifold but include the use of different definitions that have been evolving over time: under and over-reporting, different populations with different risk factors, and health practices in different regions, hospitals, and even ICUs within the same hospital. Some of the more notable studies include the one done near Seattle, which came up with an incidence of 58.7/100,000/yr and used careful screening and quality control to avoid missing patients. The COVID-19 pandemic will undoubtedly affect the incidence of ARDS for the years 2020 and 2021, but it is too early for the cases to have been counted yet.

DOI: 10.1201/9781003042136-1

A number of risk factors are well known to affect the likelihood of developing ARDS as well as outcomes. These include age, which in the Kings County, Washington, study (near Seattle) showed that patients >85 were almost 200 times more likely to have ARDS than those in their late teens. Other important risk factors for ARDS and mortality include immunodeficiency and multi-organ deficiency.

As a syndrome, ARDS is associated with no one etiology or mechanism of injury. Instead, there are dozens that have been identified, lumped broadly into pulmonary (or direct) and extra-pulmonary (or indirect) categories. The former includes pneumonia, aspiration pneumonitis, toxin inhalation, and near drowning as a few examples, whereas the latter includes sepsis, severe trauma, pancreatitis, and massive transfusion, and carries a worse prognosis because it is more often associated with multi-organ system dysfunction.

Mortality of ARDS has been less controversial than the incidence of ARDS. Earlier studies showed mortalities exceeding 50%, ranging up to 70%. Since the 1990s, overall mortality has been in the 40% range. The ALIEN study from Spain was disappointing in that the overall hospital mortality rate was nearly 48% despite the implementation of lung-protective ventilator strategies over the previous decade. The more recent LUNG SAFE trial has also shown overall hospital mortality rates in the 40% range for moderate and severe ARDS, corresponding to the ARDS category in the American European Consensus Conference (AECC) definition of ARDS, and was also disappointing in this regard. This may be related to the fact that mortality of ARDS is less often related to the respiratory failure than to other organ failures.

The LUNG SAFE study used a computer algorithm to screen for ARDS according to the Berlin definition, and the rate of clinician recognition was determined by if they included it as a potential diagnosis in their notes. Recognition was only roughly 50% in mild ARDS but nearly 89% in severe ARDS. Lack of recognition was associated with fewer interventions that have been shown to be associated with better outcomes in ARDS such as lung-protective ventilator strategies, higher levels of PEEP, and using the prone position.

Splitters often consider ARDS a "wastebasket" diagnosis which lumps too many different etiologies into the same bucket. This has complicated making sense of the epidemiology because ARDS in one study may not be defined and detected in the same way as the next. It also complicates clinical trials because of the heterogeneity of the populations enrolled. On the other hand, it has been useful for the study of therapies that address the common pulmonary pathophysiology such as using low tidal volumes or the prone position. In the not too distant future, using precision medicine, it may be possible to better delineate different mechanisms of ARDS, which should refine the classification and pave the way for trials of better targeted therapies.

ANNOTATED REFERENCES FOR DIAGNOSIS AND EPIDEMIOLOGY OF ARDS

ARDS Definition Task Force. Acute respiratory distress syndrome: the Berlin definition. *JAMA.* 2012;307:2526–2533.

Consensus conference to update the AECC definition that took place in Berlin. The participants reclassified the ALI category with PaO_2/FIO_2 ratio <300 and ≥200 as mild ARDS, PaO_2/FIO_2 <200 and ≥100 as moderate ARDS and PaO_2/FIO_2 <100 as severe. Minimum PEEP for assessing PaO_2/FIO_2 was 5 cm H_2O. Other aspects of the AECC definition were retained; acute onset, but defined as within one week, bilateral infiltrates on chest x-ray but not explained by effusions, atelectasis, or nodules, and respiratory failure not fully explained by cardiac failure or fluid overload (and no need for pulmonary artery catheterization to prove it). Four ancillary physiologic variables were considered; severity of chest x-ray abnormalities, compliance ≤40 mL/cm H_2O, PEEP ≥10 cm H_2O and minute volume ≥10 L/min, but these did not improve prediction of outcome when evaluated in a clinical dataset and were dropped.

Ashbaugh DG, Bigelow DB, Petty TL, Levine BE. Acute respiratory distress in adults. *Lancet.* 1967;2:319–323.

First description of ARDS in 12 patients with acute hypoxic respiratory failure when the authors were just starting their faculty careers. They noted that "The clinical pattern ... includes severe dyspnoea, tachypnoea, cyanosis that is refractory to oxygen therapy, loss of lung compliance, and a diffuse alveolar infiltrate seen on chest X-ray." They describe and recommend the use of PEEP to improve oxygenation.

Bellani G, Laffey JG, Pham T, et al. LUNG SAFE Investigators; ESICM Trials Group. Epidemiology, patterns of care, and mortality for patients with acute respiratory distress syndrome in intensive care units in 50 countries. *JAMA.* 2016;315(8):788–800.

Using the LUNG SAFE (Large observational study to UNderstand the Global impact of Severe Acute respiratory FailurE) database from 459 ICUs in 50 countries worldwide. Of 29,144 patients admitted to the ICUs, 10.4% met the Berlin criteria for ARDS and 23.4% of the patients were on mechanical ventilation. Thirty percent of ARDS cases were mild, 46.6% moderate and 23.4% severe. Hospital mortality was 34.9% in mild, 40.3% in moderate, and 46.1% in severe cases. Recognition of ARDS was only 51.3% in mild cases up to 78.5% in severe. Failure to recognize ARDS was associated with underutilization of lung protective ventilator strategies, lower levels of PEEP, and less use of the prone position or neuromuscular blockade.

Bernard GR, Artigas A, Brigham KL, et al. The American-European Consensus Conference on ARDS. Definitions, mechanisms, relevant outcomes, and clinical trial coordination. *Am J Respir Crit Care Med.* 1994;149:818–824.

Consensus conference convened to address problems with inconsistencies in definition of ARDS that was leading to difficulties in determining the epidemiology of ARDS. This group established the previous definition of acute lung injury (ALI) and ARDS as conditions characterized by acute onset, bilateral infiltrates on CXR, and pulmonary artery wedge pressure (PAWP) ≤18 mm Hg or no clinical evidence of left atrial hypertension. The two were distinguished by PaO_2/FIO_2 ratio ≤300 for ALI and ≤200 for ARDS.

Brun-Buisson C, Minelli C, Bertolini G, et al. Epidemiology and outcome of acute lung injury in European intensive care units. Results from the ALIVE study. *Intensive Care Med.* 2004;30(1):51–61.

> *The study identified 463 patients (7.1% of ICU admissions) with ALI (16.1% of mechanically ventilated patients). Sixty-two patients (13.4%) remained with mild ALI; the remainder had ARDS. Mortality of mild ALI was 32.7% and of ARDS was 57.9%. Risk factors for mortality included greater age, immunodeficiency, multiple organ dysfunction, and pH <7.30.*

Luhr OR, Antonsen K, Karlsson M, et al., and the ARF Study Group. Incidence and mortality after acute respiratory failure and acute respiratory distress syndrome in Sweden, Denmark, and Iceland. *Am J Respir Crit Care Med.* 1999;159:1849–1861.

> *Eight-week cohort study of 132 ICUs in Sweden, Denmark, and Iceland, using American European Consensus Conference (AECC) definitions. They found an incidence and hospital mortality of 77.9/100,000/yr and 42.2% for acute respiratory failure (ARF) including acute lung injury (ALI), 17.9/100,000/yr and 42.2% for ALI including ARDS and 13.5/100,000/yr and 41.2% for ARDS, respectively. This heralded a reduction in ARDS mortality that some doubted at the time but seems to have held up.*

Murray JF, Matthay MA, Luce JM, Flick MR. Expanded definition of the adult respiratory distress syndrome. *Am Rev Respir Dis.* 1988;138:720–723.

> *Description of the Murray Lung Injury Score incorporating ratings of severities of chest x-ray, PaO_2/FIO_2, PEEP, and compliance abnormalities. The score lost favor because of a lack of correlation with outcomes.*

Rubenfeld GD, Caldwell E, Peabody E, et al. Incidence and outcomes of acute lung injury. *N Engl J Med.* 2005;353:1685–1693.

> *Identified 1113 patients in Kings County Washington, US, receiving mechanical ventilation who met AECC criteria for ALI. Found overall incidence of 78.9/100,000/yr for ALI and 58.7/100,000/yr for ARDS. Incidence varied with age from 16/100,000/year for ages 15–19 years to 306/100,000/yr for ages 75–85 yrs. Overall mortality was 38.5%, varying from 24% for ages 15–19 to 60% for age >85 yrs. The authors had a meticulous protocol for screening patients to enhance confidence in their numbers.*

Villar J, Slutsky AR. The incidence of the adult respiratory distress syndrome. *Am Rev Respir Dis.* 1989;140:814–816.

> *Study done on the island of Las Palmas on the Canary Islands over a 3-year period. Using a definition of PaO_2 ≤75 mm Hg on FIO_2 ≥0.5, they estimated an incidence for ARDS of 3.5/100,000/yr. This illustrates the range of reported incidences related to differing definitions in the past.*

Villar J, Blanco J, Añón JM, et al. The ALIEN (Acute Lung Injury: Epidemiology and Natural history) study: incidence and outcome of acute respiratory distress syndrome in the era of lung protective ventilation. *Intensive Care Med.* 2011;37:1932–1941.

> *Prospective multicenter study of ICUs in 13 geographic regions of Spain. Two-hundred-fifty-five consecutive patients that met AECC criteria for ARDS were enrolled. Overall incidence of ARDS was 7.2/100,000/yr and hospital mortality was 47.8%. Average PaO_2/FIO_2 ratio was 114, tidal volume was 7.2 mL/kg, plateau pressure was 26 cm H_2O and PEEP was 9.3 cm H_2O. The authors speculated on possible reasons for the much higher incidences of ARDS reported from US studies compared to European ones. The authors also remarked that ARDS mortality was stable over the previous 10 years despite implementation of lung protective ventilator strategies.*

Landmark Article of the 21st Century

EPIDEMIOLOGY, PATTERNS OF CARE, AND MORTALITY FOR PATIENTS WITH ACUTE RESPIRATORY DISTRESS SYNDROME IN INTENSIVE CARE UNITS IN 50 COUNTRIES

Bellani G et al., *JAMA*. 2016;315(8):788–800

Commentary by John G. Laffey

In 2012, the Berlin definition for ARDS was developed, which heralded significant changes in how ARDS was diagnosed. I had recently taken on the role of deputy chair of the Acute Respiratory Failure section of the European Society of Intensive Care Medicine (ESICM), and together with Prof. Antonio Pesenti, the section chair, we decided to conduct a prospective cohort study to "validate" the definition and understand the "real world" management and outcomes of ARDS in the 21st century.

With relatively little direct funds, other than "in kind" support from the ESICM, St Michael's Hospital Toronto (my then institution), and University of Milan-Bicocca (A. Pesenti's and G. Bellani's institution) we engaged with the ESICM research community to enroll sites into "LUNG SAFE" as we called the study. We were astonished at the response, over 660 centers from over 50 countries on all continents indicated that they would participate. We opened the study for 3-month enrollment windows in the winter periods of both the Northern and Southern hemispheres in 2014. We asked centers to enroll for a 4-consecutive-week period. In all, we collected data on over 29,000 patients from 636 hospitals (666 ICUs) of whom over 12,000 were included in the analysis, of whom 4499 had acute hypoxemic respiratory failure, and just over 3000 of whom fulfilled the Berlin criteria for ARDS.

This primary paper described the cohort of 2377 patients that developed ARDS within 48 hours of ICU admission and required invasive mechanical ventilation. An important aspect of the design is that we didn't ask physicians to decide whether a patient had ARDS—we collected sufficient data to enable independent determination of the diagnosis. That resulted in three important findings: first, ARDS was greatly under-recognized, with only 34% recognized on day 1; second, ARDS prevalence was up to five times more frequent than previously estimated; and third, there was much less geographic variation in ARDS incidence than previously thought. ARDS accounted for 10% of all ICU admissions and 23% of patients requiring mechanical ventilation. Key evidence-based aspects of ARDS management were underused. One-third of patients with ARDS received a tidal volume over 8 of mL/kg predicted body weight, PEEP levels used were lower than expected, while prone positioning was used in a small minority of patients with severe ARDS. Clinician recognition of ARDS was associated with higher PEEP use, greater use of neuromuscular blockade, and prone positioning. Hospital mortality was 40% for all patients with ARDS.

Since this paper was published, over 25 subsequent papers have been published from the LUNG SAFE dataset, underlining the treasure trove of data therein, and giving a comprehensive picture of ARDS in the 21st century. **n = 438**

CHAPTER 2

ARDS Treatment

Review by Bruck Or, Jennifer Kodela, and Scott Kopec

In 1967, Ashbaugh and colleagues described a series of 12 patients with the acute onset of tachypnea, hypoxia, and loss of lung compliance. This paper is widely regarded as the first description of acute respiratory distress syndrome (ARDS) in the literature [1]. Since this initial report, different criteria for ARDS have been proposed, ultimately resulting in the combined effort by the European Society of Critical Care Medicine, the American Thoracic Society, and the Society for Critical Care Medicine defining ARDS into mild, moderate, and severe forms based on PaO_2/FiO_2 ratios and the requirement of a PEEP of ≥5 mm Hg [2].

Historically, mechanical ventilation strategies for ARDS utilized supraphysiologic tidal volumes which were felt to be adopted from the field of anesthesia, based on ventilation practices used during routine surgical cases to prevent atelectasis. However, multiple animal studies, some as early as the 1970s, demonstrated that supraphysiologic tidal volumes and elevated plateau airway pressures were themselves associated with the development of lung injury. There was controversy as to whether volume or pressure was the culprit. An elegant rodent study by Dreyfuss et al. demonstrated that volume was the major culprit [3]. Animals subjected to ventilation with high tidal volume and high pressure or high tidal volume and low pressure exhibited lung injury, whereas those ventilated with normal tidal volume and high pressure had no significant lung injury.

In the 1980s and 1990s, chest CT scans demonstrated that the pathologic process of ARDS was quite heterogeneous, with some areas of the lung affected, whereas other areas appeared to be free of disease. Those disease-free areas would have normal or near-normal compliance and would be more likely to be inflated during inspiration compared to diseased areas. Using supraphysiologic tidal volumes would damage those normal lung areas and worsen lung function. This lung injury would ultimately be termed ventilator-induced lung injury (VILI) and felt to be a consequence of both volutrauma from large tidal volumes and atelectrauma from repeated opening and closing of the already fragile terminal airways.

Some but not all clinical studies in the 1990s showed some benefit to a low tidal volume strategy. Amato et al. randomized ARDS patients (n = 28) to either a low tidal volume strategy (VT = 6 mL/kg with PEEP titrated to the lower inflection point of the volume pressure curve) or "conventional ventilation" (VT = 12 mL/kg with PEEP administered according to the FiO_2, hemodynamics, and $PaCO_2$) [4]. Oxygenation and weaning time improved in the low tidal volume group. There was no difference in mortality. Ranieri, et al. randomized patients (n = 48) to either standard ventilator management or a lung protection strategy where tidal volume and PEEP were applied according to volume–pressure curves [5]. They showed that plasma and bronchoalveolar lavage levels of inflammatory mediators were lower in the lung protection group. In a follow-up study, extrapulmonary organ dysfunction was less in the lung protection group. On the other hand, another study (n = 120) comparing a low tidal volume to a standard tidal volume strategy (mean 7.2 vs. 10.8 mL/kg) in patients at risk for ARDS had no effect on mortality or number of episodes of organ failure [6].

In arguably the most important study addressing the potential effects of mechanical ventilation in patients with ARDS, the ARDS Network published the seminal paper in NEJM in 2000, which showed a mortality benefit in those patients with ALI or ARDS who were treated with low tidal volumes (6 mL/kg ideal body weight [IBW]) versus those in the control group treated with tradition tidal volumes (12 mL/kg IBW) [7].

After enrolling 861 patients, the trial was prematurely discontinued after interim analysis demonstrated an 8.8% lower mortality in patients randomized to the lower tidal volume ventilation group (31% vs. 38.8%). There were also significant differences in the number of ventilator-free days (12 vs. 10), breathing without assistance at 28 days (65.7% vs. 55.0%), and less organ failure at 28 days, all favoring the low tidal volume group. There were no differences in the amount of barotrauma between the groups (10% vs. 11%).

There was some controversy generated from the ARDSnet trial as to the use of the tidal volume in the control group, which seemed excessive to some clinicians. However, one must keep in mind that ideal body weight was used to calculate the tidal volume. These tidal volumes would be similar to those used in other studies [4–6] and in clinical practice where the use of measured body weight [4–6] was standard. Furthermore, follow-up studies comparing institutions who had adopted a lung protective strategy to those that had not found a significant increase in two-year survival when a lung protection strategy was used [8].

There are non-ventilatory methods that have been proven to be effective or show promise in the treatment of ARDS. Use of the prone position will improve survival in patients with severe ARDS (P/F ratio <150) [9]. Although, use of muscle relaxants (cis-atracurium) was effective in one prospective study in improving 90-day survival, the doses that were used were quite high, and an effect on the survival curve was not apparent until day 20 [10]. The utility of corticosteroids is controversial, and data are conflicting. Interventions that should be considered rescue therapies include inhaled nitric oxide or epoprostenol and veno-venous extracorporeal life support.

In the 20 years since the publication of the ARDSnet trial, low tidal volume and lung-protective ventilation strategies have become the standard of care for managing patients with acute lung injury. Its findings have been supported in several follow-up studies, including a Cochrane meta-analysis [11]. Not only have we seen a drop in the mortality rate from around 36% to 25% for patients with acute lung injury [7], this landmark study helped open the door to further understanding of the effects of mechanical ventilation on the injured lung, and the management of patients with acute lung injury. Since its publication, other studies have demonstrated the positive effects of using higher PEEP values and maintaining lower driving pressures [12]. On the other hand, other novel ventilatory strategies, such as high-frequency oscillation, where tidal volumes should be low, have been shown to be without benefit compared to traditional low volume mechanical ventilation.

ANNOTATED REFERENCES FOR ARDS TREATMENT

1. Ashbaugh DG, Bigelow DB, Petty TL, Levine BE. Acute respiratory distress in adults. *Lancet.* 1967;290(7511):319–23.

   Although the respiratory distress syndrome had been known to occur in soldiers during war (e.g., Da Nang Lung), this paper was the first description of the respiratory distress syndrome in adult civilians. Application of PEEP improved atelectasis and hypoxemia.

2. The ARDS Definition Task Force. Acute respiratory distress syndrome: the Berlin definition. *JAMA.* 2012;307(23):2526–2533.

   The task force proposed mutually exclusive categories to characterize the severity of ARDS: mild (200 mm Hg < PaO$_2$/FiO$_2$ ≤300 mm Hg); moderate (100 mm Hg < PaO$_2$/FiO$_2$ ≤200 mm Hg); and severe (≤100 mm Hg). When analyzed against data sets from four clinical trials, these categories (mild to moderate to severe) were associated with an increase in mortality and median duration of mechanical ventilation in survivors.

3. Dreyfuss D, Soler P, Basset G, Saumon G. High inflation pressure pulmonary edema. Respective effects of high airway pressure, high tidal volume, and positive end-expiratory pressure. *Am Rev Respir Dis.* 2012;137(5):1159064.

   In a rodent model, the researchers prove convincingly that high tidal volumes rather than high pressure cause lung during mechanical ventilation.

4. Amato MB, Barbas CS, Medeiros DM, et al. Beneficial effects of the "open lung approach" with low distending pressures in acute respiratory distress syndrome. A prospective randomized study on mechanical ventilation. *Am J Resp Crit Care Med.* 1995;152:1835–1846.

   In a small randomizes trial (n = 28), the authors compared the use of a tidal volume of <6 mL/kg, PEEP applied according to the lower inflection point of the total respiratory compliance curve, and peak pressures <40 cm H$_2$O to a conventional approach of a tidal volume of 12 mL/kg and application of PEEP dictated by the FiO$_2$ and hemodynamics. PaO$_2$/FiO$_2$ ratios and compliance were higher in the lower tidal volume group.

5. Ranieri VM, Suter PM, Tortorella C, et al. Effect of mechanical ventilation on inflammatory mediators in patients with acute respiratory distress syndrome: a randomized controlled trial. *JAMA.* 1999;282:54–61.

   Patients (n = 37) with ARDS were randomized to a control group or a lung protection strategy group (lower tidal volume and plateau pressure and high levels of PEEP).

High levels of inflammatory mediators were found in the plasma and BAL of patients in the control group. A follow-up study also found a higher incidence of organ dysfunction in the control group.

6. Stewart TE, Meade MO, Cook DJ, et al. Evaluation of a ventilation strategy to prevent barotrauma in patients at high risk for acute respiratory distress syndrome. *New Engl J Med.* 1998;338:355–361.

Patients (n = 120) at high risk for developing ARDS were randomized to either a tidal volume of ≤8 mL/kg and peak inspiratory pressures of ≤30 cm of H_2O or tidal volumes of 10–15 mL/kg and peak inspiratory pressures of ≤50 cm H_2O. There was no difference in mortality nor in episodes of organ failure. Hypercarbia and need for paralytics and renal replacement therapy was greater in the low tidal volume group.

7. The Acute Respiratory Distress Syndrome Network. Ventilation with lower tidal volumes as compared with traditional tidal volumes for acute lung injury and the acute respiratory distress syndrome. *N Engl J Med.* 2000;342:1301–1308.

Patients with ARDS were randomized to tidal volumes and plateau pressures of 6 mL/kg IBW and 30 cm H2O and 12 mL/kg IBW, respectively. Mortality was significantly lower in the group treated with a VT of 6 mL/kg. In addition, days free of mechanical ventilation were greater in this group.

8. Needham DM, Colantuoni E, Mendez-Tellez PA, et al. Lung protective mechanical ventilation and two year survival in patients with acute lung injury: prospective cohort study. *Br Med J.* 2012;344:e2124.

Consecutive patients (n = 485) from 13 hospitals with acute lung injury were followed for two years. After adjusting for relevant covariates, adherence to a lung protection strategy significantly improved two-year survival.

9. Guerin C, Reignier J, Richard J-C, et al. Prone positioning in acute respiratory distress syndrome. *New Engl J Med.* 2013;368:2159–2168.

Patients with severe ARDS (P/F <150) were randomized to either the prone or supine position. Patients in the prone group had an average of four sessions, each lasting approximately 17 hours. Both 28-day and 90-day mortality were significantly lower in the prone group. Cardiac arrest was more common in the supine group.

10. Papzian L, Forel J-M, Gacouin A, et al. Neuromuscular blockers in early acute respiratory distress syndrome. *New Engl J Med.* 2010;363:1107–1116.

Patients with early ARDS were randomized to a 48-hour duration of treatment with cis-atracurium or placebo. Neuromuscular monitoring was not performed to maintain blinding. Although the crude 90-day mortality was no different between groups, the 90-day mortality rate adjusted for the P/F ratio, SOFA score, and plateau pressure, was significantly lower in the cis-atracurium group. There was no difference in ICU-acquired paresis. Curiously, the separation of the two groups in the survival curve did not start to manifest itself until around day 20.

11. Petrucci N, De Feo C. Lung protective ventilation strategy for the acute respiratory distress syndrome. *Cochrane Database Sys Rev.* 2013;(2):CD003844.

This third update of the use of lung protection strategy in treating ARDS patients shows that hospital and 28-day mortality is significantly reduced compared to the use of larger tidal volumes. Clinical heterogeneity was present based on different time lengths of follow-up and higher plateau pressures in the control groups.

12. Amato MBP, Meade MO, Slutsky AS, et al., Driving pressure and survival in the acute respiratory distress syndrome. *New Engl J Med.* 2015;372:747–755.

   Using multilever mediation analysis, the authors analyzed data from nine randomized trials of mechanical ventilation in patients with ARDS. Driving pressure (plateau pressure – PEEP) was the variable that best stratified risk of mortality (the higher the driving pressure, the higher the risk).

Landmark Article of the 21st Century

VENTILATION WITH LOWER TIDAL VOLUMES AS COMPARED WITH TRADITIONAL TIDAL VOLUMES FOR ACUTE LUNG INJURY AND THE ACUTE RESPIRATORY DISTRESS SYNDROME

ARDS Network, *N Engl J Med.* 2000;342:1301–1308

Commentary by Michael Gropper

When I was training in critical care in the early 1990s, it was common to care for patients with ARDS who had severe barotrauma, often requiring multiple tube thoracostomies to treat pneumothorax. At the time, we thought that barotrauma was simply part of the disease, and that not much could be done about it. While we were fearful of high peak and plateau airway pressures, we noted that when tidal volume was increased, there would be a transient increase in oxygenation, which we interpreted as a positive effect.

Around this time, an important pre-clinical study was published by Dreyfuss et al. (2012), showing that lung volume, rather than airway pressure, was the primary determinant of lung injury. This study, and other small clinical trials suggested that using a lung-protective strategy with low tidal volume might prevent ventilator-induced lung injury (VILI). I was fortunate to have Dr. Michael Matthay and Jeanine Wiener-Kronishs as my research mentors, and Michael invited me as a new faculty member to participate in the trial. I had met Michael and Jeanine while completing my PhD in the laboratory of Dr. Norman Staub, in the Cardiovascular Research Institute at the University of California, San Francisco. I distinctly remember the early meetings discussing the design of what became the ARDSnet trial, with considerable skepticism that simply reducing tidal volume would result in significant benefit.

When the interim analysis showed a 25% relative reduction in mortality and significant increase in ventilator-free days in the low tidal volume group, we were all surprised. One of the most important findings was that while oxygenation in the high tidal volume group was significantly better on the first two trial days, it was the same by day 4, and this group had higher mortality. This was an important lesson in trial design.

To this day, the ARDSnet Trial is the single most cited clinical trial in the history of critical care, and arguably the most important. In addition to saving countless lives, this study was one of the first to demonstrate the importance of standardized care. Until this time, critical care was much more an art than a science, with every intensivist managing patients differently. I would argue that the mortality benefit seen in this trial was greatly enhanced by the fact that ventilator management was standardized, and importantly, weaning was allowed to be performed by protocol by the bedside nurse and respiratory therapist. Unlike so many other critical care trials, this study has well withstood the test of time, and remains the standard of care. I count myself extraordinarily lucky to have been able to participate.

CHAPTER 3

Weaning from Mechanical Ventilation

Review by Nicholas A. Smyrnios

Patients who require mechanical ventilation (MV) are patients with respiratory failure. Patients who recover quickly from the original problem that led to their respiratory failure can be liberated from the ventilator easily in most cases. Examples of this category of patient include postoperative patients, patients with overdoses, and patients whose conditions cause pure lung failure that reverses rapidly. For those patients, who are estimated to comprise over 80% of mechanically ventilated patients, a period of ventilation of less than 72 hours is expected. For the smaller number of patients who do not fall into those categories, a combination of the original cause of respiratory failure and the accumulation of acquired barriers to weaning can extend the period of ventilation. Those patients experience increased morbidities, increased costs, and worse outcomes. For those patients, the 1-year survival is estimated to be 56–93% [1, 2].

The barriers to weaning that we observe frequently include: inadequate MV, cardiac disease, infection, fluid overload, nutritional deficiency, and neurological dysfunction. Mechanical ventilation that is not set appropriately for the patient, particularly for tidal volume and inspiratory flow rate, may lead to persisting respiratory muscle fatigue due to continued activation and strain of those muscles. Cardiac disease can take the form of either coronary ischemia that occurs as a result of stress due to the resumption of breathing activity or left ventricular pump failure that can lead to inadequate blood flow to the respiratory muscles. Infection can be pulmonary or non-pulmonary in origin and can raise the metabolic rate and produce circulating cytokines that adversely affect muscle function. Fluid overload may worsen oxygenation and decrease lung compliance. Nutritional deficiency may weaken the respiratory muscles and reduce their work capacity. Neurological dysfunction can take the form of neuromuscular abnormalities including critical illness neuromyopathy or altered mental status including but not limited to sedative effects.

Patients who are ready to begin liberating from MV are patients for whom the underlying reasons for MV have been stabilized, are hemodynamically stable, have adequate oxygenation (e.g., PaO_2/FIO_2 >150, PEEP ≤8 cm H_2O, FIO_2 ≤0.5), are able to initiate spontaneous breaths, do not have active coronary ischemia, and do not have CO_2 retention above their baseline level. If patients meet these criteria, a trial of spontaneous breathing or a gradual reduction of pressure support may be attempted. There is no definitive evidence proving superiority of one of these methods over the other. However, at the conclusion of a pressure support ventilation (PSV) wean, the patient ultimately is required to demonstrate spontaneous breathing with minimal pressure support.

DOI: 10.1201/9781003042136-3

Patients are usually asked to maintain stable spontaneous breathing for either 30 minutes or 120 minutes to be considered successful. Trials are generally done once daily to allow adequate time for muscle recovery. Based on a modest quality of evidence, most spontaneous breathing trials are now conducted with a low, fixed level of pressure support to overcome airflow resistance within the endotracheal tube [3].

There are no objective indices that have proven to be accurate in predicting when the patient is ready to begin weaning or when removal of the endotracheal tube is appropriate. For the former, the rapid shallow breathing index (respiratory rate/spontaneous tidal volume) does correlate with a patient's ability to sustain breathing and has been used inconsistently with a cutoff value of 100 [4]. For the latter, the cuff-leak test has been proposed as a mechanism of predicting extubation failure. Unfortunately, the cuff-leak test is limited by inconsistent standards for its interpretation. In addition, its pooled sensitivity of 0.66 and specificity of 0.88 for reintubation make it problematic for making individual patient decisions [5].

Recent efforts have focused on processes for caring for the patient after extubation to prevent reintubation. The use of non-invasive ventilation as a rescue modality in patients with respiratory failure following extubation fails to prevent reintubation and is associated with increased mortality [6]. However, extubation directly to non-invasive ventilation before any failure has occurred has been studied, and for patients with chronic obstructive lung diseases demonstrated a decrease in the rates of post-extubation respiratory failure and 90-day mortality [7]. More recently, extubation directly to a high-flow nasal cannula for patients with a high risk of post-extubation respiratory failure was found to be effective in preventing respiratory failure and in reducing the rate of reintubation [8].

Another active area of investigation is the relationship between sedation, delirium, and weaning. Following up on the work of Kress et al., Girard and colleagues randomly assigned 336 mechanically ventilated patients to a daily spontaneous awakening trial followed by a spontaneous breathing trial or to a spontaneous breathing trial and usual care. The primary endpoint was time breathing without assistance [9]. They showed that the paired awakening and breathing trials led to more days without MV, shorter ICU and hospital length of stay, and improved mortality. Since then, light sedation and "pain first" management has been formalized in the Pain, Agitation/Sedation, Delirium, Immobility and Sleep Disruption Guidelines developed by the Society of Critical Care Medicine [10].

Finally, related to sedation management is the prevention of delirium. Although the direct link between delirium and liberation from MV is not proven, the fact that delirium is associated with increased ICU and hospital length of stay suggests a possible association. There are no proven pharmacological therapies for ICU delirium. Therefore, practitioners should be vigilant about delirium prevention. Among the available options for that, avoidance of benzodiazepines, preservation of sleep cycles and early mobility seem to be the most significant. Avoidance of benzodiazepines is a primary tenet of modern sedation protocols; sleep deprivation is a well-known trigger of delirium in multiple clinical settings; and early mobility has the greatest level of evidence supporting its favorable impact on ICU delirium rates and duration [10, 11].

ANNOTATED REFERENCES FOR WEANING FROM MECHANICAL VENTILATION

1. Kurek CK, Cohen IL, Lamrinos J, Minatoya K, Booth FV, Chalfin DB. Clinical and economic outcome of patients undergoing tracheostomy for prolonged mechanical ventilation in New York State during 1993; analysis of 6,353 cases under diagnostic related group 483. *Crit Care Med.* 1997;25:983–988.

   The overall survival rate of patients who undergo tracheotomy for prolonged mechanical ventilation was 49%. Survival was inversely correlated with age. Of the survivors, 21.6% were discharged to a residential healthcare facility, but that number was also significantly affected by age, with 68.5% of the oldest cohort (>90 years of age) requiring residential placement.

2. Unroe M, Kahn JM, Carson SS, et al. One-year trajectories of care and resource utilization for recipients of prolonged mechanical ventilation. A cohort study. *Ann Intern Med.* 2010;153:167–175.

   Patients who undergo prolonged mechanical ventilation have a difficult course, often with readmission to the hospital and with multiple transitions in their care locations. Sixty-five percent of patients had a 1-year outcome of either complete functional dependency or death. The cost per year of independent function was estimated to be $3.5 million.

3. Schmidt GA, Girard TD, Kress JP, et al. Official executive summary of an American Thoracic Society/American College of Chest Physicians clinical practice guideline: liberation from mechanical ventilation in critically ill adults. *Am J Respir Crit Care Med.* 2017;195:115–119.

   This is a combined Society guideline that provides evidence-based recommendations on elements crucial to the ventilator liberation process. It provides recommendations as answers to questions regarding common dilemmas in ventilator liberation. As a clinical practice guideline, the reader should expect updates as new information becomes available.

4. Yang KL, Tobin MJ. A prospective study of indexes predicting the outcome of trials of weaning from mechanical ventilation. *N Engl J Med.* 1991;324:1445–1450.

   Probably the best study of so-called weaning parameters. The authors demonstrated a high sensitivity and moderately high specificity of the respiratory rate to tidal volume ratio (the "rapid shallow breathing index") in predicting successful weaning, defined as the ability to breathe spontaneously for 24 hours following extubation. The overall impact of the study is helped by relatively easy-to-remember cutoff value of 100.

5. Kuriyama A, Jackson JL, Kamei J. Performance of the cuff-leak test in adults in predicting post-extubation airway complications: a systematic review and meta-analysis. *Crit. Care* 2020;24(1): 640.

   An updated meta-analysis looked at the testing characteristics of the cuff-leak test for predicting post-extubation airway obstruction and reintubation. Sensitivity and specificity for predicting upper airway obstruction were 0.62 and 0.87, respectively. Sensitivity and specificity for predicting reintubation were 0.66 and 0.88, respectively. No clear standard for the performance of the cuff-leak test has been established. Therefore, different studies yield markedly different results depending on what technique is used.

6. Esteban A, Frutos-Vivar F, Ferguson ND, et al. Non-invasive positive pressure ventilation for respiratory failure after extubation. *N Engl J Med.* 2004;350:2452–2460.

Two hundred twenty-one patients who developed respiratory failure within 48 hours after planned extubation were randomly assigned to receive either non-invasive ventilation or standard therapy. Rates of reintubation were no different between the groups, but the time to reintubation was longer in the non-invasive ventilation group and the ICU mortality was higher. This study suggests that non-invasive ventilation should not be used as a rescue therapy in patients that develop respiratory failure after extubation.

7. Ferrer M, Sellares J, Valencia M, et al. Non-invasive ventilation after extubation in hypercapnic patients with chronic respiratory disorders: randomised controlled trial. *Lancet.* 2009;374:1082–1088.

One hundred six patients intubated for hypercapnic respiratory failure were randomized to receive either non-invasive ventilation or standard care immediately following planned extubation. Patients randomized to non-invasive ventilation showed lower rates of respiratory failure and 90-day mortality. The important feature was the immediate and uniform, not rescue-based use of the non-invasive ventilation.

8. Hernandez G, Vaquero C, Colinas L, et al. Effect of postextubation high-flow nasal cannula vs noninvasive ventilation on reintubation and postextubation respiratory failure in high-risk patients: a randomized clinical trial. *JAMA.* 2016;316(15):1565–1574.

Six hundred four patients considered high risk for reintubation were randomized at extubation to receive either non-invasive ventilation of high-flow nasal cannula oxygen. The two groups showed no difference in the rate of reintubation, the median time to reintubation or the incidence of respiratory failure following intubation. The study incorporated a wider range of risk factors for reintubation than other similar studies. Given the relative comfort and convenience of high flow oxygen compared to non-invasive ventilation, this study supports its use in a broad spectrum of post-extubation scenarios.

9. Girard TD, Kress JP, Fuchs BD, et al. Efficacy and safety of a paired sedation and ventilator weaning protocol for mechanically ventilated patients in intensive care (Awakening and Breathing Controlled trial): a randomised controlled trial. *Lancet.* 2008;371:126–134.

Three hundred thirty-six patients were randomly assigned to receive either a daily interruption of sedation closely followed by a spontaneous breathing trial or to receive sedation practice unrelated to the timing of the spontaneous breathing trial. Subjects in the experimental/paired group had more days breathing independently in the first 28 days after enrollment, had shorter length of ICU and hospital stay and improved mortality out to 1 year after enrollment. This study highlights the impact of sedation as a barrier to weaning and demonstrates an approach to minimize that effect.

10. Devlin JW, Skrobik Y, Gelinas C, et al. Clinical practice guidelines for the prevention and management of pain, agitation/sedation, delirium, immobility, and sleep disruption in adult patients in the ICU. *Crit Care Med.* 2018;46:e825–e873.

This is a multidisciplinary update of the 2013 Pain, Agitation and Delirium Guideline published in 2013. It has added sections related to mobility and sleep as an acknowledgment of the interrelated nature of these with sedation practice in critical care. As a clinical practice guideline, the reader should expect updates as new information becomes available.

11. Schweikert WD, Pohlman MC, Pohlman AS, et al. Early physical and occupational therapy in mechanically ventilated, critically ill patients: a randomised controlled trial. *Lancet.* 2009;373:1874–1882.

One hundred four patients were randomized to either daily interruption of sedation plus exercise and mobilization performed by physical and occupational therapists or to daily interruption of sedation without standard mobility therapy. The early mobility group showed a greater return to independent function, lower burden of delirium, and faster weaning from the ventilator. Clinical application of these findings depends on either a substantial investment in physical and occupational therapists or the incorporation of these activities into the daily responsibilities of bedside nurses and nursing assistants.

Landmark Article of the 21st Century

EFFICACY AND SAFETY OF A PAIRED SEDATION AND VENTILATOR WEANING PROTOCOL FOR MECHANICALLY VENTILATED PATIENTS IN INTENSIVE CARE (AWAKENING AND BREATHING CONTROLLED TRIAL): A RANDOMISED CONTROLLED TRIAL

Girard TD et al., *Lancet.* 2008;371(9607):126–134

Commentary by John P. Kress

In the 1990s, it was routine for almost all intubated ICU patients to be deeply sedated, or even paralyzed—an approach arising from the mindset that they should be managed like patients in the operating room. In 1996, when I started my fellowship in Pulmonary and Critical Care at the University of Chicago, our Critical Care Research team consisted of my colleagues, Anne Pohlman, RN, MSN, Michael O'Connor, MD, and mentor Jesse Hall, MD. We noticed how frequently patients would take *days* to awaken after sedatives were finally stopped. We had a policy for sedative stoppage every day, which no one followed.

We decided to do a randomized prospective study of usual care compared to daily sedative interruption. The findings were dramatic. Intervention group patients had fewer ventilator days, ICU days, benzodiazepines, tests to determine why they were not awakening (e.g., head CT), and a strong trend toward home versus alternate discharge disposition.

A few years later, colleagues from Vanderbilt and the University of Pennsylvania approached us to participate in a multicenter trial pairing daily sedative interruption with a spontaneous breathing trial. Such a pairing was not mandated in our original trial. The findings in this study mirrored those in our original trial. Ventilator, ICU, and hospital days all improved. Benzodiazepine doses were reduced. While self-extubation was higher in the intervention group, re-intubation was not. There was a strong trend towards reduction in tracheostomy rate because of failure to wean. Lastly, we noted a significant improvement in one-year survival in the intervention group.

CHAPTER 4

Pulmonary Embolism

Review by Jennifer Lynde, Ana M. Velez-Rosborough, and Enrique Ginzburg

Pulmonary embolism is diagnosed in 650,000 patients annually and proves fatal in about 100,000, most of whom are diagnosed postmortem. Incidence is generally increased in men although higher in women less than age 45 and greater than age 80. As much as 50% of venous thromboembolism (VTE) events are associated with a transient risk factor like surgery or hospital admission, 20% are associated with cancer, and the remainder has no risk factors and are considered unprovoked. The incidence of PE appears to be increasing, likely due to earlier diagnosis with spiral computed tomography (CT). More than 90% of pulmonary emboli originate from deep venous thrombosis (DVT) in the lower extremities. Risk factors include immobility, major surgery, advanced age, cancer, trauma, congestive heart failure (CHF), prior DVT/PE, pregnancy, obesity, hematologic disease, autoimmune disease, and central venous catheterization.

Upon admission to the intensive care unit (ICU), patients should undergo risk stratification as prevention is key to avoid VTE events. The Caprini risk assessment has been tested, shows reliability in predicting VTE occurrences with increasing VTE risk, and is used by facilities across the world (Obi). Another tool for VTE risk assessment is thromboelastography (TEG). TEG provides a comprehensive evaluation of clotting mechanisms from thrombin activation to fibrinolysis. Kashuk performed TEG testing on patients at ICU admission. Normal coagulability patients did not suffer thromboembolic events. After clarifying VTE and bleeding risks, intensivists should choose appropriate prophylaxis. Mechanical prophylaxis should be used in every patient without contraindication. Each patient should be assessed for chemical prophylaxis based on risk factors and clinical course. Chemical prophylaxis is low-molecular-weight heparin (LMWH) or unfractionated heparin and varies in dosage based on patient characteristics.

Clinical recognition of PE is difficult as presentation is often vague. Symptoms include dyspnea, tachypnea, chest pain, and cough. The differential diagnosis ranges from myocardial infarction to peptic ulcer to asthma. Clinical assessment alone is insufficient to diagnose or rule out PE. No single noninvasive test has both high sensitivity and specificity. Laboratory tests include D-dimer, troponin I, pro-B-type natriuretic peptide (BNP), and arterial blood gas showing hypoxemia. D-dimer alone should not be used to diagnose a recurrent VTE event as the concentration may remain elevated in patients that completed treatment. Electrocardiogram (ECG) is abnormal in 85% of patients with PE. Patients should be assessed by the intensivist and their VTE

DOI: 10.1201/9781003042136-4

19

probability calculated and the appropriate labs ordered based on the clinical picture (Goldhaber).

If suspicion for PE is high, then imaging confirmatory tests are indicated. CT angiography is the modern gold standard since its noninvasive and can diagnose other intrathoracic diseases contributing to the patient's condition. The V/Q scan is another test, but its result must be interpreted in the context of the patient's pretest clinical VTE probability. Finally, pulmonary angiography is the historical gold standard. However, it is invasive, expensive, and less readily available as compared to CT.

Emboli are characterized from small-moderate (70%) to submassive low risk (5–10%) to submassive high risk (15%) to massive (5–10%). These categories are based on a combination of the patient's clinical picture and PE characteristics. Treatment ranges from systemic anticoagulation alone to fibrinolysis to thrombectomy. Anticoagulation is the cornerstone of treatment. While in-patient, unfractionated heparin or low-molecular weight heparin (if no contraindications) may be used until oral anticoagulation therapy is appropriate. Long-term anticoagulation reduces the incidence of long-term recurrence of VTE by 80–85%. Previously anticoagulation with warfarin was standard; however, new research shows that direct oral anticoagulants (DOACs) are noninferior (Es). Consideration for extended prophylaxis should be given to patients undergoing high-risk abdominal or pelvic cancer surgery as VTE incidence is reduced with postoperative anticoagulation for up to four weeks without decreasing the safety (Bergqvist).

For submassive high risk to massive PE, anticoagulation in addition to thrombolysis or thrombectomy may be indicated. Patients that have normal systolic blood pressure but show signs of right ventricular dysfunction may benefit from thrombolysis to avoid hemodynamic decompensation (Goldhaber). Thrombolytic agents such as Tenecteplase can provide rapid resolution of emboli. However, prior to fibrinolysis, patients must undergo extensive bleeding risk assessment as use of thrombolytics has significant bleeding complications. The PEITHO trial demonstrated great efficacy at preventing hemodynamic compromise but does increase the risk of intracranial hemorrhage and major bleeding events, especially for patients over the age of 75. There is some thought that half the standard dose of Tenecteplase may decrease bleeding risks; however, more research is needed (Meyer). For massive PE or patients that require aggressive intervention for PE but are at high risk for bleeding should be considered for catheter or surgical thrombectomy. Catheter-directed thrombolysis (CDT) has shown to be effective with low bleeding risks. However, randomized controlled trials are needed to compare directly with anticoagulation or systemic thrombolytics (Bloomer). In short, treatment beyond anticoagulation requires a thorough bleeding risk assessment and discussion with the patient regarding the risks and benefits of each procedure.

Inferior vena cava (IVC) filter placement for PE and treatment of subsegmental PE are both controversial. The PREPIC2 randomized trial compared IVC filter plus anticoagulation versus anticoagulation therapy alone for treatment of acute PE. The addition of the IVC filter did not reduce the risk of symptomatic recurrent PE at 3 months (Mismetti). Small and peripheral emboli-like subsegmental PE (SSPE) are more frequently found with widespread use of CT. There is limited data regarding treatment with anticoagulation versus observation of SSPE. A 2020 Cochrane systematic review did not find any randomized trial evidence to assess efficacy or safety of anticoagulation versus control as treatment. Clinical equipoise must be used to decide upon treatment for each SSPE patient and their risk profile (Yoo).

In conclusion, the topic of pulmonary embolism is vast. Because of the low incidence and occult nature of PE, most guidelines are based on pooled data and review papers. Although not a landmark paper, this paper in *Lancet* authored by Goldhaber, one of the venerable experts in the field of thromboembolic disease, reviews the subject of pulmonary embolus including current management modalities of thrombolysis and thrombectomy. It serves as a guidepost toward diagnosis and treatment of pulmonary embolus (Goldhaber).

ANNOTATED REFERENCES FOR PULMONARY EMBOLISM

Allen CJ, Murray CR, Meizoso JP, et al. Surveillance and early management of deep vein thrombosis decreases rate of pulmonary embolism in high-risk trauma patients. *J Am Coll Surg.* 2016 Jan;222(1):65–72. doi: 10.1016/j.jamcollsurg.2015.10.014. Epub 2015 Nov 4. PMID: 26616034.

This observational study sought to compare rate of PE after implementation of a weekly venous duplex ultrasound (VDU) protocol versus symptomatic in 402 high-risk trauma patients admitted to the ICU over a 3-year period. All patients underwent screening with Greenfield's Risk Assessment Profile for VTE risk. Patients with RAP scores greater than or equal to 10 were recommended by the research team to undergo weekly bilateral VDU. There were 259 patients who underwent VDU and 143 did not. DVT rate was 11.6% in the VDU group vs 2.1% in the non-surveillance group. PE rate was 1.9% in the VDU group vs 7% in the non-surveillance group. The group concluded that high-risk trauma patients undergoing weekly VDU were diagnosed and treated for DVT earlier, leading to a lower rate of PE in that group.

Bergqvist D, Agnelli G, Cohen AT, et al. ENOXACAN II Investigators. Duration of prophylaxis against venous thromboembolism with enoxaparin after surgery for cancer. *N Engl J Med.* 2002 Mar 28;346(13):975–980. doi: 10.1056/NEJMoa012385. PMID: 11919306.

In this double-blind, multicenter, randomized controlled trial, patients undergoing planned curative open surgery for abdominal or pelvic cancer received 6–10 days of open treatment enoxaparin. Then during the double-blind treatment period, patients were randomized to enoxaparin prophylaxis versus placebo for 19–21 days. Results show a decrease in VTE rate (12.0% in placebo group vs 4.8% in enoxaparin group, p = 0.02). This difference was consistent at 3 months postoperatively and there was no difference between groups in adverse events including rate of bleeding events. VTE prophylaxis for 4 weeks post operatively is safe and reduces VTE occurrences.

Bloomer TL, El-Hayek GE, McDaniel MC, et al. Safety of catheter-directed thrombolysis for massive and submassive pulmonary embolism: Results of a multicenter registry and meta-analysis. *Catheter Cardiovasc Interv.* 2017;89(4):754–760.

Bloomer et al. reviews catheter-directed thrombolysis (CDT) data in two forms: patients diagnosed with acute PE and treated with CDT from a multicenter registry and meta-analysis of all contemporary studies utilizing CDT for pulmonary embolism (PE). Efficacy was measured by change in invasive pulmonary artery systolic pressure (PASP) and safety outcomes were listed as any major complication including fatal intracranial hemorrhage (ICH), intraocular or retroperitoneal hemorrhage or any overt hemorrhage that required blood transfusion or surgical repair. The same safety outcomes were evaluated in the registry and the meta-analysis. Results support use of CDT in PE given significant improved in PASP and its low risks. Special care must be taken since patients older than age 75 are at higher risk of ICH. However, more research is needed to compare CDT to anticoagulation alone or systemic thrombolysis.

Decousus H, Leizorovicz A, Parent F, et al. A clinical trial of vena caval filters in the prevention of pulmonary embolism in patients with proximal deep-vein thrombosis. Prévention du Risque d'Embolie Pulmonaire par Interruption Cave Study Group. *N Engl J Med.* 1998 Feb 12;338(7):409–415. doi: 10.1056/NEJM199802123380701. PMID: 9459643.

In this multicenter, randomized trial over 4 years, efficacy and safety of IVC filter placement in prevention of PE was tested in patients with known proximal DVT. Treatment groups included therapeutic unfractionated heparin, therapeutic low-molecular weight heparin (LMWH), IVC filter placement and no filter placement. Primary outcome was occurrence of symptomatic or asymptomatic PE within first 12 days after randomization. This study showed an initial efficacy in filter use for prevention of PE in patients with high-risk proximal DVT receiving anticoagulation. However, no difference in mortality was identified between filter and no filter groups. Lastly, after 2 years, filter patients developed post-phlebitic syndrome and a significant increase in recurrent DVT, possibly related to thrombosis at the filter site.

Es, NV, Coppens M, Schulman S, Middeldorp S, Buller, HR. Direct oral anticoagulants compared with vitamin K antagonist for acute venous thromboembolism: evidence from phase 3 trials. *Blood.* 2014;124(12):1968–1975.

This meta-analysis reviews six phase 3 trials comparing direct oral anticoagulants (DOACs) versus vitamin K antagonists (VKAs) in treatment of acute VTE. Over 13,500 patients were randomized to both the DOAC and VKA arms for a total of 27,023 patients. There was no difference in VTE recurrence between DOACs and VKAs. Major bleeding events including intracranial hemorrhage and gastrointestinal hemorrhage were decreased in the DOAC therapy arm. DOAC efficiency was consistent across multiple patient subgroups including weight >100 kg, cancer, moderately impaired renal clearance (CrCl 30-49 mL/min) and patients age >75. DOACs are clearly noninferior to VKA therapy for treatment of acute VTE.

Ginzburg E, Cohn SM, Lopez J, Jackowski J, Brown M, Hameed SM; Miami Deep Vein Thrombosis Study Group. Randomized clinical trial of intermittent pneumatic compression and low molecular weight heparin in trauma. *Br J Surg.* 2003 Nov;90(11):1338–1344. doi: 10.1002/bjs.4309. PMID: 14598411.

This prospective randomized trial compared intermittent pneumatic compression (IPC) devices and low-molecular weight heparin (LMWH) in trauma patients at high risk for VTE. Patients underwent admission screening DVT ultrasound of the bilateral lower extremities (popliteal, saphenous, femoral, and iliac veins) and then weekly thereafter. Patients were followed until hospital discharge or 30 days from admission or death, whichever occurred first. Rate of PE was similar in both groups and not statistically significant. The study showed comparable effects of both methods of thromboprophylaxis.

Goldhaber SZ, Bounameaux H. Pulmonary embolism and deep vein thrombosis. *Lancet.* 2012 May 12;379(9828):1835–46. doi: 10.1016/S0140-6736(11)61904-1. Epub 2012 Apr 10. PMID: 22494827.

In this review paper, Dr. Goldhaber covers the extensive topic of pulmonary embolism from epidemiology to treatment with thrombolysis and thrombectomy. His expertise on the topic is evident and this comprehensive article is an up-to-date resource and tool for physicians everywhere.

Kashuk JL, Moore EE, Sabel A, et al. Rapid thromboelastography (r-TEG) identifies hypercoagulability and predicts thromboembolic events in surgical patients. *Surgery.* 2009;146(4):764–774.

In this retrospective analysis over 7 months, 152 surgical patients in the intensive care unit were assessed as hypercoagulable or not by rapid thromboelastography (r-TEG). 67% (86 patients) were found to be hypercoagulable by r-TEG. Hypercoagulable patients had risk factors including high-risk injury, spinal cord injury, longer median ICU stay, longer median ventilatory days, and longer hospital length of stay. Nineteen percent (16 patients) in the hypercoagulable group suffered thromboembolic events and 12% (10 patients) had thromboembolic events predicted by prior r-TEG. Patients with normal coagulability did not suffer any thromboembolic events.

Meyer G, Vicaut E, Danays T, et al. Fibrinolysis for patients with intermediate risk pulmonary embolism. *N Engl J Med.* 2014;370(15):1402–1411.

The multicenter, randomized, double-blind trial compared efficacy and safety between fibrinolysis with a bolus of systemic Tenecteplase plus anticoagulation versus anti-coagulation with placebo in patients with intermediate-risk pulmonary embolism. Primary efficacy outcomes were all-cause mortality and hemodynamic decompensation. Primary safety outcomes were major bleeding events or stroke (ischemic or hemorrhagic). Results showed a single dose of Tenecteplase did reduce risk of early death or hemodynamic decompensation. However, Tenecteplase use is associated with a significant increase in intracranial hemorrhage and other major bleeding. Patients >75 did have higher risk of bleeding. Decreasing the Tenecteplase dose by half may reduce this risk, but further research is needed. Fibrinolysis is effective but comes at a cost.

Mismetti P, Laporte S, Pellerin O, et al. Effect of a retrievable inferior vena cava filter plus anticoagulation vs anticoagulation alone on risk of recurrent pulmonary embolism: a randomized clinical trial. *JAMA.* 2015;313(16):1627–1635.

This randomized trial compared treatment with inferior vena cava (IVC) filters plus anticoagulation versus anticoagulation alone on risk of recurrent pulmonary embolism. Primary outcome was death or recurrent symptomatic PE at 3 months. At that time point, in the IVC filter group, 3% (6 patients) developed recurrent PE and all cases were fatal. In the anticoagulation only group, 1.5% (3 patients) developed recurrences and 2 out of the 3 were fatal. There were no statistical differences between the groups and IVC filter placement in addition to anticoagulation did not reduce risk of recurrent pulmonary embolism.

Obi AT, Pannucci CJ, Nackashi A, et al. Validation of the Caprini venous thromboembolism risk assessment model in critically ill surgical patients. *JAMA Surg.* 2015;150(10):941–948.

This 5-year retrospective review of over 4800 critically ill patients at a tertiary academic hospital evaluated the validity of the Caprini score on venous thromboembolism (VTE) risk assessment at time of ICU admission. This is based on the 2005 Caprini RAM score. Results show increased incidence of VTE linearly with increasing Caprini score. The Caprini score is a valid and reliable tool in critically ill surgical patients.

Yoo HH, Nunes-Nogueira VS, Fortes Villas Boas PJ. Anticoagulant treatment for subsegmental pulmonary embolism. *Cochrane Database Syst Rev*. 2020 Feb 7;2(2):CD010222. doi: 10.1002/14651858.CD010222.pub4. PMID: 32030721; PMCID: PMC7004894.

This is a 2020 Cochrane review of multiple databases for randomized controlled trials assessing anticoagulation treatment versus placebo in patients with subsegmental pulmonary embolism (SSPE). However, no RCTs were identified in this area. Therefore, there is no evidence from randomized controlled trials to assess the efficacy or safety of either anticoagulation or active surveillance/observation. Clinical equipoise must be used in each patient encounter given the patient's clinical status in addition to risks and benefits of each treatment plan.

Landmark Article of the 21st Century

EFFECT OF A RETRIEVABLE INFERIOR VENA CAVA FILTER PLUS ANTICOAGULATION VS ANTICOAGULATION ALONE ON RISK OF RECURRENT PULMONARY EMBOLISM

Mismetti P et al. *JAMA*. 2015 April;313(16):1627–1635

Commentary by Suresh Agarwal

The prevention of venous thromboembolic events (VTE) has been critical to the management of surgical patients; particularly those who are at greater risk for mortality. With the creation of removable IVC filters, our practice liberalized the usage of inferior vena cava filters for the prevention of VTE in the trauma and critically ill populations, thinking that we had a panacea for their management.

The interruption of the vena cava to prevent embolic events has been described since the 1930s and has grown in popularity since the advent of transvenous placement of inferior vena cava filters (IVCF) in the 1960s. The PREPIC trial in 1998 (Prevention du Risque d'Embolie Pulmonaire par Interruption Cava Study Group) demonstrated that although there was a decrease in early pulmonary embolism, there was a subsequent significant increase in recurrent deep vein thrombosis over a two-year period, without any mortality benefit.[1] A long-term follow-up analysis (8 years) of their patients confirmed no difference in survival.[2] Subsequent meta-analyses have, similarly, been unable to advocate for the use of IVCF when anticoagulation may be safely utilized.[3,4]

Mismetti, et al. performed the PRECIP2 trial, which demonstrates that the adjunct usage of IVCF in anticoagulated patients is not warranted when full anticoagulation may be performed. This, along with other studies, have markedly changed our practice to the point where IVCF are only used in patients who cannot be anticoagulated. As all of these studies have shown, the placement and removal of IVC filters are not without consequence: the search for a panacea continues...

NOTES

1. Decousus H, Leizorovicz, et al. A clinical trial of vena cava filters in the prevention of pulmonary embolism in patients with proximal deep-vein thrombosis. *N Engl J Med.* 1998(Feb);338(7):409–415.
2. PREPIC Study Group. Eight-year follow-up of patients with permanent vena cava filters in the prevention of pulmonary embolism. *Circulation* 2005(Jul);112(3):416–22.
3. Kearon C, Akl EA, et al. Antithrombotic therapy for VTE disease: CHEST Guideline and Expert Panel Report. *CHEST* 2016(Feb);149(2):315–352.
4. Bikdeli B, Chatterjee S, et al. Inferior vena cava filters to prevent pulmonary embolism: Systemic review and meta-analysis. *J Am Coll Cardiol.* 2017(Sept);70(13):1587–1597.

CHAPTER 5

Extracorporeal Membrane Oxygenation

Review by Ronny Munoz-Acuna and Ameeka Pannu

Recent evidence from cohort studies, meta-analyses, and randomized controlled trials has shown that VV-ECMO (venovenous extracorporeal membrane oxygenation) support for patients with acute respiratory distress syndrome (ARDS) who develop refractory hypoxemia may be associated with improved outcomes [1].

ARDS is an inflammatory process in the lungs that induces non-hydrostatic pulmonary edema. The resulting decreased lung compliance, increased intrapulmonary shunt, and dead space results in profound hypoxemia. Primary mechanisms implicated include severe inflammatory injury to the alveolar-capillary barrier, surfactant depletion, and aerated lung tissue loss. The currently accepted diagnostic criteria for ARDS is provided by the Berlin definition, which combines the clinical measures of new or worsening respiratory symptoms within seven days of a known clinical insult with a combination of acute hypoxemia (PaO_2/FiO_2 ≤300 mmHg) in a ventilated patient with positive end-expiratory pressure (PEEP) of at least 5 cmH_2O and bilateral opacities on chest imaging not fully explained by heart failure or volume overload. ARDS can be further classified into mild, moderate, or severe, depending on the PaO_2/FiO_2 [2]. ARDS accounts for 10% of all admissions to the intensive care unit (ICU) and 23% of ventilated patients [3]. In addition to considerable mortality, as high as 45% in severe disease [3]. ARDS is also associated with significant morbidity, including decreased physical quality of life and increased use of health care services, even 5 years after diagnosis [4].

Despite multiple investigations into therapeutic interventions, decreasing ventilator-induced lung injury (VILI) remains the mainstay of ARDS management. Decreasing VILI includes mitigating the risk of volutrauma, barotrauma, atelectrauma, and biotrauma during mechanical ventilation, thus adopting a "lung-protective" ventilation strategy [5]. Given the results of these landmark trials, there has also been investigation into other gas exchange methods that may further protect diseased lung.

VV ECMO is an extracorporeal therapy that consists of cannulae that drain venous blood through a pump into an oxygenator allowing for gas exchange with subsequent return of oxygenated blood into a central vein. In its ideal use, VV ECMO is used as a bridge to either lung recovery or lung transplant. Using VV ECMO allows for "lung rest," that is, ultra-lung-protective ventilation can be used to minimize VILI and concomitantly allow lungs to recover from ARDS [6]. However, until recently, it was not established that patients who receive VV ECMO for ARDS have improved outcomes.

DOI: 10.1201/9781003042136-5

Published in 2009, the Conventional Ventilatory Support versus Extracorporeal Membrane Oxygenation for Severe Adult Respiratory Failure (CESAR) trial randomized 180 patients with ARDS to receive either continued conventional ventilation or transfer to an ECMO specialist center with consideration for ECMO treatment [7]. While the primary outcome of death and/or severe disability was statistically significant between groups, the trial was limited in that a large number of control patients did not receive protective ventilation, and 24% of the patients randomized to the transfer and consideration for ECMO group did not receive ECMO. Thus, while the CESAR study supported ECMO as a valid treatment option for managing patients with severe respiratory failure, it could not establish whether ECMO was a better treatment choice than protocolized lung-protective ventilation. Further evidence for the use of ECMO in ARDS came during the H1N1 pandemic, where many centers described success with the use of this modality as rescue for respiratory failure.

The ECMO to Rescue Lung Injury in Severe ARDS (EOLIA) trial published in 2018 was a prospective, multicenter, randomized controlled trial that evaluated the effect of early initiation of VV-ECMO in severe ARDS. This trial included critically ill patients with severe ARDS (average P_aO_2/F_iO_2 ratio of 72) on mechanical ventilation for less than 7 days with a SOFA score above 10, most of whom were receiving vasopressors. Notably, the ECMO approach was standardized, and ventilator management reflected the current standard of care, including neuromuscular blockade and prone positioning in addition to a low tidal-volume high PEEP strategy. Patients randomized to the early ECMO group received immediate percutaneous venovenous cannulation, while the control group patients were managed with conventional mechanical ventilation. The primary outcome, 60-day mortality, was 35% (44/124) in the ECMO group vs. 46% in the control group (57/125), RR, 0.76; 95% confidence interval [CI], 0.55 to 1.04; p = 0.09. Treatment failure, defined as the crossover to ECMO or death in the control arm, and death in the ECMO arm, was higher in the control group. The highest mortality was seen in the crossover group, where ECMO was used as rescue therapy. Patients treated with ECMO had significantly lower cardiac failure rates, renal failure, and the need for dialysis. The authors concluded that the use of ECMO did not improve 60-day survival. However, further interpretation was limited as the trial was stopped early due to predefined futility rules, and crossover may have affected the intention-to-treat analysis. Importantly, this study established the safety of routine VV ECMO use in patients with severe ARDS and provided guidance regarding ECMO cannulation criteria.

Currently, severe ARDS treatment continues to be a lung-protective ventilation strategy combined with other maneuvers like prone positioning and neuromuscular blockade. VV ECMO has now been established as a safe rescue modality in patients with severe hypoxemia refractory to the above, especially at centers that frequently use ECMO. While ECMO potentially offers a mortality benefit [1, 8], clinicians must individualize therapy to minimize adverse outcomes. Unanswered questions about the routine use of VV-ECMO include its impact on patient-centered outcomes such as: quality of life and long-term functional status, both of which are gravely impacted in severe ARDS [9]. Given the significant use of VV-ECMO during the COVID 19 pandemic [10], evidence from this experience will likely shed light on optimal patient selection and cannulation timing.

ANNOTATED REFERENCES FOR EXTRACORPOREAL MEMBRANE OXYGENATION

1. Combes A, Peek GJ, Hajage D, et al. ECMO for severe ARDS: systematic review and individual patient data meta-analysis. *Intensive Care Med.* 2020 Oct 6;1–10.

   Systematic review and individual patient data meta-analysis of two RCTs (CESAR and EOLIA) combining data from 429 patients. Showing that 90-day mortality was significantly lowered by ECMO compared with conventional management.

2. Ferguson ND, Fan E, Camporota L, et al. The Berlin definition of ARDS: an expanded rationale, justification, and supplementary material. *Intensive Care Med.* 2012 Oct 1;38(10):1573–82.

   Most current consensus on the definition of ARDS.

3. Bellani G, Laffey JG, Pham T, et al. Epidemiology, patterns of care, and mortality for patients with acute respiratory distress syndrome in intensive care units in 50 countries. *JAMA.* 2016 Feb 23;315(8):788.

   International, multicenter, prospective cohort study of patients undergoing invasive or noninvasive ventilation, conducted in 459 ICUs from 50 countries across 5 continents. Included 29,144 patients admitted to participating ICUs. The period prevalence of ARDS was 10.4% of ICU admissions. This syndrome appeared to be underrecognized and undertreated and associated with a high mortality rate.

4. Herridge MS, Tansey CM, Matté A, et al. Functional disability 5 years after acute respiratory distress syndrome. *N Engl J Med.* 2011 Apr 7;364(14):1293–304.

   Prospective, longitudinal cohort study of that evaluated 109 survivors of ARDS at 3, 6, and 12 months and at 2, 3, 4, and 5 years after discharge from the intensive care unit. Showing that physical and psychological problems developed or persisted in patients and family caregivers for up to 5 years.

5. Gattinoni L, Tonetti T, Cressoni M, et al. Ventilator-related causes of lung injury: the mechanical power. *Intensive Care Med.* 2016 Oct 1;42(10):1567–75.

   The mechanical power equation encompasses the different ventilator-related causes of lung injury and of their variations and can be easily adapted to most ventilators.

6. Abrams D, Schmidt M, et al. Mechanical ventilation for acute respiratory distress syndrome during extracorporeal life support. Research and practice. *Am J Respir Crit Care Med.* 2020 Mar 1;201(5):514–25.

   Narrative review reflecting the consensus of expert opinions of clinicians and researchers with expertise in mechanical ventilation, ARDS, and ECLS that originated from a roundtable discussion at the 4th Annual International ECMO Network Scientific Meeting in Rome, Italy in 2018, regarding mechanical ventilation for ARDS patients undergoing ECMO support.

7. Peek GJ, Mugford M, Tiruvoipati R, et al. Efficacy and economic assessment of conventional ventilatory support versus extracorporeal membrane oxygenation for severe adult respiratory failure (CESAR): a multicentre randomised controlled trial. *Lancet.* 2009 Oct 17;374(9698):1351–63.

The CESAR study was the first of the modern RCTS supporting ECMO as a valid treatment option for the management of patients with severe respiratory failure. However, it does not show that ECMO is better than conventional ventilation. It does show benefit of transferring these patients to specialized ECMO centers.

8. Goligher EC, Tomlinson G, Hajage D, et al. Extracorporeal membrane oxygenation for severe acute respiratory distress syndrome and posterior probability of mortality benefit in a post hoc Bayesian analysis of a randomized clinical trial. *JAMA.* 2018 Dec 4;320(21):2251.

Bayesian inference directly estimates the probability that a conclusion is true given the data observed in an experiment. Bayesian analyses support a consensus that ECMO lowers mortality but, at the same time, demonstrate that there remains substantial variability in the conclusions to be drawn regarding whether ECMO confers a large benefit.

9. Wilcox ME, Jaramillo-Rocha V, Hodgson C, Taglione MS, Ferguson ND, Fan E. Long-term quality of life after extracorporeal membrane oxygenation in ARDS survivors: systematic review and meta-analysis. *J Intensive Care Med.* 2020 Mar;35(3):233–43.

Systematic Review and Meta-Analysis showing greater decrements in health-related quality of life were seen for survivors of ECMO when compared to survivors of conventional mechanical ventilation, on the contrary those who received ECMO experienced significantly less psychological morbidity.

10. Schmidt M, Hajage D, Lebreton G, et al. Extracorporeal membrane oxygenation for severe acute respiratory distress syndrome associated with COVID-19: a retrospective cohort study. *Lancet Respir Med.* 2020;8(11):1121–31.

Retrospective cohort study performed in five French ICUs and included patients who received ECMO for COVID-19 associated ARDS. Showing that the estimated 60-day survival of ECMO-rescued patients with COVID-19 was similar to that of previous studies for patients with severe ARDS suggesting that ECMO can be considered for refractory respiratory failure in this cohort of patients.

Landmark Article of the 21st Century

EXTRACORPOREAL MEMBRANE OXYGENATION FOR SEVERE RESPIRATORY DISTRESS SYNDROME (EOLIA TRIAL)

Combs A et al., *N Engl J Med.* 2018;378:1965–1975

Commentary by Alan Lisbon

Design and Methods: While ECMO has been used for over 40 years in the treatment of severe acute respiratory failure, evidence of its effect on mortality is lacking. This multicenter study randomized patients with severe ARDS and intubation less than

7 days to either venovenous ECMO or continued conventional mechanical ventilation. Crossover to ECMO was allowed for refractory hypoxemia. Primary endpoint was mortality at 60 days.

Over 6 years, 249 patients were randomized but the trial was stopped after the fourth interim analysis because there was no significant difference in mortality, and there would not be within the trial design. Forty-four patients (35%) in the ECMO group and 57 (46%) in the conventional mechanical ventilation group died. Crossover to ECMO occurred in 35 (28%) in the control group. The frequency of complications was not significantly different between groups.

Limitations: This was a large, well-designed trial with standardized criteria for entry and a relatively protocolized control arm. The weaknesses of this trial are that it was underpowered and stopped after 75% enrollment, and that there was a high rate of crossover. The crossover of patients may impact upon interpretation and bias against ECMO. In addition, the need for transfer of patients to ECMO centers may be exclude the most severely ill patients (who may well have benefitted most from ECMO) from intervention/inclusion.

Conclusions: The trial showed that ECMO is relatively safe and was not associated with higher mortality than the control group. As a rescue therapy, it may be useful in patients who fail conventional therapy and continue to have severe hypoxemia.

CHAPTER 6

Perioperative Arrhythmias

Review by Jason Matos and Peter J. Zimetbaum

Postoperative atrial fibrillation (POAF) is a common complication, with an incidence ranging from 1–50% depending on the type of surgery and proximity of the procedure to the heart [1]. Atrial fibrillation after cardiac surgery has the greatest POAF risk, with approximately 30% of patients developing POAF after coronary artery bypass grafting (CABG) and 50% after valve surgery (PCSAF) [2]. Not unexpectedly, development of POAF has been linked to poor patient outcomes, including length of stay, ICU admission, stroke, heart failure, and mortality [3, 4].

Acute management of POAF involves traditional principles including either rate control and/or rhythm control to help mitigate palpitations, shortness of breath, and other manifestations of heart failure.

Anticoagulation for POAF, however, is a far more complex and nuanced topic. Anticoagulation for AF in the non-surgical setting is determined based on a patient's risk factors for thromboembolism. Most frequently, one assesses this via the CHA_2DS_2-VASc score (congestive heart failure, hypertension, age, diabetes, prior stroke/TIA, vascular disease), with a score of >1 often triggering anticoagulation. Many do not employ this risk score in the postoperative setting due to high bleeding risks and an underlying optimism that the POAF will not recur. Further, providers often decide to prescribe anti-coagulation only once the duration of AF has surpassed 48–72 hours, but these thresholds are based on minimal evidence.

There is no literature to guide anticoagulation management for POAF after non-cardiac surgery. Regarding PCSAF in particular, a seminal large retrospective study of over 16,000 patients demonstrated that, despite controlling for 32 variables, warfarin use was associated with a lower mortality compared to no anticoagulation use [5]. This work, among others, prompted the American, Canadian, and European cardiology societies to provide a weak recommendation for anticoagulation for PCSAF.

Until recently, no literature or guidance existed regarding thromboembolic risk assessment for POAF outside of the CHA_2DS_2-VASc score. This all changed after Butt et al., utilizing a comprehensive Danish nationwide database, laid the groundwork for thromboembolic risk based on the type of surgery. Compared to age, sex, and CHA_2DS_2-VASc score-matched patients in the database with non-valvular non-surgical AF (NVAF), post-CABG AF patients had lower rates of thromboembolism

DOI: 10.1201/9781003042136-6

(adjusted HR 0.55, 95%CI 0.32–0.95). Further, post-CABG AF was associated with a significantly lower risk of recurrent hospitalization for AF than NVAF (adjusted HR, 0.29; 95%CI, 0.250–0.34; P <0.001) [6]. This was the first major publication to challenge the dogma that non-surgical and surgical AF have similar thromboembolic risk.

Butt et al. published two other important works that assessed thromboembolic risk for patients with AF after valvular surgery and after non-cardiac surgery. Unlike with isolated CABG, AF in these two patient cohorts was associated with similar rates of thromboembolism compared to matched NVAF cohorts (HR 1.22, 95%CI 0.88–1.68 and HR 0.95, 95%CI 0.85–1.07, respectively) [7, 8].

This series has prompted further retrospective investigation into contemporary outcomes with anticoagulation for PCSAF. Matos et al., utilizing data from the Society of Thoracic Surgeons (STS) database found no association with anticoagulation (versus no anticoagulation) and 30-day adjusted stroke readmissions (AOR 0.87, 95%CI 0.65–1.16) among patients with new PCSAF after isolated CABG. Furthermore, there was an increase in the 30-day bleeding readmission rate among anticoagulated patients (AOR 4.30, 95%CI 3.69–5.02) [9]. Though this study only evaluated outcomes in the first 30 days after CABG, it does support the above findings of Butt et al. regarding a reconsideration of thromboembolic risk in post-CABG patients.

These crucial publications by Butt et al. have enlightened the cardiology community that PCSAF after CABG appears to be associated with lower thromboembolic risk compared to PCSAF after valvular surgery, non-cardiac surgery POAF, and non-surgical AF. Though not yet incorporated into mainstream guidelines, surgical type now should be considered when weighing risks and benefits of anticoagulation for POAF. Randomized clinical trials are underway to determine the appropriate use and timing of anticoagulation for this vulnerable population at both high stroke and high bleeding risk.

ANNOTATED REFERENCES FOR PERIOPERATIVE ARRHYTHMIAS

1. Koshy AN, Hamilton G, Theuerle J, et al. Postoperative atrial fibrillation following non-cardiac surgery increases risk of stroke. *Am J Med.* 2020;133:311–22.

   This 14 study meta-analysis of over 3 million patients demonstrated that postoperative atrial fibrillation correlates with stroke risk and this association was stronger with non-cardiac nonthoracic surgery compared with thoracic surgery.

2. Echahidi N, Pibarot P, O'Hara G, Mathieu P. Mechanisms, prevention, and treatment of atrial fibrillation after cardiac surgery. *J Am Coll Cardiol.* 2008;51:793–801.

   This comprehensive review article discusses the morbidity associated with postcardiac surgery atrial fibrillation along with various prevention and treatment modalities.

3. Villareal RP, Hariharan R, Liu BC, et al. Postoperative atrial fibrillation and mortality after coronary artery bypass surgery. *J Am Coll Cardiol.* 2004;43:742–8.

The single-center retrospective review article of over 6000 post-CABG patients demonstrated a significantly higher mortality among the 16% of patients who developed atrial fibrillation.

4. Siontis KCG, Gersh BJ, Weston, SA, et al. Association of new-onset atrial fibrillation after noncardiac surgery with subsequent stroke and transient ischemic attack. *JAMA.* 2020;324:871–8.

This retrospective cohort study of 904 patients post noncardiac surgery demonstrated a statistically significant hazard ratio (2.69) for stroke among patients who developed postoperative atrial fibrillation versus those who did not.

5. El-Chami MF, Kilgo P, Thourani V, et al. New-onset atrial fibrillation predicts long-term mortality after coronary artery bypass graft. *J Am Coll Cardiol.* 2010;55:1370–6.

This seminal large retrospective study of over 16,000 patients demonstrated that, despite controlling for 32 variables, warfarin use was associated with a lower mortality for new onset atrial fibrillation after CABG compared to no anticoagulation use.

6. Butt JH, Xian Y, Peterson ED, et al. Long-term thromboembolic risk in patients with postoperative atrial fibrillation after coronary artery bypass graft surgery and patients with nonvalvular atrial fibrillation. *JAMA Cardiol.* 2018;3:417–24.

7. *Utilizing a comprehensive Danish nationwide database, this study demonstrated that compared to age, sex, and CHA2DS2-VASc score matched patients in the database with non-valvular non-surgical AF, those with post-CABG atrial fibrillation had lower rates of thromboembolism (Adjusted HR 0.55, 95%CI 0.32–0.95).*

8. Butt JH, Olesen JB, Gundlund A, et al. Long-term thromboembolic risk in patients with postoperative atrial fibrillation after left-sided heart valve surgery. *JAMA Cardiol.* 2019;4:1139–47.

Utilizing a comprehensive Danish nationwide database, this study demonstrated that compared to age, sex, and CHA2DS2-VASc score matched patients in the database with non-valvular non-surgical AF, those with post-valvular surgery atrial fibrillation had similar rates of thromboembolism (HR 1.22, 95%CI 0.88–1.68).

9. Butt JH, Olesen JB, Havers-Borgersen E, et al. Risk of thromboembolism associated with atrial fibrillation following noncardiac surgery. *J Am Coll Cardiol.* 2018;72:2027–36.

Utilizing a comprehensive Danish nationwide database, this study demonstrated that compared to age, sex, and CHA2DS2-VASc score matched patients in the database with non-valvular non-surgical AF, those with post-noncardiac surgery atrial fibrillation had similar rates of thromboembolism (HR 0.95, 95%CI 0.85–1.07).

10. Matos JD, McIlvaine S, Grau-Sepulveda M, et al. Anticoagulation and amiodarone for new atrial fibrillation after coronary artery bypass grafting: prescription patterns and 30-day outcomes in the United States and Canada. *J Thorac Cardiovasc Surg.* 2020.

Utilizing the Society for Thoracic Surgeons database, this large retrospective study demonstrated that a majority of clinicians treat patients with amiodarone and no anticoagulation for new post-CABG atrial fibrillation at discharge. Within the first 30 days, the bleeding risk associated with anticoagulation appears to far outweigh the potential for stroke reduction.

Landmark Article of the 21st Century

BRIDGE INVESTIGATORS PERIOPERATIVE BRIDGING ANTICOAGULATION IN PATIENTS WITH ATRIAL FIBRILLATION

Douketis J, Spyropoulos A, Kaatz S et al., *N Engl J Med*. 2015;373:823–833

Commentary by Akpofure Peter Ekeh

For decades, warfarin had remained the sole oral anticoagulant drug available for chronic conditions like atrial fibrillation and atrial flutter. The need to minimize thromboembolic complications such as transient ischemic attacks (TIAs) and strokes arising from these maladies has necessitated this approach. Frequently, large proportions of this same population require varied minor and major surgical interventions. Balancing the prevention of thromboembolic events with minimizing the risks of perioperative bleeding is often a vexing conundrum. This well-designed randomized prospective, double-blind placebo-controlled multicenter trial, performed in the United States and Canada, helped to directly address this issue. It demonstrated that the practice of not "bridging" anticoagulation therapy in warfarin therapy, was not an inferior option and a viable alternative. Furthermore, their finding showing an increased risk of bleeding complications in patients who received bridging anticoagulants was insightful.

This study, however, came on the heels of a new direction in anticoagulation pharmacotherapy. After almost 60 years with warfarin as the solitary oral anticoagulant, the Food and Drug Administration started approving new classes of drugs fulfilling the same purpose but possessing characteristics more appealing to patients and providers. The introduction and increasing use of direct thrombin inhibitors (e.g., Dabigatran) and Factor Xa inhibitors (e.g., Rivaroxaban and Apixaban) has led to a gradual reduction in warfarin utilization for obvious reasons, including shorter half-lives and quicker onsets of therapeutic action. This study does not address the need for bridging of anticoagulation therapy in patients undergoing treatment for acute venous thrombosis (where continuation of anticoagulation is typically continued). Neither does this study address the occasional need for continued anticoagulation in patients with mechanical heart valves, who must be individualized on the basis of valve type and location, and the recency of valve placement. Regardless of these developments, this paper legitimately qualifies as a landmark paper that helped to modify practices and change guidelines for managing perioperative patients requiring anticoagulation for atrial arrhythmias.

CHAPTER 7

Congestive Heart Failure

Review by Brooks Willar and E. Wilson Grandin

Heart failure has become a global epidemic. Cardiogenic shock and decompensated heart failure constitute a large proportion of admissions to intensive care units [1], and rates of re-hospitalization and mortality over the subsequent year are high.

Categorizing patients with heart failure with reduced ejection fraction (HFrEF), according to a hemodynamic profile based on volume status ("wet" vs. "dry") and systemic perfusion ("warm" vs. "cold"), identifies distinct clinical phenotypes with varying risk and guides therapeutic interventions [2]. While determination of this hemodynamic profile can be made using bedside clinical assessment, if there is evidence of cardiogenic shock (CS) or patients not responding to empiric therapy, clinicians should have a low threshold to place a pulmonary artery catheter (PAC). Recent multicenter observational data have demonstrated improved outcomes for patients with CS managed with a PAC and complete hemodynamic profiling [3].

Once the hemodynamic profile is established, the mainstays of medical management for decompensated HFrEF in the ICU include decongestion, inotropic support, and systemic vasodilators. While inotropic support can increase cardiac output and systemic perfusion, it does so at the expense of increased myocardial work and oxygen demand, with potential acute and chronic detrimental effects on the heart. In contrast, systemic vasodilators reduce left ventricular afterload, decrease myocardial wall stress and, thus, can increase perfusion while decreasing myocardial oxygen demand. For patients admitted with decompensated HFrEF with low cardiac output and adequate blood pressure (e.g., mean arterial pressure >70 mmHg and systemic vascular resistance >1000 dynes-sec-cm^{-5}), systemic vasodilators are the preferred initial therapy. Sodium nitroprusside (SNP) is the most potent and effective of these agents, and while there are no randomized clinical trials of SNP in decompensated HFrEF, multiple observational studies have demonstrated clear safety, acute hemodynamic improvement, and favorable clinical outcomes [4].

While IV vasodilators like SNP are effective initial therapy for decompensated HFrEF with low cardiac output, continuation for longer periods of time can result in toxicity and tachyphylaxis. Therefore, if a patient has a favorable clinical and hemodynamic response to IV vasodilator therapy, clinicians should cross-titrate to oral vasodilators within the next 24–48 hours. Traditional oral vasodilators that are also associated with improved long-term outcomes in HFrEF include angiotensin-converting enzyme inhibitors (ACEi), angiotensin receptor blockers (ARB), and the combination of hydralazine

DOI: 10.1201/9781003042136-7

and isosorbide. More recently, ARNI therapy, which combines an ARB (valsartan) with a neprilysin inhibitor (sacubitril), has emerged as a novel vasodilator and neuro-hormonal antagonist that substantially improves clinical outcomes in HFrEF.

Inhibition of neprilysin, a neutral endopeptidase that degrades natriuretic peptides and other vasoactive peptides (e.g., angiotensin II and bradykinin), results in favor-able physiologic effects including natriuresis and systemic vasodilation. The land-mark PARADIGM-HF trial compared ARNI therapy with sacubitril-valsartan to traditional ACE inhibition with enalapril in more than 8000 ambulatory HFrEF patients [5]. Importantly, patients were required to complete a single-blind run-in phase to ensure tolerability of high-dose ACEi and ARNI before being randomized to enalapril 10 mg twice daily or sacubitril-valsartan titrated to a goal dose of 97–103 mg twice daily. The trial was stopped early due to overwhelming benefits with ARNI therapy, including a lower incidence of cardiovascular death or HF hospitalization and reduced all-cause mortality [5]. The ARNI was well tolerated except for increased rates of symptomatic hypotension, but this rarely required discontinuation of therapy. PARADIGM-HF established ARNI as superior to traditional ACEi (and by inference ARB) for ambulatory HFrEF patients, but this study enrolled very stable outpatients with robust blood pressure.

Uncertainty remained about whether ARNI therapy could be safely initiated among inpatients with decompensated heart failure, so the PIONEER-HF trial enrolled patients hospitalized with decompensated HFrEF who were hemodynamically stable [6]. A total of 881 HFrEF patients were randomized to low-dose sacubitril-valsartan (24–26 mg) or enalapril with subsequent uptitration according to a pre-specified algorithm. After 8 weeks, patients receiving ARNI had greater reductions in NT-proBNP, the primary endpoint, and the rates of adverse events were similar [6]. Importantly, a secondary analysis found that patients receiving ARNI had a substantial reduction in the risk of key composite clinical endpoints including death and re-hospitalization for HF [7]. PIONEER-HF thus established the safety and efficacy of initiating ARNI therapy among inpatients with decompensated HFrEF. ARNI therapy has not been well stud-ied in patients with advanced HFrEF or cardiogenic shock, but anecdotal experience suggests that cautious initiation is feasible and effective in these patients, and ongoing studies should provide additional data in this population [8].

Providers need to consider a few important clinical factors when initiating inpatient ARNI therapy. A 36-hour washout period from ACEi is needed prior to starting ARNI due to the significant risk of angioedema with concomitant ACE and neprilysin inhibition, both of which can potentiate bradykinin levels. For patients admitted with decompensated heart failure, particularly those who require the ICU for low cardiac output, this 36-hour washout without any ACEi/ARB/ARNI therapy should be avoided as withdrawal of that afterload reduction can be highly detrimental in these vulnerable patients. A sensible approach for patients with marginal blood pressure is starting a low-dose ARB, which, if tolerated, can be transitioned to low-dose sacubitril-valsartan (24–26 mg). The ionic form of valsartan found in sacubitril-valsartan is 40% more bioavailable than the salt used in stand-alone valsartan, so 26 mg of valsartan in sacu-bitril-valsartan is roughly equivalent to 40 mg of traditional valsartan [9]. For patients with marginal blood pressure, we suggest initiating valsartan at 20 mg twice daily and uptitrating to 40 mg twice daily before transitioning to low-dose sacubitril-valsartan. When titrating ARNI therapy in patients with marginal blood pressure, allow 48–72 hours at a stable dose before considering an increase to the next dosing level.

ARNI should generally be avoided in patients with advanced chronic kidney disease (e.g., ≥ stage IV) or severe acute kidney injury with eGFR <30 mL/min. As with ACEi/ARB, the hemodynamic effect of ARNI therapy can produce a modest (typi-cally <20%) reduction in eGFR shortly after initiation, which should not prompt discontinuation if the patient is otherwise tolerating the medication. ARNI has been shown to be safe in patients with chronic kidney disease [10], but in patients requiring renal replacement therapy, ARNI should be avoided due to the potential for accumu-lation of the sacubitril component, leading to an increased risk of hypotension and angioedema. Neprilysin inhibition increases circulating natriuretic peptide levels, which can produce a modest natriuresis, sometimes resulting in a decreased loop diuretic requirement. If patients are euvolemic at the time of ARNI initiation, the loop diuretic dose can often be reduced by 25–50% with close monitoring of clinical volume status.

In summary, patients admitted to the ICU with decompensated HFrEF should have a careful assessment of their hemodynamic profile, with a low threshold for PAC place-ment. For patients with low cardiac output and adequate blood pressure, IV vasodila-tor therapy should be favored with early overlap to oral vasodilators. ARNI therapy represents a major advance in the medical management of HFrEF, producing signifi-cant reductions in morbidity and mortality. Whenever possible, patients with decom-pensated HFrEF should be started on ARNI with close attention to volume status, blood pressure, renal function, and serum potassium. Expansion of ARNI use in this population can lead to substantial improvements in patient outcomes.

ANNOTATED REFERENCES FOR CONGESTIVE HEART FAILURE

1. Berg DD, Bohula EA, van Diepen S, et al. Epidemiology of shock in contemporary car-diac intensive care units. *Circ: Cardiovasc Qual Outcomes.* 2019 March;12(3):e005618. doi:10.1161/CIRCOUTCOMES.119.005618

   This was a cross-sectional study from 16 centers in the Critical Care Cardiology Trials Network with >3000 patients admitted to cardiac intensive care units where ~2/3 of patients had evidence of cardiogenic shock and nearly half of those were patients with decompensated HFrEF.

2. Nohria A, Tsang SW, Fang JC, et al. Clinical assessment identifies hemodynamic pro-files that predict outcomes in patients admitted with heart failure. *J Am Coll Cardiol.* 2003;41(10):1797–1804.

   This was a single-center, prospective cohort study of 452 patients admitted to Brigham and Women's Hospital with HFrEF where hemodynamic categorization based on congestion and systemic perfusion using bedside clinical assessment identified distinct profiles of risk. Patients with congestion and decreased perfusion (i.e., "cold and wet") had the highest mortality over the subsequent 18 months.

3. Garan AR, Kanwar M, Thayer KL, et al. Complete hemodynamic profiling with pulmonary artery catheters in cardiogenic shock is associated with lower in-hospital mortality. *Heart Failure*. 2020;8(11):903–913.

This was a retrospective cohort study of >1400 patients admitted with cardiogenic shock from the Cardiogenic Shock Working Group, a multicenter collaboration of academic medical centers. Patients with cardiogenic shock who were managed with a pulmonary artery catheter with complete hemodynamic profiling had a significantly lower inpatient mortality.

4. Mullens W, Abrahams Z, Francis GS, et al. Sodium nitroprusside for advanced low-output heart failure. *J Am Coll Cardiol*. 2008;52(3):200–207.

This was a retrospective, case-control study of patients admitted with decompensated HFrEF and low cardiac output at Cleveland Clinic. Compared to control patients who were managed with traditional medical therapy, patients who received sodium nitroprusside had significantly greater hemodynamic improvement, were more likely to be discharged on an oral vasodilator, and had improved long-term survival.

5. McMurray JJ, Packer M, Desai AS, et al. Angiotensin-neprilysin inhibition versus enalapril in heart failure. *N Engl J Med*. Sep 2014;371(11):993–1004. doi:10.1056/NEJMoa1409077

PARADIGM-HF was a landmark, randomized clinical trial of ARNI therapy with sacubitril-valsartan compared to traditional ACE inhibitor (enalapril) in 8442 HFrEF patients with NYHA class ≥2 symptoms, LVEF <40%, elevated BNP, and receiving stable doses of a beta-blocker and ACE inhibitor or ARB (equivalent in dose to enalapril 10 mg daily). The trial was stopped early, after a median follow-up at 27 months, due to overwhelming benefit with ARNI therapy, including a lower incidence of the primary outcome of cardiovascular death or HF hospitalization (21.8% vs. 26.5%; p <0.001, number needed to treat of 21), a significant reduction in all-cause mortality (17.0% vs. 19.8%; p <0.001, number needed to treat of 36), and better quality of life scores.

6. Velazquez EJ, Morrow DA, DeVore AD, et al. Angiotensin-neprilysin inhibition in acute decompensated heart failure. *N Engl J Med*. 02 2019;380(6):539–548. doi:10.1056/NEJMoa1812851

PIONEEF-HF was a randomized clinical trial of 881 patients admitted with decompensated HFrEF who were hemodynamically stable, defined as not requiring increasing doses of IV diuretics, vasodilators, or inotropes within 24 hours prior to randomization. Compared to patients in the control arm treated with enalapril, patients receiving ARNI therapy (sacubitril-valsartan) had significantly greater reductions in NTproBNP after 8 weeks of therapy (percent change −25.3% with enalapril versus −46.7% with sacubitril-valsartan, ratio of change 0.71, 95%CI 0.63–0.81, p <0.001).

7. Morrow DA, Velazquez EJ, DeVore AD, et al. Clinical outcomes in patients with acute decompensated heart failure randomly assigned to sacubitril/valsartan or enalapril in the PIONEER-HF Trial. *Circulation*. 2019 May;139(19):2285–2288. doi:10.1161/CIRCULATIONAHA.118.039331

This secondary analysis of the PIONEEF-HF trial demonstrated that patients randomized to sacubitril-valsartan (ARNI) compared to enalapril (ACEi) had a significantly lower rate of the combined endpoint of death, re-hospitalization for HF, left ventricular assist device implantation, or listing for cardiac transplant (hazard ratio 0.58, 95% CI 0.40–0.85, p = 0.005).

8. Mann DL, Greene SJ, Givertz MM, et al. Sacubitril/valsartan in advanced heart failure with reduced ejection fraction: rationale and design of the LIFE trial. *JACC Heart Failure.* 10 2020;8(10):789–799. doi:10.1016/j.jchf.2020.05.005

   The ongoing LIFE Trial is a 24-week, prospective, multicenter, double-blinded, double-dummy, active comparator trial of sacubitril-valsartan versus valsartan alone in patients with severe HFrEF defined as LVEF ≤35%, NYHA class IV symptoms, and at least one or more objective findings of "advanced" heart failure: 1) current inotropic support or need for inotropes within the past 6 months, 2) at least one hospitalization for heart failure in the last 6 months, 3) LVEF ≤25%, 4) peak VO2 <55% predicted or ≤16 mL/kg/min for men or ≤14 mL/kg/min for women, 5) 6-minute walk distance <300 m.

9. Gu J, Noe A, Chandra P, et al. Pharmacokinetics and pharmacodynamics of LCZ696, a novel dual-acting angiotensin receptor-neprilysin inhibitor (ARNi). *J Clin Pharmacol.* Apr 2010;50(4):401–414. doi:10.1177/0091270009343932

   This is a review of the basic pharmacokinetics and pharmacodynamics of sacubitril-valsartan.

10. Haynes R, Judge PK, Staplin N, et al. Effects of sacubitril/valsartan versus irbesartan in patients with chronic kidney disease. *Circulation.* 10 2018;138(15):1505–1514. doi:10.1161/CIRCULATIONAHA.118.034818

    The UK HARP-III study was a randomized, double-blind trial of 414 patients with chronic kidney disease and estimated glomerular filtration rate (eGFR) of 20–60 mL/min/1.73m² who were randomized to traditional ARB with irbesartan versus ARNI with sacubitril-valsartan. The primary outcome of eGFR at 12 months as well as urine albumin:creatinine was similar in both groups, and ARNI therapy was associated with significantly lower follow-up levels of troponin-I and NTproBNP.

Landmark Article of the 21st Century

ANGIOTENSIN-NEPRILYSIN INHIBITION VS ENALAPRIL IN HEART FAILURE

McMurray JJ et al., *N Engl J Med.* 2014;171:993–1004

Commentary by Alan Lisbon

Paradigm HF: Cardiovascular disease and heart failure are major causes of death, morbidity and health care costs. Blockade of the renin-angiotensin system has been shown to control blood pressure and prevent end-organ damage. Neprilysin inhibition increases levels of natriuretic peptides and has favorable effects on natriuresis and vasodilation. These peptides also oppose angiotensin II.

Design: This was a prospective, multicenter, randomized, double-blind trial of 8400 patients with class II, III, or IV heart failure with an EF <40% who received an angiotensin-neprilysin inhibitor (sacubitril-valsartan) or enalapril both twice daily.

The primary endpoint was death from cardiovascular causes or hospitalization for heart failure. The trial was also designed to detect a difference in death from CV causes.

Results: The trial was stopped early because of the overwhelming benefit of sacubitril-valsartan in the composite endpoint 21.8% vs. 26.5%, and death from CV causes 13.3% vs. 16.5%. The majority of patients had class II heart failure (70%) and 24% had class III. Renal impairment was less in the sacubitril-valsartan group. There was no difference in rates of angioedema.

Conclusions: The trial has been criticized because the dose of enalapril is different from that used in clinical practice and that an angiotensin receptor blocker was not used instead of enalapril. This study was an important change in the management of heart failure with a reduced ejection fraction.

CHAPTER 8

Perioperative Myocardial Infarction

Review by Duane S. Pinto

It is long appreciated that the physiologic stress engendered by surgery can tax the circulatory system. When coupled with altered hemostasis, blood loss, and pressure fluctuation myocardial ischemia and infarction can be provoked. Certainly, there is an interaction in a variety of patient factors such as advanced age, atherosclerosis, and the specific nature of the surgery. Obviously, procedures that result in blood loss, large fluid shifts, and hypercoagulability are of particular concern, but such complications may occur unexpectedly in many procedures, and myocardial infarction may complicate recovery even among patients deemed low risk preoperatively.

The perioperative setting poses several unique challenges in diagnosis and management compared with patients who have not recently undergone surgery. With regard to diagnosis, it is frequent that these infarctions present without chest pain; obvious ECG changes and recognition of myocardial injury may be delayed simply because the patient may be unable to accurately describe symptoms stemming from alteration in consciousness or the fact that they may be intubated. As such, the intensivist may recognize that myocardial injury is occurring only after resultant hemodynamic derangement, arrhythmia, or congestive heart failure has begun to develop. It is not surprising that there is substantial mortality associated with perioperative myocardial infarction.

An important determination is that of the underlying pathophysiology of acute coronary syndrome. Is the ischemia caused by an ulcerated thrombotic coronary plaque or embolism, a so-called Type I infarction according to the universal definition of myocardial infarction, or is the syndrome related to a supply/demand mismatch, called "Type II" infarction? These are related to the increased demand of infection or metabolic demand oftentimes in conjunction with reduced supply from chronic fixed coronary disease, systemic hypotension, or anemia. While cardiac biomarkers such as creatine kinase-MB and cardiac troponin will be elevated in both scenarios, the management of these entities is quite different. Management of the Type II infarction involves rather than focusing upon interventions involving anticoagulation or coronary revascularization. Interventions targeting atherothrombosis are utilized for Type I infarctions including anticoagulants, antiplatelet agents and, in some cases, coronary intervention. Sometimes the ability to make the distinction is unclear, and in those cases, clinical judgement supervenes balancing the risk and benefits of anticoagulants, angiography, and

DOI: 10.1201/9781003042136-8

revascularization. It is estimated that Type II infarctions account for at least 75% of perioperative myocardial infarctions.

For all myocardial infarctions, optimal management includes attempting to reduce myocardial demand, often using beta-blockers as well as agents aimed at reducing pain and blood pressure. Myocardial oxygen supply is increased with the administration of nitroglycerine and by alleviating hypoxemia and anemia. Routine oxygen administration to patients who are not hypoxic has not been shown to be beneficial. Unfortunately, all of these agents cannot uniformly be applied in the perioperative setting since patients may be hypotensive or on vasopressors. Calcium channel blockers are primarily negative inotropes and should be avoided given lack of benefit in randomized trials. Control of tachycardia in the perioperative setting merits specific consideration; fever, anemia, pain, and heart failure are often coexisting conditions, where agents aimed at controlling the heart rate in an effort to reduce myocardial demand may be ineffective or deleterious. The most prudent course of action is to address the underlying stimulus for tachycardia, if possible.

With regard to specific therapies in Type I infarction, these are managed according to established standards for acute coronary syndromes, which involve first risk assessment with regard to the chances of recurrent MI, shock, or death. Patients at an increased risk are selected for more aggressive measures. The presence of ST segment deviation on the 12-lead electrocardiogram, elevated cardiac biomarkers, congestive heart failure, ventricular arrhythmia, or hemodynamic derangement stemming from myocardial dysfunction signify patients at increased risk. Standard interventions include administration of 325 mg of aspirin, unfractionated heparin bolus (50 units/kg up to 5000 units) and drip (12 units/kg/h).

The intensivist makes an enormous contribution in this setting. In recognizing and understanding the short term risk of full anticoagulation with regard to bleeding and the medium-term risk of administration of potent antiplatelet therapies, a balanced decision can be made with regard to ischemic risk, as well as the decision on whether or not the patient can be treated for their infarction. If the patient cannot receive aspirin and anticoagulation, they must be managed noninvasively; if the patient cannot receive aspirin with clopidogrel after the procedure, then coronary intervention will not likely be possible. Depending upon the type of surgery, potential location of bleeding, and resultant complications, a decision to proceed despite the high risk of bleeding with sustained anticoagulation and administration of antiplatelet agents may be necessary in a patient with profound cardiovascular compromise. By contrast, a patient with a small infarction, where the consequences of bleeding may be devastating, is best managed conservatively. It should be noted, that even amongst patients with high-risk infarctions, the magnitude of difference between a patient managed invasively compared with one managed conservatively is moderate.

If a decision is made to proceed with invasive intervention, the timing of intervention depends upon two factors; whether it is believed that the culprit vessel is totally occluded and how ill the patient is with regard to cardiovascular hemodynamics. If it is likely that the culprit vessel is totally occluded, invasive evaluation is emergent. While infrequent, accounting for <20% of myocardial infarctions, ST segment elevation on the 12-lead ECG is the most reliable clue that the vessel may be totally occluded, also if there is the presence of ongoing chest pain that cannot be relieved. If the vessel is thought to be patent, then the invasive investigation can occur urgently within 24–48 hours. Other patients, regardless of ECG findings that may require more urgent invasive evaluation, are those where advancing cardiogenic shock, refractory ventricular tachyarrhythmias, or coronary revascularization may be part of the management strategy; however, percutaneous mechanical circulatory support (intra-aortic balloon counterpulsation, microaxial flow pump insertion) may become necessary. Recurrent episodes of ischemia, especially if associated with dynamic ECG changes or heart failure, may require more urgent evaluation. Increasing biomarker levels without any of these associated findings does not necessarily warrant emergent evaluation and is to be expected as part of the natural history of myocardial infarction.

Again, decisions in the perioperative setting are more challenging where determination of whether the patient is having refractory chest symptoms can be difficult in the setting of pain from the surgical wounds, administration of narcotics, or intubated status. The patient may have hemodynamic derangement from other cardiac or cardiac causes or some element of volume overload simply related to resuscitative measures. In such settings, it may be useful to assess cardiac function with echocardiography. If infarction is occurring, but there is very little contractile dysfunction, the care team will feel more confident in a conservative strategy. Cardiac tamponade, unrecognized profound right or left ventricular dysfunction, or valvular heart disease can aid in the management of unexplained hypotension. Again, relatively preserved myocardial functions may support a conservative approach with the myocardial infarction and/or direct further workup and management to other disorders.

ANNOTATED REFERENCES FOR PERIOPERATIVE MYOCARDIAL INFARCTION

Collett JP, Thiele H, Barbato E, et al. 2020 ESC Guidelines for the management of acute coronary syndromes in patients presenting without persistent ST-segment elevation: the Task Force for the management of acute coronary syndromes in patients presenting without persistent ST-segment elevation of the European Society of Cardiology (ESC). *Eur Heart J.* 2021;42(14):1289–1367.

This is the most recent societal guideline summarizing evidence and recommendations for the various aspects of management of myocardial infarction with ST-segment elevation. This comprehensive document can serve as a reference for the practicing intensivist.

Ferreira, T, Arede, MJ, Oliveira, F, et al. Myocardial infarction after noncardiac surgery, a 10 year experience. *Eur J Anaesthesiol.* 2013;30:72.

This analysis provides special context for differences in the presentation of perioperative vs. spontaneous myocardial infarction as well as the frequency and associated mortality.

Freemantle N, Cleland J, Young P, Mason J, Harrison J. Beta Blockade after myocardial infarction: systematic review and meta regression analysis. *Br Med J.* 1999;318(7200):17.

This review summarizes over 20 years of randomized trials evaluating the benefits and risks of beta-blockade after myocardial infarction. A 23% reduction in the odds of death in long term trials (95% confidence interval 15% to 31%), and a 4% reduction in the odds of death in short term trials ([-]8% to 15%). In long term trials, the number needed to treat for 2 years to avoid a death is 42.

Hofmann R, James, SK, Jernberg, T, et al. Oxygen therapy in suspected acute myocardial infarction. *N Engl J Med.* 2017;377(13):1240–1249.

The Determination of the Role of Oxygen in Suspected Acute Myocardial Infarction (DETO2X-AMI) was a multicenter, randomized control trial with a total of 6629 patients assigned to either oxygen or ambient-air group. All-cause mortality at 1 year was similar in the oxygen and ambient air groups (5.0% vs. 5.1%; HR 0.97; p = 0.80), as was MI rehospitalization at 1 year (3.8% vs. 3.3%; HR p = 0.33). The trial suggests avoiding routine use of oxygen among patients with normoxia and MI or findings concerning for MI.

Mehta SR, Granger CB, Boden WE, et al. Early versus delayed invasive intervention in acute coronary syndromes. *N Engl J Med.* 2009;360(21):2165–2175.

A number of randomized trials demonstrated the benefit of early invasive intervention with angiography in high-risk patients with unstable angina (UA) and NSTEMI. This trial evaluated timing of this intervention. The trial randomized 3031 patients with unstable angina or NSTEMI to either early-intervention (as early as possible and <24 hours) or delayed-intervention (minimum delay of 36 hours). At 6 months, the primary outcome (composite of death, new MI, or stroke) occurred in 9.6% of patients in the early-intervention group compared to 11.3% in the delayed-intervention group (HR 0.95; 95% CI 0.68 to 1.06; p = 0.15). A prespecified subgroup analysis showed the highest risk patients undergoing early intervention had a significantly lower rate of the primary outcome compared to those in the delayed intervention arm (13.9% vs. 21.0% HR 0.65, CI 0.48 to 0.89, p = 0.006). When this same subgroup analysis was applied to low- to moderate-risk patients, there was no significant difference in the primary outcome between early or delayed intervention. This trial informs perioperative management decisions with regard to timing in the perioperative setting where the magnitude of benefit according to risk can be balanced against the harms associated with performing angiography and administering anticoagulants.

Thygesen K, Alpert JS, Jaffe AS, et al. Fourth universal definition of myocardial infarction. *J Am Coll Cardiol.* 2018;72(18):2231–2264.

This consensus document outlines the definitions and pathophysiologic differences in the various forms of myocardial infarction. Of particular interest to intensivists are the distinctions between spontaneous, Type I infarctions, and Type II infarctions secondary to supply/demand mismatch. Infarctions related to stent thrombosis, sudden death, and after coronary artery bypass surgery are also discussed.

Landmark Article of the 21st Century

POSTOPERATIVE PROPHYLACTIC ADMINISTRATION OF β-ADRENERGIC BLOCKERS IN PATIENTS AT RISK FOR MYOCARDIAL ISCHEMIA

Urban M, Markowitz S, Gordon M et al., *Anesth Analg*. 2000;90:1257–1261

Commentary by Claire Larson Isbell

As a surgical intern, it was deemed crucial to write postoperative β-blocker orders for our "at-risk" surgical patients. During that time, I frequently did what I was told without questioning "why?," and it was not until much later that I developed a healthy respect for β-blockers and why and when they should be used.

β-Blockers were first employed in the 1960s but were not a mainstay of perioperative care. Prior to this publication, the benefit of β-blockade in the postoperative surgical patient was not yet recognized. Now, most of my surgical ICU patients receive scheduled doses of β-blockers. This study was one of the first to investigate β-blocker use in postoperative patients, and revealed that myocardial ischemia is present in subjects with coronary artery disease (CAD) risk factors following non-cardiac surgery. The authors attempted to control for hemodynamic instability induced by general anesthesia by studying β-blocker effects in patients undergoing the same procedure under regional anesthesia. Although several limitations exist, this work represents a springboard by which surgical intensivists began to better understand their role in optimizing cardiac health following non-cardiac surgery.

Full appreciation for the authors' forward-thinking is now evident, and most intensivists can agree on the following: the decision to treat a patient with β-blockade during the postoperative period is one that requires careful consideration of patient CAD risk factors and history, as well as their hemodynamic status following surgery (including the potential effects of anesthesia) to mitigate further risk of myocardial ischemia.

CHAPTER 9

Blood Pressure Control in Acute Stroke

Review by Stephen Heard

Arterial blood pressure is often elevated during acute ischemic stroke and is postulated to be protective as hypertension may maintain perfusion in the penumbra surrounding the stroke. One factor which may contribute to this hypertension is the stress response to the stroke itself. There appears to be a U-shaped blood pressure response to stroke. Those patients with exceedingly high or low blood pressure on hospital admission have an increased 30-day risk of death [1].

Whether or not hypertension should be treated in acute stroke and how low the pressure should be decreased, if at all, are controversial. Data from randomized controlled trials do not provide much guidance. The MAPAS trial randomized patients to one of three groups based on targeted blood pressure control within 12 hours of stroke onset [2]. There was no difference among the groups in the percentage of good clinical outcome measured at 90 days, although patients in the higher systolic blood pressure range had an increased rate of symptomatic intracranial hemorrhage. However, a logistic regression analysis adjusted for confounders found that the maintenance of systolic blood pressure in the range of 161–180 mm Hg was associated with improved outcomes compared to the other two groups. A randomized controlled prehospital trial comparing transdermal nitroglycerin (NTG) to placebo administered within 4 hours of stroke onset found that NTG had statistically significant but clinically modest effects on lowering blood pressure. Ninety-day functional outcome was not different between groups. The trial included patients with ischemic stroke, transient ischemic attack, and intracerebral hemorrhage [3]. Data from other large trials do not provide much guidance as enrollment of patients was allowed up to 30–48 hours following stroke onset and some also enrolled patients with intracerebral hemorrhage. Finally, a number of meta-analyses have failed to demonstrate convincingly a beneficial effect on outcome.

Recent guidelines from the American Heart Association and American Stroke Association recommend that blood pressure should not be treated in patients who will not undergo thrombolytic therapy unless the systolic or diastolic blood pressure is >220 mm Hg or >120 mm Hg, respectively [4]. For those patients who are treated with a thrombolytic, the systolic and diastolic blood pressures should be ≤185 mm Hg and ≤110 mm Hg. Following therapy, the blood pressure should be around 180/105 for 24 hours. If blood pressure reduction is deemed necessary, labetalol (combined alpha and beta blocker), nicardipine, or clevidine (the latter two being dihydropyridine calcium channel blockers) should be used to avoid rapid decline in blood pressure. Nitroprusside can increase

DOI: 10.1201/9781003042136-9

intracranial pressure by vasodilation and should not be considered as a first line agent. Although observational studies have shown conflicting results on the association of lower blood pressure and outcome, and there are no clinical studies which have examined the utility of treating hypotension in acute ischemic stroke, the guidelines recommend either crystalloid or colloid therapy for treatment of hypotension. The amount and duration of such therapy as well as the use of vasopressors are unanswered questions.

Blood pressure management during mechanical thrombectomy and type of anesthesia is also controversial. Because general anesthesia (GA) might have a greater propensity to cause a lower blood pressure and retrospective studies have shown that patients receiving GA have worse neurological outcomes compared to patients who have received conscious sedation (monitored anesthesia care, MAC), many neuro-interventional radiologists prefer MAC for these procedures. However, the SIESTA trial randomized patients with an acute ischemic stroke in the anterior circulation to MAC or GA [5]. Early outcome (24 hours) was no different between the two group although complications including hypothermia, delayed extubation, and pneumonia were more frequent in the GA group. There was no difference in mortality between the two groups at 3 months but more patients in the GA group were functionally independent at that time. In a small, single-center prospective trial comparing MAC to GA, there was no difference in neurological impairment (modified Rankin Scale score) at 3 months and no difference in hospital mortality despite a greater percentage of patients with a mean arterial blood pressure (MAP) 20% lower than the baseline MAP in the GA group [6]. A greater percentage in patients in the GA group required vasopressor support to maintain the MAP.

Similar to patients with acute ischemic stroke, blood pressure is often elevated in patients with spontaneous intracerebral hemorrhage and may cause expansion of the hematoma with an increase in intracranial pressure. Lowering blood pressure may limit hematoma expansion but may also result in worsening of ischemia and neurological outcome. However, some data suggest that lowering blood pressure does not impair regional blood flow around the hematoma. Several prospective randomized trials have attempted to provide guidance. The INTERACT2 trial was a large, randomized trial of patients with ICH [7]. Treatment within 6 hours of stroke onset to one of two systolic blood pressure (SBP) goals (<180 or <140 mm Hg) did not result in any difference in death or severe disability. However, overall improved measures of disability were better in the lower target SBP group. The ATACH-2 trial randomized, scute ICH patients within 4.5 hours to targeted treatment SBP ranges of 110–139 or 140–179 mm Hg [8]. No difference in mortality or disability rates were observed. Consensus guidelines recommend that patients with acute ICH and in whom the SBP is between 150 and 220 mm Hg be treated with antihypertensives to reduce the SBP to 140 mm Hg [9]. For those who present with an SBP of >220 mm Hg, more aggressive SBP control is recommended with a continuous infusion of an antihypertensive agent. Recommended medications include labetalol, nicardipine, clevidine, esmolol, enalaprilat, fenoldopam, and/or phentolamine.

It should be made clear from the discussion above that consensus guidelines provide SBP targets that require aggressive ICU management (vasodilators, vasopressors via central lines, etc.) despite the fact that there is little data to support these thresholds and little evidence of patient benefit. Protocols should be based upon solid evidence as the consequences of overly rigid "guidelines" is extremely resource intensive (prolonged stay in the ICU) and can be injurious to the patient (i.e., volume overload, end organ ischemia).

ANNOTATED REFERENCES FOR HYPERTENSIVE EMERGENCIES

1. Filho JO, Mullen MT. Initial assessment and management of acute stroke. http://www. uptodate.com. Accessed 12/26/2020

   Overview of the management of both ischemic and hemorrhagic stroke.

2. Nasi LA, Martins SCO, Gus M, et al. Early manipulation of arterial blood pressure in acute ischemic stroke (MAPAS): results of a randomized controlled trial. *Neurocrit Care.* 2019;30:372–70. PMID: 30460598

   A relatively small prospective evaluating the effect of three different targets for blood pressure control. Good clinical outcome was not different among the three groups. However, symptomatic intracranial hemorrhage was more common in the higher blood pressure group. Adjusted logistic regression suggested the odds of having a good clinical outcome was higher in the group where a blood pressure range of 161–180 mm Hg was attained.

3. Bath PM, Scutt P, Anderson CS, et al. Prehospital transdermal glyceryl trinitrate in patients with ultra-acute presumed stroke (RIGHT-2): an ambulance-based, randomized, sham-controlled, blinded, phase 3 trial. *Lancet.* 2019;393(10175):1009–20. PMID: 30738649

   Prehospital administration of transdermal nitroglycerin did not improve the modified Rankin scores in stroke patients compared to placebo. In addition, there was no difference in secondary outcomes and death. Almost half did not have an ischemic stroke and included hemorrhagic stroke, transient ischemic attack and non-stroke mimic.

4. Powers WJ, Rabinstein AA, Ackerson T, et al. Guidelines for the early management of patients with acute ischemic stroke: 2019 update to the 2018 guidelines for the early management of acute ischemic stroke: a guidelines for healthcare professionals from the American Heart Associate/American Stroke Association. *Stroke.* 2019;50:3344–e418. PMID: 31662037

   Consensus guidelines for the early management of acute ischemic stroke.

5. Schonenberger S, Uhlmann L, Hacke W, et al. Effect of conscious sedation versus general anesthesia on early neurological improvement among patients with ischemic stroke undergoing endovascular thrombectomy: a randomized clinical trial. *JAMA.* 2016;316:1986–96. PMID: 27785516

   Prospective, single-center, randomized, parallel-group, open-label treatment trial comparing the effect of GA versus MAC on outcome following endovascular thrombectomy in patients with anterior circulation ischemic strokes. A total of 150 patients were randomized. There was no difference in the 24 hour National Institutes of Health Stroke Scale (NIHSS) score between the groups. Most secondary outcomes were not different either. However, patient movement was less in the GA group whereas hypothermia, delayed extubation, and pneumonia were more common. At 3 months, more GA patients were functionally independent based on the modified Rankin Scale but there was no difference in mortality.

6. Henden PL, Rentzos A, Karlsson J-E, et al. General anesthesia versus conscious sedation for endovascular treatment of acute ischemic stroke. The AnStroke Trial (anesthesia during stroke). *Stroke.* 2017;48:1601–07. PMID 28522637

Prospective, randomized, single-center study comparing general anesthesia (GA) to conscious sedation during endovascular treatment of ischemic stroke. There were 45 patients in each group. There was no difference in the modified Rankin Scale score at 3 months. Mean arterial blood pressure was significant lower in the GA group and use of vasopressor support was more common.

7. Anderson CS, Heeley E, Huang Y, et al. Rapid blood-pressure lowering in patients with acute intracerebral hemorrhage. *N Engl J Med.* 2013;368:2355–65. PMID: 23713578

Large multicenter, randomized trial comparing two systolic BP goals (<140 [intensive treatment] versus <180 mm Hg) within one hour in patients suffering from a hemorrhagic stroke. At 90 days, those in the intensive treatment group had a lower modified Rankin Scale as determined by ordinal analysis but there was no difference in mortality between the groups.

8. Qureshi AI, Palesch YY, Barsan WG, et al. Intensive blood-pressure lowering in patients with acute cerebral hemorrhage. *N Engl J Med.* 2016;375:1033–43. PMID 27276234

Prospective, randomized trial comparing intensive systolic BP control (SBP, 110–139 mm Hg) to standard SBP control (140–179 mm Hg) within 4.5 hours of symptom onset in patients with intracerebral hemorrhage. At 3 months, there was no difference in the modified Rankin Scale or mortality between the groups. Serious adverse events within the first 72 hours after randomization were no different although adverse renal events were noted in the intensive treatment group in the first 7 days.

9. Hemphill JC III, Greenberg SM, Anderson CS, et al. Guidelines for the management of spontaneous intracerebral hemorrhage: a guideline for healthcare professionals from the American Heart Association and American Stroke Association. *Stroke.* 2015;46:2032–60. PMID: 26022637

Consensus guidelines which include guidance for blood pressure control in patients with spontaneous intracerebral hemorrhage.

Landmark Article of the 21st Century

EFFECTS OF IMMEDIATE BLOOD PRESSURE REDUCTION ON DEATH AND MAJOR DISABILITY IN PATIENTS WITH ACUTE ISCHEMIC STROKE THE CATIS RANDOMIZED CLINICAL TRIAL.

He et al., *JAMA.* 2014;311(5):479–489

Commentary by Stephen Heard

This study was a single-blind, multicenter, blinded endpoints, randomized clinical trial of patients with acute ischemic stroke without thrombolytic therapy and with acute hypertension. They sought to determine if reduction of systolic blood pressure (SBP) within 48 hours of symptom onset would decrease death and disability at 14 days or hospital discharge.

Patients in the intervention group received antihypertensive treatment to lower SBP by 10–25% within 24 hours of randomization and to reach a goal pressure <140/90 mm Hg. The control group had all antihypertensive agents stopped.

Within 24 hours of randomization, mean SBP in the intervention group was reduced by 12.7%, whereas SBP decreased by 7.2% in the control group. The endpoint of death and disability (modified Rankin Scale) did not differ between the two groups at 14 days or hospital discharge or at the 3-month follow-up.

Weaknesses of the study include the wide time interval in which patients could be treated. It is difficult to ascertain how initiation of antihypertensive treatment close to 48 hours after the onset of a stroke could be beneficial. In addition, patients in the control group could have been treated with antihypertensive agents for a significant period of time before they were discontinued. The mean time from stroke onset to antihypertensive treatment was 15 hours and suggests the inclusion of "immediate" in the title is a misnomer. Finally, the difference in the reduction in blood pressure noted in the two groups was statistically significant but quite minor (9.1 mm Hg) and clinically irrelevant.

This is another investigation which failed to demonstrate that treatment of the acute onset of systolic hypertension in patients with acute ischemic stroke results in improved outcomes such as reduced mortality and disability.

CHAPTER 10

Mechanical Circulatory Support

Review by Megan Lynn Krajewski

The foundation of modern mechanical circulatory support (MCS) dates to the first use of cardiopulmonary bypass for open heart surgery in the 1950s. As case complexity grew, interest in applying bypass technology to post-cardiotomy shock developed, as did enthusiasm for developing a device capable of extended cardiac support. Over the next several decades both implantable artificial hearts and extracorporeal left ventricular assist devices (LVADs) were developed [1]. LVADs became the dominant focus for durable support, and with subsequent reduction in size and internalization of devices, long-term treatment is now possible. A spectrum of MCS devices exists, ranging from temporary percutaneous support for patients in cardiogenic shock to long-term surgically implanted devices for patients with advanced heart failure.

TEMPORARY MCS

Temporary MCS devices provide a range of hemodynamic support through different mechanisms, augmenting cardiac output and maintaining end organ perfusion [2]. Common indications for temporary MCS include cardiogenic or post-cardiotomy shock, support during high risk procedures, and cardiac arrest. By supporting organ function, temporary MCS provides a bridge to recovery or potentially to durable support. Temporary MCS options can support the left ventricle, right ventricle, or both, and includes the intra-aortic balloon pump, percutaneous catheter-based VADs, and venoarterial extracorporeal membrane oxygenation (ECMO). In the absence of high quality data supporting the use of temporary MCS, clinical experience and physiologic principles largely guide decision-making.

DURABLE MCS

Due to the significant morbidity and mortality associated with advanced heart failure, durable MCS has become an increasingly important therapy. LVADs, the most commonly implanted durable devices, improve both survival and quality of life. The first generation intracorporeal LVADs, designed to mimic the pulsatility of the heart, were originally used in the 1990s as a transition therapy in patients awaiting heart transplant. In 2001, the REMATCH trial demonstrated a survival benefit with LVAD treatment compared to optimal medical therapy in patients who were not candidates for transplantation [3]. This study opened the door for LVADs to be used not only as a bridge to transplant (BTT), but also as a treatment strategy for patients ineligible for

DOI: 10.1201/9781003042136-10

transplant, i.e., destination therapy (DT). However, the poor durability and complications of the first-generation devices limited the therapeutic potential for DT patients. Second-generation devices implemented significant design changes, shifting from pulsatile pumps to axial continuous-flow pumps, resulting in a smaller profile and improved durability. DT patients treated with the HeartMate II (Abbott) experienced greater survival, free from disabling stroke and reoperation for device malfunction as compared to those treated with a pulsatile device [4]. However, adverse events remained common, and later pump thrombosis emerged as a significant problem [5].

Like their second generation predecessors, the current third generation LVADs have continuous flow pumps, but with important design changes. The newer devices use centrifugal pumps, and instead of mechanical bearings, employ either a combination of hydrodynamic and magnetic forces (HeartWare HVAD, Medtronic) or fully magnetic forces (HeartMate 3, Abbott) to suspend the impeller. In the ENDURANCE trial, the HVAD was non-inferior to the HeartMate II with respect to the composite outcome of survival free from disabling stroke or reoperation for device malfunction; however, the HVAD group did have higher rates of stroke and right ventricular failure [6]. HVAD received FDA approval for BTT in 2012 and DT in 2017. MOMENTUM 3, the largest randomized LVAD trial, randomized patients to treatment with the HeartMate 3 or the commercially available HeartMate II. The HeartMate 3 group had higher survival, free from disabling stroke or need for reoperation for device malfunction (largely due to reduction in pump thrombosis). There was also benefit with respect to reducing hemocompatibility-related adverse outcomes (pump thrombosis, stroke of any size, and bleeding events). If real world and long-term experience confirm a reduction in adverse events, this may shift the risk-benefit balance when considering LVAD therapy for greater numbers of advanced heart failure patients. HeartMate 3 received FDA approval for BTT in 2017 and DT in 2018. For new implantations, third generation centrifugal-flow devices have supplanted second generation axial-flow devices [7].

Due to the technological progress achieved by continuous-flow pumps, one-year survival now exceeds 80% and is similar to that of cardiac transplant [7]. Five-year survival of patients receiving LVADs is 47%, while that of cardiac transplantation is 74% [7], however, it will be several years before we have longer term data from newly implanted third generation devices. Historically, the major cause of early mortality is multisystem organ failure; stroke is the primary cause of death in long term. The leading indication for LVAD implantation is now destination therapy, highlighting the importance of not only survival, but also freedom from serious complications including gastrointestinal bleeding, stroke, device-related infection, and right heart failure. Despite the progress that has been made, these adverse events cause real limitations.

The acuity of patients being considered for MCS is classified according to the Intermacs profiles, ranging from profile 7, an ambulatory patient with New York Heart Class III symptoms, to profile 1 representing critical cardiogenic shock [8]. In recent years, over half of the patients undergoing primary isolated LVAD implantation met criteria for Intermacs profile 1 or 2, and nearly 35% of patients undergoing isolated

LVAD implantation were receiving temporary MCS. Risk factors for early mortality include older age, higher Intermacs profile acuity, need for temporary MCS, higher creatinine or pre-implant dialysis, and prior cardiac surgery [7, 9]. Need for right ventricular assist device (RVAD) is associated with markedly reduced survival compared to isolated LVAD implantation, and outcomes are worse with delayed RVAD implantation [9]. Accurate prediction of right ventricular failure remains elusive, but there is enthusiasm for the potential role of percutaneous MCS options in the management of right ventricular failure following LVAD implantation.

With the proliferation of new MCS technologies in recent years, it is important to understand the long-term clinical impact of these interventions and identify management strategies or modifications necessary to reduce significant complications. The landscape of temporary MCS requires efforts to better define which patients derive the most benefit and the optimal timing to initiate these therapies. Innovation with durable LVADs continues, from minimally invasive implantation techniques via thoracotomy, to growing off-label use of durable bi-ventricular assist devices, to the task of developing fully implantable wireless devices. The achievements are remarkable and will continue to positively impact management of the growing population with advanced heart failure.

ANNOTATED REFERENCES FOR MECHANICAL CIRCULATORY SUPPORT

1. Helman DN, Rose EA. History of mechanical circulatory support. *Prog Cardiovasc Dis.* 2000;43(1):1–4.

   This review article provides a detailed history of the early development of mechanical support devices through the late 1990s.

2. Combes A, Price S, Slutsky AS, Brodie D. Temporary circulatory support for cardiogenic shock. *Lancet.* 2020;396(10245):199–212.

   A comprehensive review article focused on temporary mechanical circulatory support devices.

3. Rose EA, Gelijns AC, Moskowitz AJ, et al. Long-term use of a left ventricular assist device for end-stage heart failure. *N Engl J Med.* 2001;345(20):1435–1443.

   A multicenter, randomized, controlled trial of patients with end-stage heart failure ineligible for transplantation, comparing treatment with LVAD (n = 68) to optimal medical therapy (n = 61). Treatment with a first generation LVAD (HeartMate XVE) reduced all-cause mortality as compared to treatment with optimal medical therapy alone. Mortality was reduced at one year (52% vs. 25%, p = 0.002), but not at 2 years (25% vs. 8%, p = 0.09). Infection and device failure drove mortality in the device group. Patients treated with an LVAD were more likely to have an adverse event than those receiving medical therapy. The device group demonstrated improved quality of life. This study established the benefit of LVADs for destination therapy, leading to FDA approval for this indication in 2002.

4. Slaughter MS, Rogers JG, Milano CA, et al. Advanced heart failure treated with continuous-flow left ventricular assist device. *N Engl J Med.* 2009;361(23):2241–2251.

A multicenter, randomized, controlled trial of patients with advanced heart failure ineligible for transplantation treated with either a second-generation axial continuous-flow device (HeartMate II, n = 134) or the device approved at the time, a first generation pulsatile-flow device (HeartMate XVE, n = 66). In the continuous-flow group, 46% of patients reached the primary composite endpoint of survival free from disabling stroke or need for reoperation for device replacement or repair, as compared to 11% in in the pulsatile-flow group (p <0.001). Failure to reach the primary outcome was driven by need for reoperation and death. Adverse events including infection, right heart failure, and rehospitalization were reduced in the continuous-flow group. There was no reduction in stroke or bleeding. Both groups demonstrated improvement in quality of life metrics.

5. Starling RC, Moazami N, Silvestry SC, et al. Unexpected abrupt increase in left ventricular assist device thrombosis. *N Engl J Med.* 2014;370(1):33–40.

   A retrospective study examining data from 837 HeartMate II patients at three institutions. This study demonstrated an increased rate of pump thrombosis associated with substantial mortality if not treated with device replacement or transplantation. A marked increase in lactate dehydrogenase levels often preceded new pump thrombosis.

6. Rogers JG, Pagani FD, Tatooles AJ, et al. Intrapericardial left ventricular assist device for advanced heart failure. *N Engl J Med.* 2017;376(5):451–460.

   A multicenter, randomized, controlled trial of patients with advanced heart failure ineligible for transplantation comparing a centrifugal continuous-flow LVAD with hydrodynamic and magnetic levitation (HeartWare HVAD, n = 297) to the commercially available axial continuous-flow LVAD (HeartMate II, n = 148). The study showed non-inferiority of the centrifugal-flow device relative to the axial-flow device with respect to the primary composite endpoint of two-year survival free from disabling stroke or need for reoperation due to pump malfunction or failure. Strokes of any severity and RV failure were more frequent in patients in the centrifugal-flow group; patients receiving the axial-flow device more frequently required reoperation. Both groups had improved quality of life metrics. Post-hoc analysis of the centrifugal-flow group demonstrated patients with mean arterial pressure <90 mmHg had lower incidence of stroke.

7. Teuteberg JJ, Cleveland JC, Jr., Cowger J, et al. The society of thoracic surgeons Intermacs 2019 annual report: the changing landscape of devices and indications. *Ann Thorac Surg.* 2020;109(3):649–660.

   The Interagency Registry for Mechanically Assisted Circulatory Support (Intermacs) is a North American registry that prospectively collects data on all patients who received a Food and Drug Administration-approved mechanical circulatory support device. This annual report provides longitudinal granular data including clinical characteristics and outcomes according to device type. This is the most recent annual report at the time of this writing, and examines data from the period of January 2014 through September 2019, reflecting contemporary experience.

8. Stevenson LW, Pagani FD, Young JB, et al. INTERMACS profiles of advanced heart failure: the current picture. *J Heart Lung Transplant.* 2009;28(6):535–541.

   A classification system according to illness severity for advanced heart failure patients being considered for mechanical circulatory support.

9. Goldstein DJ, Meyns B, Xie R, et al. Third annual report from the ISHLT Mechanically Assisted Circulatory Support Registry: a comparison of centrifugal and axial continuous-flow left ventricular assist devices. *J Heart Lung Transplant.* 2019;38(4):352–363.

The International Society for Heart and Lung Transplantation (ISHLT) Mechanically Assisted Circulatory Support (IMACS) Registry collects global data on patients receiving durable mechanical support devices. Intermacs (reference 7) contributes data to this registry, as do registries from Europe, Japan, and the UK. Twenty-four additional hospitals also provide data to the registry. The report includes longitudinal granular data including clinical characteristics and outcomes according to device types. The report includes data from the time of the registry inception in 2013 through the end of 2017.

Landmark Article of the 21st Century

A FULLY MAGNETICALLY LEVITATED LEFT VENTRICULAR ASSIST DEVICE—FINAL REPORT

Mehra MR et al., *N Engl J Med.* 2019 Apr 25;380(17):1618–1627

Commentary by Alan Lisbon

The use of a mechanical left ventricular assist device as a treatment for severe heart failure has been sought for 50 years and has been complicated by thrombosis, stroke, bleeding complications, and infections. This trial compared a magnetically levitated, centrifugal flow device (HeartMate 3) to an axial continuous-flow pump (HeartMate 2) as left ventricular support in patients with advanced stage heart failure as either a bridge to transport or destination therapy. The primary endpoint was survival at 2 years free of disabling stroke or reoperation to remove/replace a malfunctioning device. Secondary endpoint was replacement of the device at 2 years.

Results: The study enrolled 1028 patients. At the end of 2 years, 397 patients (76.9%) in the centrifugal pump group compared to 332 (64.8%) in the axial flow group were alive and free from disabling stroke or reoperation. Pump replacement was less common in the centrifugal pump group 2.3% vs. 11.3%. Strokes, major bleeding, and GI hemorrhage were also lower in the centrifugal pump group.

Comment: While this study shows superiority of the HeartMate 3 device in patients with severe heart failure followed for 2 years, the adverse event profile for these devices is significant. These complications include pump thrombosis, stroke (10%), bleeding, as well as right ventricular failure (34%) and significant infections (58%). A completely internal device without external drivelines is needed. While these devices are improving, they are still far from perfect.

CHAPTER 11

Severe Electrolyte Disturbances

Review by Melanie P. Hoenig and Jeffrey H. William

Hyponatremia, defined as a blood sodium concentration of <135 mmol/L is the most common electrolyte abnormality observed in the intensive care unit (ICU). When hyponatremia is severe, patients may be admitted to the ICU for close monitoring since overly rapid correction can lead to the osmotic demyelination syndrome. Recommendations for the treatment of severe hyponatremia have evolved considerably over the past 20 years.

First, treatment should be initiated with consideration of the cause; patients with the syndrome of inappropriate diuresis (SIAD) are unlikely to experience rapid correction; whereas, those who have volume depletion with retention of dilute fluids may experience a rapid increase in the serum sodium after volume resuscitation, when the stimulus for vasopressin is no longer present and water is rapidly excreted.

In the setting of SIAD, the serum sodium will rise slowly with water restriction and ongoing insensible losses, but this will occur very slowly if the urine osmolality is very high. If the patient is symptomatic, traditionally, 3% saline at a slow infusion rate is recommended to provide solute which can be readily excreted by the kidney with the excess water. Many now favor small bolus infusions of 3% saline of 100–150 mL which may be repeated, and this practice has been endorsed for symptomatic patients by both European and US guidelines on the treatment of hyponatremia [1]. This strategy was examined recently with a multi-centered open label randomized trial in the Republic of Korea that compared slow continuous infusion of 0.5 mmol/kg/h with rapid bolus of 3% saline of 2 mL/kg every 6 hours. The primary outcome was overly rapid correction which was defined as >12 mmol/L in 24 hours or >18 mmol/L in 48 hours. Both arms of the study led to improvement in symptoms and correction of the hyponatremia, but approximately half of all patients required an intervention to limit the rate of rise of the serum sodium [2]. It is important to note that both arms of the trial employed more aggressive prescriptions for the 3% saline than current guidelines.

The target rate of correction has become more conservative in recent years based on the observation that even small increases in the serum sodium can alleviate symptoms such that the daily increase in the serum sodium should be just 4–6 mmol/L rather than targets of <12 mEq/L recommended in years past.

DOI: 10.1201/9781003042136-11

With such small targets in vogue, overly rapid correction has become a larger concern and patients may require an intervention to slow the correction. This can be achieved with infusion of desmopressin to limit further water losses along with infusion of 3% saline to control the rate of correction or along with dilute fluids to lower the sodium after overly rapid correction [3]. To explore this practice, a retrospective study of patients with severe hyponatremia was performed from 2004 to 2014 at two large academic centers in Canada. Investigators observed a substantial increase in the use of desmopressin in patients with hyponatremia during the study. Desmopressin use was associated with more severe hyponatremia and a lower rate of safe correction though this likely reflects the retrospective nature of the report [4].

Hypernatremia, defined as a serum sodium concentration >145 mmol/L, is also commonly encountered in patients in the intensive care unit setting. Hypernatremia may be present on admission or develop during the ICU stay [5]. When hypernatremia develops, there is movement of water out of cells into the extracellular fluid and a decrease in cell size results. If severe and acute, hypernatremia leads to a decrease in brain volume which can cause cerebral vein rupture, focal hemorrhage, and potentially irreversible neurologic damage. Osmotic demyelination has also been reported in patients who have developed hypernatremia abruptly in the setting of severe hyperglycemia or diabetes insipidus. In contrast, if hypernatremia develops slowly, neurons can increase their solute concentration to allow water to return to the cells and increase cell size back toward normal.

Hypernatremia may be caused by water loss or sodium gain. Water loss can develop from gastrointestinal losses from emesis, diarrhea, or surgical drainage of gastrointestinal fluids. Urinary losses can occur either from a solute diuresis induced by mannitol, a high protein diet or hyperglycemia, or from a water diuresis as observed with diabetes insipidus. Water losses from skin as with sweat with fever or loss of the skin barrier function from severe burns may also cause hypernatremia. Sodium gain is a less common cause of hypernatremia, particularly prior to hospital admission but has been described with ingestions of seawater in near drowning, gargling, or dangerous behaviors such as soy sauce or pickle juice ingestion. During hospitalization, sodium gain can occur with the use of hypertonic fluids such as repeated administration of intravenous sodium bicarbonate ampules.

Persistent hypernatremia in the ICU setting has been associated with mortality in the 20–40% range [6, 7]. This high mortality is likely because persistent hypernatremia is a marker for the severity of the underlying disorders. Indeed, individuals who are awake experience extreme thirst when the serum sodium is elevated and if able, would normally drink until resolution of the hyperosmolar state. Thus, persistent hypernatremia only occurs in those who do not experience thirst, are too ill to tolerate enteral fluid intake, and/or have severe persistent losses. Nevertheless, it is also possible that hypernatremia directly contributes to morbidity and mortality in the ICU.

Given the high mortality of hypernatremia, treatment is important and includes limiting further loss of water or gain of sodium, along with the replenishment of water.

The rapidity of development of hypernatremia should determine the pace of treatment. Abrupt onset merits rapid attention whereas rapid correction of chronic hypernatremia can lead to cerebral edema.

Despite these concerns and caveats, there is neither consensus nor are there controlled studies to guide clinicians on the safest pace of correction for hypernatremia. In contrast, there are numerous guidelines, yet also no controlled studies, on the appropriate rate of correction of the serum sodium in the setting of hyponatremia. Historically, for hyponatremia, a rate of no greater than 10–12 mEq/L/24 h (0.5/L/h) was embraced based on catastrophic outcomes in patients who corrected more rapidly than these limits. Recently, a more conservative approach to hyponatremia has been endorsed with target changes of only 6–8 mEq/L each day, and experts have advocated for the use of vasopressin to slow rapid correction. Although many consider hypernatremia the "flip side" of hyponatremia, adverse events from overly rapid treatment of hypernatremia are even more scarce than that of hyponatremia [8]. Indeed, there are only anecdotal reports or very small series of seizure or neurological consequences in infants and very young children who received rapid treatment for hypernatremia (>0.5 mEq/L/h), but there are no similar reports of adverse outcomes for rapid treatment of chronic hypernatremia in adults [9]. Nevertheless, despite the absence of data, the limits for the treatment of hyponatremia have been readily applied to the treatment of hypernatremia.

In addition, it is worth noting that although hyponatremia can correct rapidly if the kidneys excrete a large water load, hypernatremia is only corrected by the addition of water, which can be controlled easily in a hospital setting. In fact, the opposite issue is common in hypernatremia; patients with hypernatremia frequently have ongoing losses and require significant intake of dilute fluids to simply address losses and require more still to correct the serum sodium downwards toward normal.

Recently, treatment for hypernatremia was investigated in a retrospective study that explored a large database of ICU patients at Beth Israel Deaconess Medical Center, the Medical Information Mart for Intensive Care-III [2]. The rate of correction of hypernatremia (>155 mEq/L) was examined in 122 patients who were admitted with hypernatremia and 327 with hospital-acquired hypernatremia, the largest cohort described to date. Investigators performed manual chart review for evidence of neurologic consequences and used the database to calculate the rate of change in sodium. Analysis of the data found no differences in outcome in those who had an improvement in the serum sodium that was more rapid >0.5 mEq/L/hr (>12 mEq/L/day) compared to those who had slower correction in the serum sodium. In addition, patients who had more rapid correction had a shorter length of stay, a finding mirrored in several other small series. This observation may capture patients who have severe ongoing losses or are too sick to tolerate replenishment of the water deficit.

Care of patients with hypernatremia should include calculation of the water deficit and consideration of ongoing losses [10]. Once treatment with dilute fluids begins, further evaluation and reassessment should be routine. In children, the rate of correction of

<0.5 mEq/L/h (12 mEq/L/day) is advised, whereas for adult care, a more rapid rate appears to be safe. Furthermore, since adverse events have been described in adults from the rapid rise in serum sodium but not from the correction, undue caution regarding the rate of correction should be held in check.

ANNOTATED REFERENCES FOR SEVERE ELECTROLYTE DISTURBANCES

1. Verbalis JG, Goldsmith SR, Greenbrg A, et al. Diagnosis, evaluation, and treatment of hyponatremia: expert panel recommendations. *Am J Med.* 2013;126(10 Suppl 1):S1–42.

   https://pubmed.ncbi.nlm.nih.gov/24074529/

   United States expert guidelines on hyponatremia include a recommendation to increase the serum sodium only 4–6 mmol/L/24 h for severe hyponatremia.

2. Baek SH, Jo YH, Medina-Liabres K, Oh YK, Lee JB, Kim S. Risk of overcorrection in rapid intermittent bolus vs. slow continuous infusion therapies of hypertonic saline for patients with symptomatic hyponatremia: the SALSA randomized clinical trial. *JAMA Intern Med.* 2021 Jan 1;181(1):81–92.

3. Rafat C, Schortgen F, Gaudry S, Miguel-Montanes R, Bertrand F, Dreyfuss D. Use of desmopressin acetate in severe hyponatremia in the intensive care unit. *Clin J Am Soc Nephrol.* 2014;9(2):229–237.

   https://www.ncbi.nlm.nih.gov/pmc/articles/PMC3913226/

   A retrospective review of 20 patients who received desmopressin as part of their treatment for severe hyponatremia found that desmopressin is effective in slowing the rise of plasma sodium concentration in severe hyponatremia from a mean of 0.8 mmol/L to 0.02 mmol/L.

4. MacMillan TE, Cavalcanti RB. Outcomes in severe hyponatremia with and without desmopressin. *Am J Med.* 2018;131(3):317.e1–317.e10.

   https://pubmed.ncbi.nlm.nih.gov/29061503/

   A retrospective review of 254 admissions for severe hyponatremia in which desmopressin was used to help slow the rise in serum sodium in a reactive or proactive strategy or for rescue if the serum sodium corrected too quickly.

5. Palevsky PM, Bhagrath R, Greenberg A. Hypernatremia in hospitalized patients. *Annals Int Med.* 1996;124:197–203.

   A prospective series of just over 100 patients with a serum sodium of 150 or greater, admitted over a 3-month period at a single urban university hospital. Eighteen patients presented with hypernatremia, whereas the rest had hospital-acquired hypernatremia. Those with hypernatremia on presentation were older (mean age 76 vs. 59), more likely to be from a nursing home (61% vs. 9%) and had more severe hypernatremia than those who developed hypernatremia in the ICU.

6. Linder G, et al. Hypernatremia in the critically ill is an independent risk factor for mortality. *Am J Kidney Dis.* 2007;50(6):952–7.

   https://pubmed.ncbi.nlm.nih.gov/18037096/

   In a retrospective series of nearly 1000 ICU patients, 9% had hypernatremia (2% on admission and 7% developed hypernatremia during their ICU stay). The mortality for these patients was significantly higher (39% and 43%, respectively) compared to ICU patients without hypernatremia (24%).

7. Alshayeb HM, et al. Severe hypernatremia correction rate and mortality in hospitalized patients. *Am J Med Sci.* 2011;341(5):356–60.

   https://pubmed.ncbi.nlm.nih.gov/21358313/

   This retrospective review of 131 patients with hypernatremia (>155 mEq/L) found that 90% of patients had a correction rate of <0.5 mEq/L/h but less than 1/3 achieved a serum sodium of <145 after 72 hours of treatment. The overall mortality rate was 37% and multivariate analysis found that slower correction of the serum sodium was an independent predictor of 30-day mortality.

8. Sterns RH. Evidence for managing hypernatremia: is it just hyponatremia in reverse? *Clin J Am Soc Nephrol.* 2019;14(5):645–7.

   https://pubmed.ncbi.nlm.nih.gov/31064771/

   A well-known expert in the "dysnatremias" explores the evidence for the management of hypernatremia with this cogent editorial of the landmark paper. Dr. Sterns contrasts hypernatremia with hyponatremia and refutes the "quest for symmetry" that many consider in the care of patients with hypernatremia.

9. Kahn A, Brachet E, Blum D. Controlled fall in natremia and risk of seizures in hypertonic dehydration. *Intensive Care Med.* 1979;5:27–31.

   https://pubmed.ncbi.nlm.nih.gov/35558/

   A retrospective series of 47 infants who were admitted for dehydration and were treated with intravenous fluids. Nine of these infants experienced seizures (all with a rate of correction >0.7 mEq/h) This report has been heralded as proof that the rate of correction should be <0.5 mmol/h.

10. Adrogue HJ, Madias NE. Hypernatremia. *N Engl J Med.* 2000;342:1493–99.

    https://www.nejm.org/doi/10.1056/NEJM200005183422006

    A popular review of hypernatremia that also outlines the use of an equation which predicts the serum sodium after a liter of IV fluid.

Landmark Article of the 21st Century

RATE OF CORRECTION OF HYPERNATREMIA AND HEALTH: OUTCOMES IN CRITICALLY ILL PATIENTS

Chauhan K et al., *Clin J Am Soc Nephrol.* 2019;14:656–663

Commentary by Stephen Heard

The authors performed a retrospective logistic regression analysis of patients who were admitted ($n = 122$) with severe hypernatremia (>155 mmol/L) or who acquired ($n = 327$) severe hyponatremia during hospitalization and the effect of rate of correction on various outcomes. Data for the years 2001–2012 were obtained from the Medical Information Mart for Intensive Care-III (MIMIC-III) which is a publicly available database from a single hospital. They found that regardless of the rate of correction (>0.5 mmol/L/h or <0.5 mmol/L/h), there was no difference in 30-day mortality. In addition, morbidities such as worsening mental status, seizures, or cerebral edema could not be attributed to rapid correction of hypernatremia.

This study is provocative and challenges the orthodoxy of cautious correction (<0.5 mmol/L/h) of severe hypernatremia. However, before there is wholesale change in the way severe hypernatremia is treated, more data are needed. The study is retrospective, and the data were obtained from one medical center. The number of patients in the admission group with severe hypernatremia is small. Furthermore, of that number, only 32 were treated at a rate >0.5 mmol/L/h. The number of patients with chronic hypernatremia treated at rates >0.5 mmol/L/h was half that of those treated more conservatively. As is typical for retrospective data collection, the clinical indication for the rapid or slow correction is not stated; therefore, we are uncertain as to the concomitant problems that may have lead the healthcare staff to determine the aggressiveness of care. Finally, although the authors performed manual reviews of imaging reports, progress notes, and discharge summaries, not all documents were available.

CHAPTER 12

Acute Kidney Injury

Review by Jeffrey H. William and Melanie P. Hoenig

Acute kidney injury (AKI) was first described by William Heberden in 1802, then referred to as *ischuria renalis* (literally, reduction in the flow of urine). A century later, William Osler's *Textbook of Medicine* details this pathologic state as a "consequence of toxic agents, pregnancy, burns, trauma or operations on the kidneys." In developed countries, AKI is estimated to occur in up to 15% of hospitalized patients and up to 60% of critically ill patients. While the pathophysiology of AKI is complex, alterations in blood flow from volume depletion, hemorrhage, or third-spacing of fluids result in renal hypoperfusion and a decrease in the glomerular filtration rate with preserved, non-ischemic renal parenchyma, a condition termed "pre-renal AKI" [1]. When the etiology of the AKI is hypothesized to be related to these alterations in blood flow that have not yet resulted in ischemic damage to the organ itself, fluid resuscitation is a cornerstone of treatment.

Prior to the cholera epidemic of 1832, it is estimated that 76 treatments had been attempted before fluids were administered directly into a vein. In their analyses of the blood of patients with cholera and yellow fever, scientists noted the loss of its "fluidity" and believed that the thickening of the blood led to its stagnation and decreased circulation. Dr. William Brooke O'Shaughnessy, a recent graduate of Edinburgh Medical School at the time, hypothesized that restoring the blood of its "deficient saline matters" would be critical in treating patients with cholera. Only 7 weeks after publication of these ideas, Dr. Robert Lewins and Dr. Thomas Latta described the results of intravenous administration of an alkalinized salt solution to six patients as "restoring the natural current in the veins and arteries, of improving the color of the blood, and recovering the functions of the lungs." In a rather prescient statement, they also recommended that repeated injections of large quantities of this solution be guided by the patient's pulse and symptoms, thereby giving birth to the modern-day treatment of critically ill patients with resuscitative fluids and goal-directed therapy.

As the cholera pandemic waned, intravenous saline in its current form experienced both a reckoning and renaissance with the advancement in our understanding of circulatory physiology and the treatment of patients with trauma or hemorrhage. In 1885, Dr. Sydney Ringer further developed "physiologic saline" in his efforts to maximize the function of isolated frog nerves and muscles. Having noticed that a salt solution made from pipe water seemed to work much better than distilled water, he determined that the inorganic constituents of the pipe water may be important as well. Ringer's solution, the first "balanced solution," was later improved upon by Dr. Alexis

DOI: 10.1201/9781003042136-12

Hartmann, who added sodium lactate (which is metabolized by the liver to bicarbonate) to reduce the acidosis seen in infants with diarrhea, most analogous to our modern-day lactated Ringer's solution [2].

Asanguinous, or crystalloid, fluid resuscitation is now universally utilized in patients with critical illness in the ICU. A concentration of 0.9% NaCl, or "normal saline," is normal (i.e., similar to blood plasma) with respect to the cation (sodium) concentration, but is not normal with respect to the anion. The relative surplus of chloride in this fluid can lead to hyperchloremia when large volumes are infused. The ubiquity of 0.9% NaCl has led to a greater understanding of some of its serious adverse effects, including hyperchloremic metabolic acidosis. Despite the known high prevalence of AKI in the critically ill patient population, the selection of resuscitative crystalloid fluids remains controversial. There is a wide variation in clinical practice with respect to which fluids should be used for resuscitation, driven mostly by regional and clinician preferences. Consensus statements from medical societies about the use of fluid in specific patient populations have been based largely on expert opinion or low-quality evidence. Systematic reviews of randomized, controlled trials through 2012 have consistently shown little evidence for the selection of one type of resuscitative fluid over another in terms of mortality reduction, improved effectiveness, or increased safety [3].

The spirited debate of whether to use 0.9% saline or balanced crystalloid solutions was renewed in 2012 with an observational trial employing a "chloride-restrictive" fluid resuscitation strategy. The authors showed an impressive decline in the incidence of acute kidney injury and the need for renal replacement therapy in the chloride-restricted fluid cohort versus those in the chloride-liberal fluid cohort [4]. A few years later, a small randomized, double-crossover controlled trial in multiple ICUs in New Zealand showed that the use of a buffered crystalloid solution compared with saline did not reduce the risk of AKI [5].

Due to the ongoing controversy, the SMART (Isotonic Solutions and Major Adverse Renal Events Trial) investigators published the largest randomized controlled trial of its kind, comparing balanced crystalloids and 0.9% saline as resuscitative fluids in nearly 16,000 critically ill adults, with a primary outcome designated as "major adverse kidney events" (MAKE)—the composite of death, new receipt of renal-replacement therapy, or persistent renal dysfunction. In this critically ill adult population, administration of balanced crystalloids resulted in a lower rate of the composite outcome [6]. Another trial by the same investigators (SALT-ED) conducted in parallel with the SMART trial included nearly 14,000 non-critical patients and showed a similar modest reduction in the pre-defined composite outcome in those who received balanced crystalloids [7]. Though the treatment effects in the SMART trial are relatively small, intravenous fluids are provided to millions of patients globally and therefore may still represent a large population-level effect.

A recent meta-analysis of 21 randomized controlled trials, including a few ongoing studies, confirmed that in-hospital mortality is similar with the use of 0.9% saline or balanced crystalloids. However, the certainty of evidence that balanced crystalloids and 0.9% saline were no different with respect to prevention of acute kidney injury was low. Therefore, the authors concluded that additional high-quality research is needed to resolve this debate [8].

Until then, as large confirmatory randomized controlled trials are ongoing, the SMART trial remains a landmark study in that it is the most convincing data available to guide our selection of fluid resuscitation in the critically ill with respect to the risk of the development of AKI.

ANNOTATED REFERENCES FOR ACUTE KIDNEY INJURY

1) Makris K, Spanou L. Acute kidney injury: definition, pathophysiology and clinical pheno-types. *Clin Biochem Rev.* 2016;37(2):85–98.

   https://www.ncbi.nlm.nih.gov/pmc/articles/PMC5198510/

   This straight-forward review article focuses on the complicated history of defin-ing AKI, multifactorial etiologies of AKI, and our evolving understanding of the pathophysiology.

2) Awad S, Allison SP, Lobo DN. The history of 0.9% saline. *Clin Nutr.* 2008;27(2):179–188.

   https://www-sciencedirect-com.ezp-prod1.hul.harvard.edu/science/article/pii/S0261561408000289

   The authors provide a detailed and exhaustive review of the origins and development of 0.9% saline, including the historical fictions that have been propagated over time and the most important figures in the development of derivative intravenous fluids.

3) Myburgh JA, Mythen MG. Resuscitation fluids. *N Engl J Med.* 2013;369:1243–1251.

   https://www.nejm.org/doi/full/10.1056/nejmra1208627

   The authors provided a detail review of the available resuscitative fluids in the current armamentarium, comparing the evidence for their use. This review article covers a brief history of intravenous fluids, physiology of fluid resuscitation, and a comparison of the intravenous fluids available for the acutely ill patient.

4) Yunos NM, Bellomo R, Hegarty C, Story D, Ho L, Bailey M. Association between a chloride-liberal vs chloride-restrictive intravenous fluid administration strategy and kidney injury in critically ill adults. *JAMA.* 2012;308(15):1566–1572.

   https://pubmed.ncbi.nlm.nih.gov/23073953/

   This observational pilot study evaluated the use of chloride-liberal solutions (0.9% saline, 4% succinylated gelatin solution, or 4% albumin solution) versus chlo-ride-restrictive solutions (Hartmann solution, Plasma-Lyte 148, or chloride-poor 20% albumin). Analysis of 1533 ICU patients concluded that a chloride-restrictive fluid strategy was associated with a decrease in the incidence of AKI and the use of renal replacement therapies.

5) Young P, Bailey M, Beasley R, et al. for the SPLIT Investigators and the ANZICS CTG. Effect of a buffered crystalloid solution vs. saline on acute kidney injury among patients in the intensive care unit. The SPLIT randomized clinical trial. *JAMA.* 2015;314(16):1701–1710.

   https://jamanetwork.com/journals/jama/fullarticle/2454911?guestAccessKey=899f99d9-b1ce-4e49-80b4-85da816d8dfe

This double-blind, cluster randomized, double-crossover trial of saline versus buffered crystalloid solutions evaluated renal complications of ICU patients in four different units in New Zealand. Analysis of 2278 patients did not show any benefit of the use of buffered crystalloid solutions in reducing the incidence of AKI.

6) Semler MW, Self WH, Wanderer JP, et al.; the SMART Investigators and the Pragmatic Critical Care Research Group. Balanced crystalloids versus saline in critically ill adults. *N Engl J Med.* 2018;378:829–839.

   https://www.nejm.org/doi/pdf/10.1056/NEJMoa1711584

   The SMART trial randomized 15,802 critically ill adults to receive either 0.9% saline or balanced crystalloids. The use of balanced crystalloids showed slightly more favorable results in a composite outcome of all-cause mortality, new renal replacement therapy, and persistent kidney dysfunction, though the individual outcomes did not reach statistical significance.

7) Self WH, Semler MW, Wanderer JP, et al. Balanced crystalloids versus saline in noncritically ill adults. *N Engl J Med.* 2018;378(9):819–828. doi:10.1056/NEJMoa1711586

   https://www.nejm.org/doi/10.1056/NEJMoa1711586?url_ver=Z39.88-2003&rfr_id=ori:rid:crossref.org&rfr_dat=cr_pub%20%200pubmed

   The SALT-ED trial was run by the same investigators of, and in parallel with, the SMART trial. In a total of 13,347 non-critically ill patients, the number of hospital-free days was similar among those who received 0.9% saline versus balanced crystalloids, but there was a lower incidence of major adverse kidney events with balanced crystalloids (over 30 days of follow-up).

8) Antequera Martín AM, Barea Mendoza JA, Muriel A, et al. Buffered solutions versus 0.9% saline for resuscitation in critically ill adults and children. *Cochrane Database Syst Rev.* 2019;7(7):CD012247. Published 2019 Jul 19. doi:10.1002/14651858.CD012247.pub2

   https://www.cochranelibrary.com/cdsr/doi/10.1002/14651858.CD012247.pub2/full

   Using strict inclusion criteria, this Cochrane Review meta-analyzed 21 randomized controlled trials of providing 0.9% saline or balanced crystalloids in adults and children in the critical care setting. The authors concluded that there was no effect of in-hospital mortality between 0.9% saline and crystalloids, with high-certainty of evidence. While the prevention of acute kidney injury was also similar among both types of crystalloid, the evidence was of lower certainty and they suggest further research could provide more helpful information in drawing a conclusion.

Landmark Article of the 21st Century

BALANCED CRYSTALLOIDS VERSUS SALINE IN CRITICALLY ILL ADULTS

Semler MW et al., *N Engl J Med.* 2018;378:829–839

Commentary by Daniel J. Bonville

The empiric choice of intravenous fluid for resuscitation has been debated for decades. Until recently, much of the debate had centered around dogma. Semler et al. report 15,802 adults randomized to normal saline (0.9% NaCl) or balanced crystalloids (lactated Ringer's [LR] solution or Plasma-Lyte A).

Background: Several prior studies revealed a relationship between saline administration and hyperchloremic acidosis, acute kidney injury, and even death [1–6]. However, others failed to show any difference in outcomes [7–8].

Assessment: This large cluster randomized trial hypothesized that the use of balanced crystalloids would result in a lower incidence of death, new renal replacement therapy (RRT), and persistent renal dysfunction than saline. Each group was well matched in this well organized and powered study. The balanced crystalloids group had a lower rate of death, RRT, or persistent renal dysfunction than the saline group. Overall, the effect size was modest at 1.1% in favor of balanced fluids. However, given the fact that over 5 million patients are admitted to ICUs every year, the reduction in patients with this outcome using this data could be over 50,000/year. This difference appears to have been most pronounced in sepsis, septic shock cohorts.

Limitations: The results cannot be used to provide guidance on the use of balanced fluids in patients with traumatic brain injury. The clinical conduct at a single center may not be generalizable to other centers. Clinicians were not blinded; the outcomes of death and creatinine level are objective, but the decision to initiate renal replacement therapy may be susceptible to bias.

REFERENCES

1. Yunos NM, Kim IB, Bellomo R, et al. The biochemical effects of restricting chloride-rich fluids in intensive care. *Crit Care Med.* 2011;39:2419–2424.
2. Yunos NM, Bellomo R, Hegarty C, Story D, Ho L, Bailey M. Association between a chloride-liberal vs chloride-restrictive intravenous fluid administration strategy and kidney injury in critically ill adults. *JAMA.* 2012;308:1566–1572.
3. Raghunathan K, Shaw A, Nathanson B, et al. Association between the choice of IV crystalloid and in-hospital mortality among critically ill adults with sepsis. *Crit Care Med.* 2014;42:1585–1591.
4. Rochwerg B, Alhazzani W, Sindi A, et al. Fluid resuscitation in sepsis: a systematic review and network meta-analy-sis. *Ann Intern Med.* 2014;161:347–355.
5. Shaw AD, Raghunathan K, Peyerl FW, Munson SH, Paluszkiewics SM, Schermer CR. Association between intravenous chloride load during resuscitation and in-hospital mortality among patients with SIRS. *Intensive Care Med.* 2014;40:1897–1905.
6. Shaw AD, Bagshaw SM, Goldstein SL, et al. Major complications, mortality, and resource utilization after open abdominal surgery: 09% saline compared to Plasma-Lyte. *Ann Surg.* 2012;255:821–829.
7. Young P, Bailey M, Beasley R, et al. Effect of a buffered crystalloid solution vs saline on acute kidney injury among patients in the intensive care unit: the SPLIT randomized clinical trial. *JAMA.* 2015;314:1701–1710.
8. Semler NW, Wanderer JP, Ehrenfeld JM, et al. Balanced crystalloids versus saline in the intensive care unit: the SALT randomized trial. *AM J Respir Crit Care Med.* 2017;195: 1362–1372.

Continuous versus Intermittent Renal Replacement Therapy

Review by Kenneth Ralto and Matthew J. Trainor

Acute kidney injury (AKI) remains a common and morbid complication affecting 57% of critically ill patients, 23.5% of whom will require renal replacement therapy (RRT) [1]. Despite the frequency of AKI, there is significant variation in availability and utilization of different RRT modalities. Intermittent hemodialysis (IHD) is widely available and is most commonly performed by dedicated dialysis nurses. This form of RRT can be performed through either a hemodialysis catheter or a more permanent vascular access such as an arteriovenous fistula or graft as found in patients with end stage renal disease (ESRD). Due to hemodynamic instability, many intensive care unit (ICU) patients are started on continuous renal replacement therapy (CRRT), which is available only at larger hospitals, requires a hemodialysis catheter, and is typically performed by ICU nursing staff. There are several different types of CRRT available which can use dialysate to achieve diffusive clearance as with continuous venovenous hemodialysis (CVVHD), or replacement fluid can be utilized for convective clearance with continuous venovenous hemofiltration (CVVH). These two modalities can also be performed simultaneously as continuous venovenous hemodiafiltration (CVVHDF).

There are numerous theoretical benefits to CRRT in a critically ill patient, including improved hemodynamic tolerance, more effective volume management, and reduced risk for cerebral edema in high risk patients. The rapid solute clearance achieved with IHD is often associated with hypotension due to several factors. First, as uremic toxins are removed from the plasma, there is a reduction in serum osmolality which creates an osmotic gradient promoting the movement of water from the vascular space to the interstitial space. For this reason, the rapid solute removal with IHD can exacerbate cerebral edema due to the osmotic movement of water into brain tissue, which is a particular risk for patients with neurologic injury [2] or fulminant liver failure [3]. The relatively short duration of IHD also requires high ultrafiltration rates (sometimes exceeding 1000 mL/h) in order to maintain volume balance, which further reduces vascular volume and promotes hypotension. Lastly, cardiac dysfunction is a common comorbidity in patients requiring IHD and blunts the physiologic responses to the above hemodynamic stressors.

CRRT addresses many of these clinical concerns by performing both solute clearance and ultrafiltration at a slower rate. For this reason, CRRT is the preferred therapy for

DOI: 10.1201/9781003042136-13

patients at high risk for cerebral edema. However, this gentler solute removal comes at the cost of more slowly correcting metabolic derangements and CRRT may not be the appropriate initial therapy for patients with acutely life-threatening hyperkalemia or acidemia. An additional advantage of CRRT is improved volume management due to the higher daily ultrafiltration volumes that can be achieved due to the continuous nature of this therapy.

Despite these theoretical advantages for CRRT in critically ill patients, several randomized trials have not shown a mortality benefit for this therapy when compared to IHD. Vinsonneau and colleagues conducted the Hemodiafe study which was a randomized trial of 360 critically ill patients with AKI and multiple organ dysfunction syndrome from 21 French hospitals. Patients were assigned to receive either IHD or CRRT and the primary end point was 60-day survival. At the end of the study, there was no significant difference in 60-day survival: 32% in the IHD group and 33% in the CRRT group. This study reached the same conclusion as several other trials comparing CRRT to IHD, which showed no evidence of improved mortality with continuous RRT modalities in critically ill patients [4–6]. One such trial actually showed higher in-hospital mortality with CRRT in comparison to IHD [7], however some of this difference has been attributed to the higher severity of illness (particularly the higher percentage of patients with liver failure) who were randomly assigned to the CRRT arm.

Despite the results of these studies, CRRT continues to be performed in the intensive care units of virtually every major medical center. The Hemodiafe trial, as well of the other studies described above, had methodological issues which limit their generalizability to clinical practice. Most notably, these trials had relatively small sample sizes with low power to detect a different in mortality, non-standardized criteria for the initiation of RRT, and CRRT prescriptions that were below the modern standard of care for adequate dialysis dosing. Subsequent studies have shown that while a very high dialysis dose does not improve outcomes [8], there is a lower limit of dialysis dosing at which adequate metabolic control is not achieved for critically ill patients. Compounding this issue is the fact that due to interruptions in treatments, the delivered dose of CRRT averages 15% lower than prescribed [9]. Another factor that limits the application of these results to clinical practice is that the IHD arm in several of these trials more closely resembled slow low efficiency dialysis (SLED), which is characterized by slower, longer, and more frequent hemodialysis treatments.

What is notable from these trials of IHD vs. CRRT is that the majority of critically ill patients were still able to tolerate IHD, albeit with a modified dialysis prescription and more frequent treatments. In the Hemodiafe trial, 87% of patients were on vasopressors and 96% required mechanical ventilation. Despite this, only six patients crossed-over from IHD to CRRT and there was no difference in the rate of hypotension between the two dialysis modalities. This suggests that with careful attention to the IHD prescription, even hemodynamically unstable patients can often tolerate this therapy. These modifications to the IHD prescription include lower blood and dialysate flow rates, cooler dialysate temperature, longer treatment time, and a higher dialysate sodium concentration.

The main take away point from the Hemodiafe trial, and the other above mentioned trials comparing CRRT to IHD, should be that IHD remains a reasonable option for most critically ill patients in the intensive care unit. Given the heterogeneity and complexity of critically ill patients, the decision to initiate CRRT or IHD should remain an individualized clinical decision that incorporates patient factors (hemodynamics, volume status, available vascular access, presence of immediate life-threatening metabolic derangements), institutional expertise, as well as staff and equipment availability. Unlike when patients are randomized in trials, the decision on RRT modality in clinical practice is not binary, with many patients transitioning between IHD, CRRT, as well as hybrid modalities (SLED or accelerated venovenous hemofiltration) as their condition evolves. It is unlikely that any single trial comparing CRRT to IHD will be able to conclusively show superiority of one modality over the other in a diverse population of critically ill patients.

ANNOTATED REFERENCES FOR CONTINUOUS VERSUS INTERMITTENT RENAL REPLACEMENT THERAPY

1. Hoste EA, et al. Epidemiology of acute kidney injury in critically ill patients: the multinational AKI-EPI study. *Intensive Care Med.* 2015;41(8):1411–1423.

   This cross-sectional study examined the incidence of AKI by examining over 1800 patients at 97 different medical centers from 33 different countries during the first week of ICU admission. Over 57% of patients developed AKI, with 18.4%, 8.9%, and 30.0% developing KDIGO stage 1, 2, and 3 AKI, respectively. Of the patients who developed AKI, 23.5% required renal replacement therapy during their first week in the ICU. The risk of death increased with greater severity of AKI and patients with stage 3 AKI had a greater than 7-fold increased risk of death compared to ICU patients without AKI. This study highlights the high burden and morbidity of AKI in critically ill patients.

2. Davenport A. Renal replacement therapy in the patient with acute brain injury. *Am J Kidney Dis.* 2001;37(3):457–466.

   This review covers the best practices in managing renal replacement for patients with acute neurologic injury. Conventional HD can lower cerebral perfusion pressure both through a reduction in mean arterial pressure as well as an increase in cerebral edema due to osmotic shifts from rapid solute removal. CRRT is the preferred modality for patients with acute neurologic injury who are at risk for cerebral edema. Peritoneal dialysis also allows for slow solute removal and has minimal effects on intracranial pressure, however this therapy is more challenging to initiate in critically ill patients.

3. Davenport A. The clinical application of CRRT—current status: continuous renal replacement therapies in patients with liver disease. *Sem Dialysis.* 2009;22(2):169–172.

   Patients with both acute and chronic liver failure present a challenge when the need for RRT arises. They are often hypotensive due to high levels of nitric oxide and other endogenous vasodilators. Patients with fulminant liver failure often have elevated ammonia levels and are at risk for increased intracranial pressure with IHD. Similar to patients with neurologic injury, this is due both to decreased mean arterial pressure as well as rapid lowering of the serum osmolality and osmotic movement of water into brain tissue. CRRT is preferred for patients with fulminant liver failure or severe hyperammonemia.

4. Augustine JJ, et al. A randomized controlled trial comparing intermittent with continuous dialysis in patients with ARF. *Am J Kidney Dis.* 2004;44(6):1000–1007.

Eighty critically ill patients with AKI and a requirement for RRT were randomized to either IHD or continuous venovenous hemodialysis (CVVHD). The IHD group received thrice weekly dialysis with standard blood and dialysis flow rates of 300 and 500 mL/min, respectively. Patients in the CVVHD group had greater volume removal and less hypotension than patients in the IHD group, however this did not translate to an improvement in clinical outcomes. There was no difference for in-hospital mortality or recovery of renal function when comparing IHD to CVVHD.

5. Lins RL, et al. Intermittent versus continuous renal replacement therapy for acute kidney injury patients admitted to the intensive care unit: results of a randomized clinical trial. *Nephrol Dialysis Transplant.* 2009;24(2):512–518.

This was a multicenter RCT of 316 critically ill patients with AKI who developed a need for RRT and were randomized to continuous venovenous hemofiltration (CVVH) or IHD. The IHD group in this study received treatments that more closely resembled SLED—daily hemodialysis with low blood and dialysate flows, and a long duration of 4–6 hours. There was no difference in the outcomes of in-hospital mortality, ICU, or hospital length of stay, or renal function at follow-up. There were also no differences in mortality when examining pre-specified subgroups including patients with sepsis, elderly patients (over 70 years old), or patients requiring mechanical ventilation.

6. Uehlinger DE, et al. Comparison of continuous and intermittent renal replacement therapy for acute renal failure. *Nephrol Dialysis Transplant.* 2005;20(8):1630–1637.

This single center trial randomized 125 critically ill patients with AKI requiring RRT to either continuous venovenous hemodiafiltration (CVVHDF) or IHD. The patients in the IHD group received standard intensite treatments over 3 to 4 hours as deemed appropriate by the treating nephrologist, however the median number of IHD treatments was high at 5 per week. There were no differences for in-hospital mortality, hospital length of stay, or duration of RRT when comparing CVVHDF to IHD.

7. Mehta RL, et al. A randomized clinical trial of continuous versus intermittent dialysis for acute renal failure. *Kidney Int.* 2001;60(3):1154–1163.

A multicenter trial (four medical centers in California) which randomized 166 ICU patients with AKI requiring RRT to either IHD or continuous renal replacement therapy. Notably some of the patients in the CRRT group received continuous arteriovenous hemodiafiltration (CAVHDF) and some received continuous venovenous hemodiafiltration (CVVHDF). This was the only major trial of CRRT vs. IHD which showed a significant difference between the two groups: in-hospital mortality was 65.5% in the CRRT group and 47.6% in the IHD group. Part of this difference appears to be due to unequal randomization of patients with severe illness between the two groups. In the CRRT group, 42.9% had liver failure compared to 29.3% in the IHD group. The APACHE III score was also higher in the CRRT group. Both of these differences were statistically significant and would be expected to affect mortality, independent of the assigned RRT modality.

8. Palevsky PM, et al. Intensity of renal support in critically ill patients with acute kidney injury. *N Engl J Med.* 2008;359(1):7–20.

This study's aim was to assess whether the intensity of RRT affected outcomes for critically ill patients with AKI. At 27 hospitals there were 1124 patients randomized to high intensity (IHD/SLED 6 days per week or CVVHDF with an effluent rate of 35 mL/kg/h) or low intensity RRT (IHD/SLED 3 days per week or CVVHDF with an effluent rate of 20 mL/kg/h). There was no difference in the primary endpoint of 60-day mortality: 53.6% in the high intensity group and 51.5% in the low-intensity group. There were higher rates of hypotension and electrolyte disturbances in the high-intensity group. This study does not support the use of higher intensity RRT.

9. Evanson JA, et al. Prescribed versus delivered dialysis in acute renal failure patients. *Am J Kidney Dis.* 1998;32(5):731–738.

This study assessed the prescribed vs. delivered dose of dialysis in 40 hospitalized patients who experienced AKI requiring IHD. Forty-nine percent of the patients were prescribed a dialysis treatment which was below the guideline-recommended minimum adequate dose (a Kt/V of 1.2). Additionally, 68% of patients had an inadequate delivered dose of IHD. This study highlights the difference between prescribed and delivered dose of IHD in hospitalized patients with AKI, and also emphasizes the frequency of inadequate dialysis prescriptions.

Landmark Article of the 21st Century

CONTINUOUS VENOVENOUS HAEMODIAFILTRATION VERSUS INTERMITTENT HAEMODIALYSIS FOR ACUTE RENAL FAILURE IN PATIENTS WITH MULTIPLE-ORGAN DYSFUNCTION SYNDROME: A MULTICENTER RANDOMISED TRIAL

Vinsonneau C et al., *Lancet.* 2006;368(9533):379–385

Commentary by Christophe Vinsonneau

Intermittent hemodialysis (IHD) was the only one method available to treat acute renal failure (AKI) in the intensive care unit (ICU) until 1990s. This method needed to be implemented by expert nurses trained in the dialysis unit. Most ICUs were unable to develop this type of renal support and patients needed to be transferred to other units. In addition, the expertise of nephrologists was mandatory to manage the IHD machines. These requirements limited the development of this kind of care. Early in the 90s, continuous dialytic methods based on convection (continuous venovenous hemofiltration, CVVH) were proposed and soon after, specific automated machine were developed. The learning curve for the doctor and nurse was very short and the nephrologist was no longer mandatory. Therefore, this new method rapidly became very popular in most ICUs all over the world, particularly where IHD was not developed. It was thought that this method was superior compared to IHD because of its prolonged duration and the slow solute and fluid removal. Albeit the lack of comparative studies, this method became the gold standard to treat AKI in the ICU. As we

used IHD in the ICU of Cochin Hospital (Paris Descartes University, Paris, France)
we decided to conduct a French study to compare the continuous method to IHD.
I started my fellowship in 1998 and was assigned to conduct this multicenter study
under the supervision of Professor Dhainaut. We enrolled 360 patients with AKI and
multiple organ failure in 21 centers. At this time, no prospective randomized study
was conclusive and many observational studies reported conflicting results. Our study
showed no differences in terms of mortality or renal recovery. In addition, the rate of
hypotension was similar in the two groups. This study was the first to demonstrate
that IHD was not inferior to continuous methods. Subsequently, several studies have
shown similar results whereas no one has demonstrated the superiority of continuous
methods over IHD. Currently, most experts agree that IHD may be used in ICUs to
treat AKI, and the choice of the method is based more on team experience and technical considerations.

CHAPTER 14

Colloid versus Crystalloids

Review by Peter Rhee and Stephen Heard

For the patient with hypotension due to hypovolemia, one of the first therapeutic interventions is fluid replacement. The options for replacement include crystalloids or colloids. The three main crystalloids are hypertonic saline, normal (0.9%) saline (NS), and balanced (buffered) salt solutions. The most commonly used balanced salt solution in the United States is lactated Ringer's (LR). The colloids include albumin, starch, and gelatin solutions.

The dose and duration of treatment with either crystalloids or colloids depends on the degree of hypovolemia and response to therapy. Blood pressure, heart rate, and urine output are traditional signs that are monitored. The blood pressure goal is generally a mean arterial blood pressure (MAP) of 65 mm Hg. Urine output should be >0.5 mL/kg/h. Lactate levels and base deficit are additional valuable parameters that can be followed to determine the adequacy of resuscitation. More recently, additional means to detect hypovolemia in intubated and mechanically ventilated patients, such as systolic blood pressure or stroke volume variation, hold the promise of providing guidance on appropriate fluid replacement and reducing the risk of fluid overload. However, use of tidal volumes greater than 8 mL/kg obfuscate the reliability of these monitors. Focused bedside ultrasonography and echocardiography can give clues about volume status (flattened inferior vena cava [IVC] versus a dilated IVC) and heart function.

Although hypertonic saline may be of value in treating patients with intracranial hypertension or symptomatic severe hyponatremia, its utility in traditional resuscitation has not been shown conclusively to be of benefit compared to other fluids. Normal saline is traditionally used in medical intensive care units. The side effect profile of NS, such as hyperchloremic acidosis and potential renal injury, tempers enthusiasm by some intensivists for its use. LR and similar solutions are the most common crystalloids used to treat hypovolemia. Infusing one liter of isotonic fluids will result in 100–200 mL of intravascular volume expansion. Several prospective, randomized studies have compared the use of buffered solutions to NS. Some have shown a lack of difference between the two groups in composite outcomes (death, need for renal replacement therapy [RRT], or incidence of acute kidney injury [AKI]). More recent large investigations of ICU or emergency department (ED) patients have demonstrated modest reductions in composite outcomes (30-day

DOI: 10.1201/9781003042136-14

mortality, need for RRT, and persistent renal insufficiency) associated with bal-anced salt solutions. Finally, a meta-analysis of 21 randomized controlled tri-als failed to discern any benefit of the use of balanced salt solutions over NS. Nonetheless, knowing that NS reliably causes hyperchloremic acidosis and possibly hypernatremia, many clinicians will opt for a buffered solution such as LR. LR has a sodium and potassium concentrations of 130 mEq/L and 4 mEq/L, respectively. Hyponatremia is a theoretical concern as is hyperkalemia. However, the potassium load per liter is low and large volumes would be required to affect plasma potas-sium concentrations. Since NS can cause an acidosis, the risk of hyperkalemia is likely higher in patients with renal failure. Other balanced salt solutions have electrolyte concentrations similar to that seen in plasma, but these solutions tend to be more expensive.

Albumin is the most common colloid used in resuscitation and is available in the United States in two concentrations: 5% and 25%. Twenty-five percent albumin is commonly used to maintain plasma volume during therapeutic paracentesis. Five percent albumin should be used for volume resuscitation. One liter of 5% albumin can be expected to result in a plasma volume expansion of 500–1000 mL. Less administration of fluid can be expected and perhaps resuscitation endpoints can be realized more quickly. However, albumin will eventually reach the interstitial space and result in edema. Due to uncertainty as to the benefit of the use of albumin over crystalloid, a prospective, randomized multi-center trial was performed comparing 4% albumin to NS when fluid administration was determined to be necessary to maintain or increase intravascular volume. There was no difference in 28-day mor-tality, hospital length of stay or organ dysfunction as measured by the SOFA score. Subgroup analysis suggested that use of albumin in trauma patients with traumatic brain injury had an increased risk of death compared to the NS group. This finding was confirmed in a follow-up publication. However, in patients with severe sepsis, there was a trend towards increased survival in the albumin group. A very recent retrospective study of two independent cohorts comparing 5% albumin plus NS to NS alone in over 18,000 ICU patients demonstrated by multivariate regression that 5% albumin was associated with lower 30-day mortality. The incidence of acute kidney injury was higher in the albumin group but did not translate into persistent renal insufficiency. It is unclear how to interpret these results as regression analysis shows correlation not causation.

Artificial colloids such as 6% hydroxyethyl starch (HES) should be avoided. In one prospective randomized study comparing HES to NS, the incidence of AKI necessitat-ing RRT was higher in the HES group. There was no difference in mortality. A meta-analysis comparing HES to other standard resuscitation regimens found that HES was associated with higher mortality and need for RRT. Notably, seven trials associated with scientific misconduct were excluded from that study. Those seven trials reported favorable effects of HES. HES is still on the market, but its use has plummeted as a consequence of these and other unfavorable data.

ANNOTATED REFERENCES FOR COLLOID VERSUS CRYSTALLOIDS

Annane D, Siami S, Jaber S, et al. Effects of fluid resuscitation with colloids vs. crystalloids on mortality in critically ill patients presenting with hypovolemic shock: the CRISTAL randomized trial. *JAMA* 2013;310:1809–17. PMID 24108515

The investigators performed a randomized, multicenter clinical trial stratified by case mix on 2857 patients admitted to one of 57 ICUs. Patients were randomized to receive either colloids or crystalloids. There was no difference in mortality at day 28 (primary outcome); however, survival was higher in the colloid group by day 90. There was no difference in the need for renal replacement therapy. Days alive without mechanical ventilation or vasopressor therapy at days 7 and 28 were greater in the colloid group. The authors concluded their results should be considered preliminary.

Finfer S, Bellomo R, Boyce N, et al. A comparison of albumin and saline for fluid resuscitation in the intensive care unit. *N Engl J Med.* 2004;350:2247–56. PMID 15163774

The investigators conducted a randomized, multicenter, double-blind trial to determine the effect of either 4% albumin or NS on mortality of ICU patients who needed fluid resuscitation. There was no difference in 28-day mortality between patients (n = 3497) who received albumin compared to those (3500) who received NS. Furthermore, there was no difference organ failure, ICU or hospital length of stay, duration of mechanical ventilation or renal replacement therapy.

Gattas DJ, Dan A, Myburgh J. Fluid resuscitation with 6% hydroxyethyl starch (130/0.4 and 130/0.42) in acutely ill patients: systemic review of effects on mortality and treatment with renal replacement therapy. *Intensive Care Med.* 2013;39:558–68. PMID 23423413

Two meta-analyses demonstrate that resuscitation with HES is associated with the need for RRT. Moreover, mortality is higher when HES is used although in one study, the statistical significance is borderline.

Gomez H, Priyanka P, Bataineh A, et al. Effects of 5% albumin plus saline versus saline alone on outcomes from large-volume resuscitation in critically ill patients. *Crit Care Med.* 2021;49:79–90. PMID 33165027.

Using two ICU databases that covered 14.5 years, the authors performed a retrospective cohort study evaluating the effects of 5% albumin plus NS versus NS on outcomes in critically ill patients. Albumin treated patients had lower mortality rates at 30, 90, and 365 days. There was a higher risk of acute kidney in the albumin group that did not result in chronic renal insufficiency.

Mandell J, Palevsky PM. Treatment of severe hypovolemia or hypovolemic shock in adults. In: www.uptodate.com. Accessed 2/3/2021

Contemporary review of the approach to the treatment of patients with hypovolemia.

Martin AMA, Mendoza JAB, Muriel A, et al. Buffered solutions versus 0.9% saline for resuscitation in critically ill adults and children. *Cochrane Database Syst Rev.* 2019;7:CD012247. PMID 31334842

The authors performed a meta-analysis evaluating the effect of BSS versus NS on hospital mortality and acute kidney injury (AKI). Twenty-one randomized controlled trials with a total of 19,054 patients were used. No difference between BSS and NS in either outcome variable was observed. The certainty of evidence for mortality was high, whereas it was low for AKI.

Myburgh JA, Finfer S, Bellomo R, et al. Hydroxyethyl starch or saline for fluid resuscitation in intensive care. *N Engl J Med.* 2012;367:1901–11. PMID 23075127

The authors randomly assigned ICU patients (n = 7000) to either 6% hydroxyethyl starch (HES) or NS for fluid resuscitation. There was no significant difference in mortality at 90 days (primary outcome). Although more patients in the NS group had evidence of kidney injury, more patients in the HES group required renal replacement therapy (RRT).

Perner A, Haase N, Guttormsen AB, et al. Hydroxyethyl starch 130/0.42 versus Ringer's acetate in severe sepsis. *N Engl J Med.* 2012;367:124–34. PMID 22738085

The investigators performed a randomized, multicenter, blinded, parallel-group study evaluating treatment of either 6% HES 130/0.42 or Ringer's acetate (RA) in patients (n = 804) with severe sepsis. Ninety-day mortality and need for RRT were greater in the HES-treated patients.

Semler MW, Self WH, Wanderer JP, et al. Balanced crystalloids versus saline in critically ill adults. *N Eng J Med.* 2018;378:829–39. PMID: 29485925

A pragmatic, cluster randomized, multiple-crossover trial was conducted in five intensive care units. Patients (n = 15,802) were treated with normal saline or balanced salt solutions (LR and Plasma-Lyte-A [PLA]) based on a randomization scheme according to which unit the patient was admitted. Patients in the balanced salt solution (BSS) group had fewer major adverse kidney events than the NS group. There was a trend towards lower need for renal replacement therapy and 30-day mortality BSS group. There was no difference in persistent kidney dysfunction.

The SAFE study investigators. Saline or albumin for fluid resuscitation in patients with traumatic brain injury. *N Engl J Med.* 2007;357:874–84. PMID 17761591

The authors performed a post-hoc analysis of patients with traumatic brain injury who had been enrolled in the SAFE study (n = 6890). Of those patients with a Glasgow Coma Scale of <9 who received albumin, 41.8% died. The corresponding death rate in the saline group was 22.2%.

Zarychanski R, Abou-Setta AM, Turgeon AF, et al. Association of hydroxyethyl starch administration with mortality and acute kidney injury in critically ill patients requiring volume resuscitation: a systematic review and meta-analysis. *JAMA.* 2013;309:678–88. PMID 23407978

Landmark Article of the 21st Century

A COMPARISON OF ALBUMIN AND SALINE FOR FLUID RESUSCITATION IN THE INTENSIVE CARE UNIT

Finfer S et al., *N Engl J Med.* 2004;350(22):2247–2256

Commentary by Matthew J. Dolich

When I was a surgical resident, references to the "battle" between crystalloid and colloid solutions for volume resuscitation of critically ill patients were abundant. Proponents for each side touted various advantages of their intravenous fluid of choice, and there was indeed no paucity of data that everyone could tap to advance their own beliefs. At the time, I must confess that my own personal bias was that albumin as a resuscitative fluid was simply not cost-effective in most circumstances.

Needless to say, in 2004 I was beside myself with excitement when the SAFE study was published. In this landmark study, almost 7000 ICU patients were randomized to receive either 4% albumin or normal saline as a resuscitative fluid, with the primary outcome being all-cause mortality during the 4-week study period. The investigators found no significant difference in mortality, and additionally there were no differences in ICU length of stay, hospital length of stay, organ failure incidence, duration of mechanical ventilation, or duration of renal replacement therapy. Their conclusion: "... albumin and saline should be considered clinically equivalent treatments for intravascular volume resuscitation in a heterogeneous population of patients in the ICU."

Boom. Question asked and answered. Let's move on.

Well, it's 17 years later and here we are. At our institution, and many other US medical centers, albumin use continues to account for hundreds of thousands of dollars (or more) each year. Albumin resuscitation is given "to reduce the amount of crystalloid," because "the patient is hypoalbuminemic," or with furosemide with the concept of "push/pull" without compelling evidence to support these approaches. Although the SAFE study was not designed to be a cost-effectiveness study, it seems clear that, in most circumstances, using a product that costs 20–50 times more than its clinically equivalent alternative is neither rational nor cost-effective.

CHAPTER 15

Gastrointestinal Bleeding

Review by Bruce Crookes

Upper gastrointestinal bleeding (UGIB) is defined as intra-luminal hemorrhage from a bleeding diathesis proximal to the ligament of Treitz, whereas lower gastrointestinal bleeding (LGIB) is bleeding distal to the ligament. UGIB occurs at a rate of 40–150 episodes per 100,000 persons per year, results in 300,000 US hospital admissions per year, and is a common cause for admission to the intensive care unit (ICU). LGIB occurs at a rate of 36 episodes per 100,000 persons per year and accounts for 3% of surgical hospital admissions. Over 85% of UGI bleeds and LGIB stop spontaneously, but when bleeding continues or when the bleed occurs in a high-risk patient, decisive management is required. Outcomes are dependent upon rapid identification of the hemorrhage's etiology, implementation of appropriate pharmacologic and procedural therapies, and prevention of re-bleeding. UGIBs rarely require surgery, and less than 6% of LGIB require an operation, making it imperative that intensivists are cognizant of the options for management.

The majority (80–90%) of UGIB are due to non-variceal causes, with ulcer disease accounting for the majority of non-variceal bleeds. Other etiologies of UGIB include esophageal varices, Mallory–Weiss syndrome, vascular lesions, and inflammatory states of the upper GI tract. LGIB results from diverticulosis, ischemic colitis, hemorrhoids, and carcinomas.

In general, LGIB will present with hematochezia, but about 10% of UGIB will present in a similar fashion. While insertion of an NGT with lavage has been used to differentiate UGIB from LGIB, the sensitivity of the test is so low as to obviate its use. In all cases of hematochezia, upper and lower GI endoscopy should be utilized as the primary means of identifying the etiology of the hemorrhage.

Advances in pharmacologic, endoscopic, and radiographic therapies have helped UGIB mortality rates to decrease, most significantly in patients >65 years of age. Surgery, while once the mainstay of treatment, has become unnecessary.

Most UGI bleeds stop spontaneously. Clinicians, however, can optimize patient outcomes through both pharmacologic and procedural interventions. As ulcer disease is the cause of the majority UGIB, providers must first identify the etiology of the ulceration, with three causes being the most prevalent: stress-related mucosal damage (SRMD), NSAID use, and *Helicobacter pylori* infection.

DOI: 10.1201/9781003042136-15

UGIB caused by ulcer disease is treated with acid suppression, just as in prevention. PPIs have been found to be superior to H_2RA agents, and they have become first line therapeutic agents. The identification of *H. pylori* as a contributing factor to peptic ulcer disease has further revolutionized care, and treatment paradigms are now well-established.

Medical treatment of variceal bleeding differs from that of the bleeding ulcer, as the therapeutic agents used are different in their mechanisms of action: mainstays of the pharmacologic treatment of variceal bleeding are vasoconstrictive and vasoactive drugs. Vasopressin and terlipressin are vasoconstrictors which have been shown to decrease active variceal bleeding. Octreotide, a hormone analogue of somatostatin, is the main vasoactive drug used to treat variceal bleeding. Multiple studies have demonstrated superior efficacy of octreotide over vasopressin for stopping active bleeding and preventing re-bleeds. Banding ligation, however, is the most effective therapy for variceal bleeding and should be the primary intervention for controlling hemorrhage.

Endoscopy is beneficial in UGI bleeds because it can be simultaneously diagnostic and, occasionally, therapeutic. Ulcer bleeding can be stopped or reduced with medical treatment as discussed previously, but studies have shown that endoscopy prevents re-bleeding. Endoscopic findings of active bleeding or a visible vessel require treatment due to their high rates of re-bleeding. While endoscopy is used for the treatment of ulcer disease, it can be used for both the treatment of active bleeding and prophylaxis in patients with varices. Options for endoscopic management of varices include injection sclerotherapy and banding ligation. Both techniques have been used for the control of acute hemorrhage: multiple studies, however, have found that ligation is superior to sclerotherapy. Regardless of cause, patients admitted with an UGIB benefit from endoscopic intervention within the first 24 hours of admission.

While there are many reports on the use of angiography for the identification and control of UGI bleeding from more obscure bleeding sources (small bowel diverticula, mesenteric aneurysms), data for its use in the control of typical UGI hemorrhage is weak. The advent of "super selective" angioembolization for UGIB seems to show a fairly high immediate success rate, but re-bleed rates are high. Most studies indicate that embolization should be used in patients with massive ongoing hemorrhage who cannot tolerate surgery due to medical co-morbidities.

LGIB is initially evaluated with both upper and lower GI endoscopy. The timing of this intervention remains controversial: randomized controlled trials show no difference in outcome when colonoscopies are done within 24 hours of admission or thereafter. Regardless, colonsocopy has a diagnostic yield of 90% and a complication rate of 0.6%. Colonoscopic interventions for hemorrhage include argon beam coagulation, YAG laser, thermal coagulation, injection with epinephrine, endoclips, and band ligation.

Radiographic evaluation of LGIB does not supersede colonoscopy as a tool for diagnosis or management. Scintigraphy has a sensitivity ranging from 23% to 97%, making it an accessory tool, at best. CT angiography can detect bleeding at rates of 0.3 mL/min, has a sensitivity of 79–100%, and can function as a selection tool for angiographic intervention; its role has yet to be fully defined. Angiography can detect bleeding rates as low as 0.5 mL/min, and can be used to control hemorrhage through embolization, but its invasive nature, complications, and re-bleeding rates (up to 20%) render it a secondary tool to endoscopy. Overall, angiography adds little clinically useful information in patients with acute LGIB. Finally, surgery is rarely required, and carries with it a 15.9–17% mortality.

Clearly, over the course of the past two decades there has been a revolution in the management of GIB, much to the benefit of patients. The studies included below are a sample of the seminal papers that have served as a foundation for treatment.

ANNOTATED REFERENCES FOR GASTROINTESTINAL BLEEDING

Chan FK, Wong VW, Suen BY, et al. Combination of a cyclo-oxygenase-2 inhibitor and a proton-pump inhibitor for prevention of recurrent ulcer bleeding in patients at very high risk: a double-blind, randomised trial. *Lancet.* 2007;369:1621–6. 28

Four-hundred-forty-one patients who were taking non-selective NSAIDs and had a history of hospital admission for upper-gastrointestinal bleeding (H. pylori negative) were randomized to receive either celecoxib and placebo or celecoxib and esomeprazol. Patients were then followed for 12 months, with the primary endpoint being recurrent ulcer bleeding. Combination treatment was more effective than celecoxib alone for prevention of ulcer bleeding in patients at high risk.

Cook D, Guyatt G, Marshall J, et al. A comparison of sucralfate and ranitidine for the prevention of upper gastrointestinal bleeding in patients requiring mechanical ventilation. Canadian Critical Care Trials Group. *N Engl J Med.* 1998;338:791–7. 21

In this multi-center, randomized, blinded, placebo-controlled trial, members of the Canadian Critical Care Trials Group compared sucralfate with the H_2-receptor antagonist ranitidine for the prevention of UGIB. Twelve hundred critically ill patients on mechanical ventilation were enrolled, and those who received ranitidine had a significantly lower rate of clinically relevant gastrointestinal bleeding. There were no significant differences in the rates of ventilator-associated pneumonia, the duration of the stay in the ICU, or mortality.

Graham DY, Lew GM, Evans DG, Evans DJ, Klein PD. Effect of triple therapy (antibiotics plus bismuth) on duodenal ulcer healing. A randomized controlled trial." *Ann Intern Med.* 1991 August;115(4):266–9. 82

In this study of 105 VA patients with UGI ulcers, patients were randomized to receive either ranitidine or ranitidine plus "triple therapy" (tetracycline, metronidazole, bismuth subsalicylate). "Triple therapy" was administered for the first 2 weeks of ulcer treatment only. Patients then underwent endoscopy after 2, 4, 8, 12, and 16 weeks of therapy. "Triple therapy" was superior to ranitidine alone for duodenal ulcer healing, as evidenced by more rapid ulcer healing on endoscopy.

Groszmann RJ, Garcia-Tsao G, Bosch J, et al. Beta-blockers to prevent gastroesophageal varices in patients with cirrhosis. *N Engl J Med.* 2005;353:2254–61. 47

Nonselective beta-adrenergic blockers are known to decrease portal pressure, but their effectiveness in preventing varices was unknown at the time of this study. Two-hundred-thirteen patients with cirrhosis and portal hypertension were randomly assigned to beta-blocker or placebo, with the primary end point being the development of gastroesophageal varices or variceal hemorrhage. There were no significant differences in the rates of variceal bleeds, nor were there significant differences in the rates of ascites, encephalopathy, liver transplantation, or death. Adverse events were more common among patients in the beta-blocker group than among those in the placebo group.

Hwang SJ, Lin HC, Chang CF, et al. A randomized controlled trial comparing octreotide and vasopressin in the control of acute esophageal variceal bleeding. *J Hepatol.* 1992;16:320–5. 49

This randomized controlled trial was conducted to compare the efficacy of intravenous infusion of octreotide with vasopressin. Forty-eight cirrhotic patients with endoscopically proven bleeding esophageal varices were randomized to one of the two treatment arms. Octreotide infusion was more effective, and had fewer side effects, than vasopressin in initially controlling acute esophageal variceal bleeding, until definitive treatment (endoscopic sclerotherapy) could be performed.

Jensen D, Mahicado G, et al. Urgent colonoscopy for the diagnosis and treatment of severe diverticular hemorrhage. *N Engl J Med.* 2010;342(2):78–82. 83

One-hundred-twenty-one patients were enrolled in this study examining the role of colonoscopy in patients with hematochezia and diverticulosis. One fifth of patients had definitive diverticular hemorrhage; colonoscopic intervention prevented the need for surgical intervention.

Khuroo MS, Yattoo GN, Javid G, et al. A comparison of omeprazole and placebo for bleeding peptic ulcer. *N Engl J Med.* 1997;336:1054–8. 35

The role of medical treatment for patients with bleeding peptic ulcers was uncertain at the time of this double-blind, placebo-controlled trial. Two-hundred-twenty patients with duodenal, gastric or stomal ulcers, and signs of recent bleeding, confirmed by endoscopy, were enrolled and randomly assigned to receive 5 days of omeprazole or placebo. The outcome measures studied were further bleeding, surgery, and death. Treatment with omeprazole decreased the rate of further bleeding and the need for surgery.

Laine L, Shah A. Randomized eternal of urgent vs. elective colonoscopy in patient hospitalized with lower GI bleeding. *Am J Gastroenterol.* 2010;105:2636–41.

Eighty-five eligible patients had urgent upper endoscopy; 13 (15%) had an upper source. The remaining 72 were randomized to urgent or elective colonoscopy. There was no significant difference between the two groups in further bleeding, units of blood transfused, hospital days, subsequent diagnostic or therapeutic interventions, and hospital charges. Note that this study was limited by its failure to reach the pre-specified sample size. The authors conclude that patients with clinically serious hematochezia should have upper endoscopy initially to rule out an upper GI source, and that there was no difference between urgent colonoscopy and routine elective colonoscopy.

Lau JY, Sung JJ, Lam YH, et al. Endoscopic retreatment compared with surgery in patients with recurrent bleeding after initial endoscopic control of bleeding ulcers. *N Engl J Med.* 1999;340:751–6. 18

In this prospective, randomized study, the authors compared endoscopic re-treatment with surgery after initial endoscopy for control of bleeding peptic ulcers. Endoscopic re-treatment reduced the need for surgery without increasing the risk of death. Endoscopic therapy was also associated with fewer complications than surgery.

Lau J, Yu Y, Tang R, et al. Timing of endoscopy for acute upper gastrointestinal bleeding. *N Engl J Med.* 2020;382:1299–1308. 16

In this single center, randomized, patients presenting to the ER underwent UGI endoscopy within 6 hours of admission (urgent endoscopy group) or 6–24 hours after admission (delay-endoscopy group). Note that the patients were screened using the Glasgow-Batchford scoring system, and thus the patients who were enrolled were at high risk for bleeding or death. Patients who were in hypotensive shock were excluded. 516 patients were enrolled, and there was no difference between groups with respect to mortality, further bleeding episodes within 30 days, or the presence of ulcers, but the rate of endoscopic hemostatic treatments was higher in the urgent-endoscopy group. The authors conclude that there was no difference in mortality between endoscopy before 6 hours, or between 6–24 hours after admission.

Poultsides GA, Kim CJ, Orlando R, 3rd, Peros G, Hallisey MJ, Vignati PV. Angiographic embolization for gastroduodenal hemorrhage: safety, efficacy, and predictors of outcome. *Arch Surg.* 2008;143:457–61. 71

Fifty-seven patients were referred to a tertiary referral center for management after failed endoscopic treatment of UGIB. Surgery was not immediately considered in these patients because of poor surgical risk, patient refusal to consent, or endoscopist's decision. Angiographic embolization for gastroduodenal hemorrhage was associated with in-hospital re-bleeding in almost half of these patients. Angiographic failure was associated with delay to embolization, blood transfusion of more than 6 units of packed red blood cells, or re-hemorrhage from a previously suture-ligated duodenal ulcer.

Sarin SK, Lamba GS, Kumar M, Misra A, Murthy NS. Comparison of endoscopic ligation and propranolol for the primary prevention of variceal bleeding. *N Engl J Med.* 1999;340:988–93. 55

The authors compared propranolol therapy and endoscopic ligation for the primary prevention of bleeding from esophageal varices. This prospective, controlled trial enrolled patients who had large varices (>5 mm in diameter) that were considered to be at high risk for bleeding. The patients were assigned to either propranolol therapy or weekly variceal ligation. After 18 months, the probability of bleeding was 43% in the propranolol group and 15% in the ligation group. Endoscopic ligation of the varices was proven to be safe and more effective than propranolol for the primary prevention of variceal bleeding.

Villanueva C, Minana J, Ortiz J, et al. Endoscopic ligation compared with combined treatment with nadolol and isosorbide mononitrate to prevent recurrent variceal bleeding. *N Engl J Med.* 2001;345:647–55. 56

One-hundred-forty-four patients with cirrhosis who were hospitalized with esophageal variceal bleeding were randomized to receive treatment with endoscopic ligation or the medical therapy with nadolol and isosorbide mononitrate. Ligation sessions were repeated every two to three weeks until the varices were eradicated. The primary end points were recurrent bleeding, complications, and death. Combined therapy with nadolol and isosorbide mononitrate was more effective in preventing recurrent hemorrhage than endoscopic ligation, and was associated with a lower rate of major complications.

Landmark Article of the 21st Century

TIMING OF ENDOSCOPY FOR ACUTE UPPER GASTROINTESTINAL BLEEDING

Lau JYW et al., *N Engl J Med.* 2022;382:1299–308

Commentary by James Y.W. Lau

Acute upper gastrointestinal bleeding is often self-limiting. In the majority of patients, urgent endoscopy is not warranted. There is little controversy that endoscopic hemostatic treatment should be made available to those with exigent bleeding and hypotension. In those who are stable or respond to volume resuscitation, the role of urgent endoscopy is less well defined. Early randomized controlled trials that compared urgent (within 6–12 hours of admissions) to early endoscopy (generally the next morning) consisted of small numbers of patients and were without risk categorization. Observational studies, with their inherent bias, produced conflicting results. A large cohort study from Europe showed a higher mortality in those who underwent endoscopy within 6 hours irrespective of their hemodynamic status. To detect a small difference in clinical outcomes, a large trial size is required. Only high-risk patients should be included in such a trial. Urgent endoscopy in low risk patients would likely lead to their early discharge, reduce hospital resource utilization, and have no impact on clinical outcomes. The strengths of the study are: 1) a randomized trial; 2) predicted high risk patients who were not too sick (those with ongoing bleeding and shock refractory to volume resuscitation excluded); 3) the use of a validated risk score (the Glasgow Blatchford score has been extensively validated and shown to be better than other risk scores in the prediction in the need for intervention); 4) an intention-to-treat analysis; and 5) mortality as the primary outcomes. There are, however, limitations when we interpret trial results. The reported mortality in the trial was lower than that in a validation cohort, and the waiting time in ER before trial inclusion suggest that the trial selected a lower risk group. The low proportion of patients with esophagogastric varices also limits its generalizability to areas with high prevalence of liver cirrhosis. In patients with stable hemo-dynamics, but at predicted high risk of further bleeds and deaths, we can safely initiate medical therapy and perform endoscopy the next morning.

CHAPTER 16

Acute Pancreatitis

Review by Umar F. Bhatti and Hasan B. Alam

Herophilus was the first to appreciate the pancreas in the early medieval period. Rufus devised the name which in the Greek language meant "all flesh." Gladen proposed that the pancreas served as a protective cushion to the underlying vasculature, and this false belief was first challenged in the 1600s when Wirsüng discovered the pancreatic duct. Physiology of the pancreas was better understood by the 19th century and in the 1880s, Fitz demonstrated the clinical features of acute pancreatitis (AP). He thought that it stemmed from gastroduodenitis. Senn was first to suggest a surgical intervention to manage AP albeit, the dawn of the 20th century saw mixed views and pancreas was regarded as an organ ill-disposed to surgery. Today, the optimum treatment for AP is subject to debate (Lankisch, 2010).

AP is the most frequent gastrointestinal cause of hospital admissions in the United States, affecting 13–45/100,000 individuals annually. It is distributed equally between males and females; however, the gender demographic varies significantly with etiology—alcoholism being the most common risk factor in males and gallstones in females. Recently, there has been an increase in incidence among the pediatric population (Yadav & Lowenfels, 2013).

Abdominal pain that radiates to the back, serum amylase/lipase level greater than three times the upper limit, and evidence of pancreatitis on abdominal imaging are the three most important diagnostic features. Presence of any two of these establishes a diagnosis (Tenner et al., 2013). Although the levels of both amylase and lipase are raised in the serum, the lipase level is not only superior for ruling out the disease, but it also provides a larger diagnostic window due to its longer half-life. Prognostic indices like the Ranson criteria, the Acute Physiology and Chronic Health Evaluation II (APACHE II) and the Bedside Index of Severity in Acute Pancreatitis (BISAP) are commonly used to evaluate the severity. While all scoring systems have limitations, BISAP is regarded as a reliable and easy-to-use tool to classify disease severity (Papachristou et al., 2010). Ultrasonography is valuable in cases with gallstone etiology. Since necrosis takes time to become obvious, CT and MRI have limited utility in the first 48–72 hours of symptom onset unless the diagnosis is uncertain. Contrast-enhanced CT is performed in patients with severe pancreatitis to rule out acute necrotizing pancreatitis. Use of MRI is emerging due to its ability to better identify gallstones and characterize the contents of fluid collections seen on CT.

DOI: 10.1201/9781003042136-16

AP is an inflammatory pathology mediated by auto-digestion of the pancreas due to abnormal activation of pancreatic enzymes—most notably trypsinogen. Based on the presence or absence of necrosis, the Atlanta classification divides AP into two distinct subtypes: the interstitial edematous pancreatitis and necrotizing pancreatitis (Sarr, 2013). Regardless of the severity of disease, critical to the management of AP is the assessment of hemodynamic status and early intravenous fluid resuscitation with crystalloids to account for fluid losses due to third spacing. Pain is managed with intravenous analgesics. If tolerated well, an oral low-fat soft or solid diet is initiated. Parenteral modes of nutrition are reserved in cases where enteral routes are inadequate to meet the caloric requirement. An early naso-enteric tube feeding in patients that are at high risk of complications doesn't provide additive benefit over oral feeds (Bakker et al., 2014). Patients require intensive care due to an increased susceptibility to complications like shock and multi-organ failure (MOF).

Since the etiology is not bacterial, use of antibiotics is generally not indicated. Antibiotic prophylaxis does not prevent progression in severe acute necrotizing pancreatitis, and treatment with antibiotics does not improve outcomes in AP (Dellinger et al., 2007). An early cholecystectomy (within 48 hours of admission) is ideal for mild biliary pancreatitis because it is associated with decreased length of stay (LOS). According to the pancreatitis of biliary origin, optimal timing of cholecystectomy (PONCHO) trial for mild biliary pancreatitis, same-admission cholecystectomy (within 1 day of randomization) is superior to interval cholecystectomy (within 27 days of randomization) because of the decreased risk of mortality or readmissions for biliary complications (5% in same-admission vs. 17% in interval) (da Costa et al., 2015). However, implementing this approach can be challenging because it warrants a shift from elective to acute care surgery which requires different skillset and infrastructure.

Endoscopic retrograde cholangiopancreatography (ERCP) with stent placement is useful in cases of biliary pancreatitis with concomitant cholangitis. In patients with mild to moderate biliary AP, post-operative ERCP is superior to pre-operative ERCP due to shorter LOS and lower total expenditure (Chang et al., 2000). Symptomatic parapancreatic fluid collections like pseudocysts or walled-off pancreatic necrosis should be drained endoscopically when anatomically feasible.

A discord exists regarding the management of acute necrotizing pancreatitis (20% of the total cases) which carries a high risk of death (8% to 39%). A secondary infection of necrotic tissue in patients with necrotizing pancreatitis (5% of all cases of AP) almost always warrants an intervention. Efforts are made to first wall-off the necrotic debris by delaying the intervention for 4 weeks. While open necrosectomy is traditionally the standard for treating necrotizing pancreatitis with infectious necrosis, a minimally invasive step-up approach has been shown to decrease the rate of major complications like MOF and death, and the incidence of long-term complications like new-onset diabetes and incisional hernias according to a well-designed randomized trial (van Santvoort et al., 2010). This in part is because the drainage of infected debris in the step-up approach eliminates the infectious nidus, and the minimally invasive technique elicits significantly less surgical trauma. In addition to better outcomes, it is believed that the step-up approach can reduce the annual healthcare costs in the United States by $185 million which makes it a very compelling alternative to the more invasive open necrosectomy.

ANNOTATED REFERENCES FOR ACUTE PANCREATITIS

Bakker OJ, et al. Early versus on-demand nasoenteric tube feeding in acute pancreatitis. *N Engl J Med.* 2014;371(21):1983–1993.

In this randomized controlled trial, the authors compared the outcomes of an early (within 24 hours of randomization) naso-enteric tube feeding to the outcomes of an oral diet initiated 72 hours after presentation, and found that opposite to the popular belief, naso-enteric tube feeding has no additive benefit over oral feeding in reducing the rate of infection or death in patients with AP who are at a high risk of complications.

Chang L, et al. Preoperative versus postoperative endoscopic retrograde cholangiopancreatography in mild to moderate gallstone pancreatitis: a prospective randomized trial. *Ann Surg.* 2000;231(1):82–87.

A randomized control trial was conducted on patients with mild to moderate biliary pancreatitis to see whether pre-operative ERCP has an advantage over selective postoperative ERCP. It was concluded that in cases with mild to moderate pancreatitis without concomitant cholangitis, postoperative ERCP does not only reduce the LOS and total cost of treatment, but it also decreases unnecessary ERCPs that would otherwise be performed preoperatively.

Da Costa DW, et al. Same-admission versus interval cholecystectomy for mild gallstone pancreatitis (PONCHO): a multicentre randomised controlled trial. *Lancet.* 2015;386(10000):1261–1268.

In this multicenter, parallel-group, assessor-masked, randomized controlled trial, the authors investigated the optimal timing of cholecystectomy for mild biliary pancreatitis. Same-admission cholecystectomy was associated with significantly lower risk of mortality and biliary complications (same-admission vs. interval cholecystectomy; 5% vs. 17%, p=0.002). The risk of recurrent pancreatitis and biliary colic was also significantly lower with same-admission cholecystectomy.

Dellinger EP, et al. Early antibiotic treatment for severe acute necrotizing pancreatitis: a randomized, double-blind, placebo-controlled study. *Ann Surg.* 2007;245(5):674–683.

The authors conducted a double-blinded, randomized, placebo-controlled trial to study the role of antibiotic treatment and prophylaxis in 100 patients with clinically severe acute necrotizing pancreatitis. The study was conducted at 32 centers in North America and Europe. It was concluded that treatment with meropenem does not confer an advantage over placebo in reducing the risk of developing pancreatic or peri-pancreatic infections, mortality or requirement of surgical intervention. It was also concluded that there is no benefit of antibiotic prophylaxis in patients with acute necrotizing pancreatitis.

Lankisch PG. Treatment of acute pancreatitis: an attempted historical review. *Pancreatology.* 2010;10(2-3):134–141. doi:10.1159/000255465

This article is a fine attempt at a historical review on treatment of acute pancreatitis. It sheds light on how the past research impacts our current understanding of the topic. The author utilizes the well-known online medical libraries and their personal library collected over a period of 40 years as a pancreatologist to produce this excellent report.

Papachristou GI, Muddana V, Yadav D, et al. Comparison of BISAP, Ranson's, APACHE-II, and
   CTSI scores in predicting organ failure, complications, and mortality in acute pancreatitis.
   Am J Gastroenterol. 2010;105(2):435–441; quiz 442. doi:10.1038/ajg.2009.622

   *The authors perform a detailed comparison of various prognostic scoring systems for
   AP, including the more recent BISAP score. They deduce that BISAP score is reliable and
   easier to use because it has lesser components, however, it doesn't improve the predictive accuracy when compared to the conventional scoring systems like APACHE II and
   Ranson's score. The study puts emphasis on the need of devising novel models of scoring
   to improve the accuracy of predicting the severity of AP.*

Sarr MG. 2012 revision of the Atlanta classification of acute pancreatitis. *Pol Arch Med Wewn.*
   2013;123(3):118–124.

   *An excellent account on the revised Atlanta classification of acute pancreatitis that fea-
   tures the changes from the older classification.*

Tenner S, et al.. American College of Gastroenterology guideline: management of acute pancreatitis. *Am J Gastroenterol.* 2013;108(9):1400–1415; 1416.

   *ACG guidelines on the management of patients with AP. These guidelines take into
   account the recent advances and development in the understanding of diagnosis, etiology,
   and management of AP.*

Yadav D, Lowenfels AB. The epidemiology of pancreatitis and pancreatic cancer.
   Gastroenterology. 2013;144(6):1252–1261. doi:10.1053/j.gastro.2013.01.068

   *The authors detail the descriptive epidemiology of pancreatic disease demonstrating the
   incidence, prevalence, and trends of acute pancreatitis with respect to patient demographics. The authors also elucidate the etiology of acute pancreatitis and provide an insight on
   disease progression and mortality.*

Landmark Article of the 21st Century

A STEP-UP APPROACH OR OPEN NECROSECTOMY FOR NECROTIZING PANCREATITIS

Vansantvoort HC et al., *N Engl J Med.* 2010;362:1491–1502

Commentary by Hjalmar C. van Santvoort

Around 30% of patients with necrotizing pancreatitis develop secondary bacterial infection of the pancreatic and peripancreatic necrosis [1]. Infected necrosis causes sepsis
with associated multiple-organ failure and is therefore an indication for invasive intervention [2]. The historical treatment was primary open necrosectomy: a laparotomy with
complete debridement of the infected necrosis. Open necrosectomy was associated with
a high risk of complications (34%–95%) and death (11%–39%) [3, 4]. The alternative
"step-up approach" aims at reducing the pro-inflammatory response of major surgery by
control of the source of infection, rather than complete removal of the infected necrosis.
The first step is percutaneous or endoscopic catheter drainage to mitigate sepsis; this
may postpone or even obviate surgical necrosectomy. If drainage does not lead to clinical
improvement, the next step is video-assisted retroperitoneal debridement (VARD) [5].

In the 2010 PANTER trial, 88 patients from 19 hospitals of the Dutch Pancreatitis Study Group with (suspected) infected necrotizing pancreatitis were randomized to primary open necrosectomy ($n = 45$) or the step-up approach ($n = 43$) [6]. The step-up approach reduced the primary end point of major complications (i.e., multiple-organ failure, bleeding, enteric perforations) and death (69% vs. 40%, $p = 0.006$). Of the patients assigned to the step-up approach, 35% were treated with catheter drainage only. Patients assigned to the step-up approach also had a lower rate of incisional hernias (7% vs. 24%, $p = 0.03$) and new-onset diabetes (16% vs. 38%, $p = 0.02$).

Patients with infected necrotizing pancreatitis should be treated with a step-up approach, consisting of catheter drainage, followed, if necessary, by minimally invasive necrosectomy.

REFERENCES

1. van Santvoort HC, Bakker OJ, Bollen TL, et al. Dutch Pancreatitis Study Group. A conservative and minimally invasive approach to necrotizing pancreatitis improves outcome. *Gastroenterology*. 2011;141(4):1254–1263.
2. APA Acute Pancreatitis Guidelines. IAP/APA evidence-based guidelines for the management of acute pancreatitis. *Pancreatology*. 2013;13(4):e1–e15.
3. Beger HG, Buchler M, Bittner R, Oettinger W, Block S, Nevalainen T, et al. Necrosectomy and postoperative local lavage in patients with necrotizing pancreatitis: results of a prospective clinical trial. *World J Surg*. 1988;12:255–262.
4. Traverso LW, Kozarek RA. Pancreatic necrosectomy: definitions and technique. *J Gastrointest Surg*. 2005;9:436–439.
5. Horvath KD, Kao LS, Ali A, Wherry KL, Pellegrini CA, Sinanan MN, et al. Laparoscopic assisted percutaneous drainage of infected pancreatic necrosis. *Surg Endosc*. 2001;15(7):677–682.
6. van Santvoort HC, Besselink MG, Bakker OJ, et al. A step-up approach or open necrosectomy for necrotizing pancreatitis. *N Engl J Med*. 2010;362(16):1491–1502.

CHAPTER 17

Abdominal Compartment Syndrome

Review by Peter P. Lopez and Edward Lineen

Abdominal compartment syndrome (ACS) is when a patient has intra-abdominal hypertension (IAH) that reduces blood flow to their abdominal organs leading to dysfunction in their pulmonary, cardiovascular, renal, and gastrointestinal systems. The World Society of the Abdominal Compartment Syndrome (WSACS; www.WSACS.org) defines ACS as a sustained IAH greater than 20 mm Hg (with or without an abdominal perfusion pressure [APP] less than 60 mm Hg) that is associated with new organ dysfunction/failure [1]. ACS can develop in a host of surgical and non-surgical conditions requiring aggressive fluid resuscitation including sepsis, burns, and pancreatitis. If left untreated ACS leads to fulminant multiple organ failure and death. Early recognition and treatment of IAH/ACS are critical in order to decrease morbidity and mortality.

Primary ACS arises from injury or disease within the abdominopelvic cavity. Secondary ACS, which is more common, manifests from conditions that originated outside the abdominopelvic cavity. Recurrent ACS is the persistence of ACS despite medical and surgical management. The development of ACS depends on both the elevation in pressure and the rate at which the pressure rises. Patients who require large volume resuscitation or massive transfusion, who are oliguria, hypotensive, hypothermic, acidotic, or who have acute respiratory failure with elevated intrathoracic pressures, major trauma or burns, hemoperitoneum, ileus, ascites, or sepsis, should be screened and followed for the development of IAH or ACS. The incidence of IAH and ACS in any given surgical-medical ICU/trauma ICU patient population varies from 31–58.8%/2–50% for IAH and 0.5–8%/1–15% for ACS [2, 10, 11]. Timely recognition of IAH/ACS can lead to early medical and surgical treatment with improved outcomes.

Intra-abdominal pressure is the steady state concealed within the abdominal cavity. IAP is primarily determined by the intra-abdominal volume which is the volume abdominal viscera and the intra-compartment fluid volume. It varies with respiration; increasing with respiration and decreases with expiration. The normal IAP is 0–5 mm Hg. Intra-abdominal hypertension is when the patient has an elevated intra-abdominal compartment pressure of equal or greater than 12 mm Hg. IAH has been broken down into four groups defined by increasing pressure: Grade I: 12–15 mm Hg, Grade II: 16–20 mm Hg, Grade III: 21–25 mm Hg, Grade IV: >25 mm Hg. Abdominal perfusion pressure (APP) is defined by the mean arterial pressure minus IAP (MAP–IAP = APP). APP equal or greater than 50 mm Hg has been shown to correlate with survival in patients with IAH and ACS [3].

DOI: 10.1201/9781003042136-17

Marey first described the respiratory effects caused by elevated IAP in 1863 [4]. Kron et al. first described ACS and the technique used to measure IAP [5]. The modified Kron technique of intra-vesical measurement of IAP "bladder pressure" is the most common way to measure IAP [4]. The technique measures the pressure in the bladder in a supine patient at the end of expiration. Fifty milliliters of saline are introduced into the foley catheter, the foley is clamped and the resulting pressure in the bladder is transduced at the level of the patient's mid-axillary line at the level of the iliac crest [2]. This pressure measurement correlates to IAP. However, this measurement is in cm H_2O not mm Hg. To convert cm H_2O to mm Hg, multiply the value by 0.74. In 1989, Fietsam et al. reported on four patients who developed intra-abdominal compartment syndrome after repair of their ruptured abdominal aortic aneurysm [6].

The pathophysiology of IAH and ACS is multifactorial and leads to organ dysfunction. No matter the cause of shock, impaired capillary blood flow leads to development of capillary leak, intravascular fluid shifts leading to interstitial edema, which leads to the release of inflammatory mediators and more shock. Increased swelling and edema of the abdominal viscera and retroperitoneal space leads to increased IAP. The abdominal wall fascia is relatively non-compliant with the intra-abdominal contents reaching a maximum after which IAP begins to rise.

Oliguria progressing to anuria is usually the first sign of IAH/ACS. Decreases in preload and cardiac output with an increase in afterload result from IAH/ACS. This is manifested as hypotension. The pulmonary insult caused by IAH/ACS presents clinically as hypoxia, hypercapnia, and elevated airway pressures. Basal atelectasis, reduced lung compliance, increased pulmonary dead space, and increased ventilatory pressures all occur with IAH/ACS. The clinical neurologic effects of IAH/ACS are directly related to the increase in intracranial pressure and a decrease in cerebral perfusion pressure. Gastrointestinal effects of IAH/ACS are decreased metabolite clearance and energy substrate production by the liver, intestinal hypomotility, intestinal ischemia, and bacterial translocation. Venous stasis also occurs in patients with IAH/ACS making them more susceptible to venous thromboembolism [7, 9].

Medical and surgical management of IAH/ACS are used to reduce the IAP before irreversible organ damage occurs. Early recognition and prevention of those at risk should lead to appropriate IAP monitoring. Delays in managing IAH/ACS increases the risk of morbidity and mortality. Medical management focuses on reducing intra-abdominal volume and or increasing the abdominal wall compliance [2]. Abdominal wall tension can be relieved by controlling pain and anxiety with analgesia, anxiolytics, and muscle relaxants. Gastric decompression, prokinetics, and colonic stimulates are all used to increase bowel motility and decompress the bowel. Restarting enteral feeding as soon as possible helps maintain bowel integrity, which reduces alteration in bowel flora and bacterial translocation. Fluid management is paramount. Balance between resuscitation and third space overload should be directed by aggressive hemodynamic monitoring. Additional indicators of adequate or inadequate fluid resuscitation recommended by Carr are base excess, pH, and lactate [8]. Pharmacologic diuresis in conjunction with renal replacement therapy may be beneficial in reducing IAH. Paracentesis can be used to manage ascites [1, 2, 4]. Surgical management with decompressive laparotomy and temporary closure of the open abdomen is the only definitive treatment of ACS. A midline incision from xyphoid sternum to the symphysis pubis is made with the immediate release of pressure causes a dramatic improvement in visceral perfusion and end organ function. Recurrent ACS can occur after surgical decompression if the underlying pathology responsible has not been treated.

Decompressive laparotomy while being potentially lifesaving, the resulting open abdomen can be associated with significant morbidity and should be used when medical treatment has failed. Reperfusion injury, massive protein loss, hypercatabolic state, fascial retraction, ventral hernia, frozen abdomen, infection, and enterocutaneous fistulas can all complicate the patient with an open abdomen [2, 7, 8]. The open abdomen is managed with a variety of temporary abdominal closure techniques and often requires several explorations of the abdominal cavity. Despite the many different temporary abdominal closure techniques, the open abdomen can be closed in up to 70–90% of patient within 7–9 days [2]. Large ventral hernias remain a problem for patients who fully recover from ACS once the abdomen is closed.

Abdominal compartment syndrome remains a severe complication resulting from a sustained increase in intra-abdominal pressure causing significant morbidity and mortality. When managing patients at risk for developing IAH/ACS appropriate monitoring and measuring of IAP will lead to early intervention and better outcomes in patients with IAH/ACS.

ANNOTATED REFERENCES FOR ABDOMINAL COMPARTMENT SYNDROME

1. Kirkpatrick AW, Roberts DJ, De Waele J, et al. Intra-abdominal hypertension and the abdominal compartment syndrome: updated consensus definitions and clinical practice guidelines from the World Society of the Abdominal Compartment Syndrome. *Intensive Care Med.* 2013;39:1190–1206.

   The second consensus conference report and expert panel on IAH and ACS by the WSACS. This report expands and updates on the 2006 WSACS consensus publication on IAH and ACS. The report uses the GRADE system to rate the quality of evidence and strength of management recommendations.

2. Hecker A, Hecker B, Hecker M, et al. Acute abdominal compartment syndrome: current and therapeutic options. *Langenbecks Arch Surg.* 2016;401:15–24.

   Recent review of current diagnostic and therapeutic options of IAH, ACS and open abdomen.

3. Cheatham ML, White M, Sagraves S, Johnson J, Block E. Abdominal perfusion pressure: a superior parameter in the assessment of intra-abdominal hypertension. *J Trauma Acute Care Surg.* 2000;49(4):621–627.

   Study using APP as a parameter to monitor the clinical effects of IAH.

4. Sosa G, Gandham N, Landeras V, Calimag AP, Lerma E. Abdominal compartment ayndrome. *Disease-a-Month.* 2019;65.

   Good overall review of ACS with a brief mention of historical milestones.

5. Kron IL, Harman PK, Nolan SP. The measurement of intrabdominal pressure as a criterion for abdominal re-exploration. *Ann Surg.* 1984;199:28–30.

The paper was the first to describe abdominal compartment syndrome and described a technique how to measure intra-abdominal pressure.

6. Fietsam J, Villalba M, Glover J, Clark K. Intra-abdominal compartment syndrome as a complication of ruptured abdominal aorta aneurysm repair. *Am Surg.* 1989;55(6):396–402.

First to introduce the term intra-abdominal compartment syndrome.

7. An G, West MA. Abdominal compartment syndrome: a concise clinical review. *Crit Care Med.* 2008;36(4):1304–1310.

A concise review of ACS.

8. Carr JA. Abdominal compartment syndrome: a decade of progress. *J Am Coll Surg.* 2013;216:135–146.

Another good review of ACS.

9. Cheatham ML. Abdominal compartment syndrome: pathophysiology and definitions. *Scand J Trauma Resusc Emerg Med.* 2009;17(1):10.

Another good physiologic review of ACS.

10. Hong JJ, Cohn SM, Perez JM, Dolich DO, Brown M, McKenney MG. Prospective study of the incidence and outcome of intra-abdominal hypertension and the abdominal compartment syndrome. *Brit J Surg.* 2002;89:591–596.

Prospective study to describe a low incidence of IAH/ACS in trauma patients.

11. Meldrum DR, Moore FA, Moore EE, Franciose RJ, Sauaia A, Burch JM. Prospective characterization and selective management of the abdominal compartment syndrome. *Am J Surg.* 1997;174:667–672.

Prospective study identifying trauma patients with ACS and their treatment.

Landmark Article of the 21st Century

IS THE EVOLVING MANAGEMENT OF INTRA-ABDOMINAL HYPERTENSION AND ABDOMINAL COMPARTMENT SYNDROME IMPROVING SURVIVAL?

Michal L, Cheatham, MD, Karen Safcsak RN, *Crit Care Med.* 2010;38(2):402–407

Commentary by Michael L. Cheatham and Karen Safcsak

Young surgeons unfamiliar with the history of intra-abdominal hypertension (IAH) and abdominal compartment syndrome (ACS) management may take for granted damage control laparotomy as a valuable tool in the acute care surgeon's armamentarium. Just over two decades ago, IAH and ACS were essentially unrecognized causes of morbidity and mortality among the critically ill. Abdominal decompression was regarded with skepticism and reserved as a highly morbid last resort for patients who had failed contemporary resuscitation. ACS mortality was exceedingly high with some surgeons arguing that abdominal decompression was futile. As the new millennium approached, however, surgeon attitudes toward decompression softened as studies demonstrated improved survival through *preventing* rather than *reacting* to IAH/ACS.

We began prospectively studying our open abdomen patients in 1997, ultimately creating the largest single-center IAH/ACS database in the world. Our survival rate was initially a dismal 35%. By employing an evidence-based management algorithm that included serial intra-abdominal pressure (IAP) measurements, goal-directed resuscitation using judicious crystalloid volumes and massive transfusion protocols, multi-modality medical IAP management, and especially prophylactic abdominal decompression, we increased our survival rate to 72% a decade later with an enviable primary fascial closure rate of 81%. We found ACS to be independently associated with a five-fold increase in mortality and prophylactic decompression to have a three-fold increase in survival compared to a reactive decompression strategy.

Thankfully, IAH/ACS is not seen with the frequency it once was. The evolution of IAH/ACS management serves to remind us of the value of constantly pursuing better strategies for patient survival.

CHAPTER 18

Mesenteric Ischemia

Review by Abdul Alarhayem and Sungho Lim

Acute mesenteric ischemia (AMI) is a challenging and potentially fatal condition that requires a high index of suspicion, early diagnosis, and prompt restoration of blood flow to avoid fulminant bowel necrosis and death. Delays in diagnoses have been associated with a mortality of up to 80% (Mamode et al., 1999; Clair and Beach, 2016). Intestinal ischemia is broadly categorized according to the segment of bowel to which blood flow is compromised and the acuity of onset. The presentation management strategies and outcomes of these entities varies widely; accurate diagnosis is thus paramount (Lim et al., 2019). Whereas, colonic ischemic (ischemic colitis) is limited to the colon, mesenteric ischemia primarily affects the small bowel. And while patients with chronic mesenteric ischemia exhibit episodic or recurrent intestinal angina and "food fear" and can be managed in a less urgent manner, acute mesenteric ischemia requires immediate intervention.

Thromboembolic occlusion of the superior mesenteric artery is the most common cause of acute mesenteric ischemia (Acosta et al., 2005). Less frequent etiologies include venous thrombosis and non-occlusive hypoperfusion. Embolism is seen in patients with cardiac arrhythmias, recent myocardial infarction, cardiac valvular disease, infective endocarditis, aortic atherosclerosis, or aneurysmal disease. Embolism usually involves the SMA just distal to the origin of the middle colic and jejunal arteries. Compared to the celiac artery and the IMA, the SMA has a less acute angle of takeoff from the aorta. The SMA's diameter also decreases beyond the middle colic artery, resulting in a classical duodenal and transverse colon sparing distribution of ischemia.

Thrombotic occlusion occurs (acute-on-chronic mesenteric ischemia) in patients with risk factors for atherosclerosis (especially smoking) and an antecedent history of chronic mesenteric ischemic symptoms (postprandial abdominal pain, food fear, and weight loss). It usually presents with more proximal occlusion and results in greater bowel involvement as it represents spillover atherosclerotic disease from the aorta. Elderly patients and those with low cardiac output states are also at higher risk of thrombosis.

Mesenteric venous thrombosis accounts for less than 10% of all cases of acute mesenteric ischemia. It usually arises in patients with heritable or acquired thrombophilias; however, it may occur independently of this in the setting of local intra-abdominal

DOI: 10.1201/9781003042136-18

inflammatory pathology (perforated appendicitis, diverticulitis, etc.). Venous or out-flow thrombosis results in increased resistance in the capillary bed decreasing perfusion pressure. This results in bowel wall edema and perpetuates a vicious cycle which ultimately results in bowel wall necrosis.

Bowel ischemia is seen in about 20% of small bowel obstructions (SBOs) (hernia, adhesive disease, etc.). While SBO can be associated with bowel necrosis, it does not typically fall under the umbrella of mesenteric ischemia, a term reserved for when perfusion compromise involving the major vessels (arteries or veins) is the inciting event, and not secondary to progressive bowel dilatation from obstruction.

The primary pathophysiological mechanism at the base of all forms of mesenteric ischemia is a supply demand mismatch. Insufficient delivery of oxygen and nutrients usually due to an abrupt cessation of blood flow at the capillary level, which ultimately results in cellular hypoxia and death. This can lead to full-thickness bowel wall necrosis with a massive systemic release of the by-products of ischemic injury and free radicals, resulting in multi-organ dysfunction and death.

Diagnosis of mesenteric ischemia can prove challenging. Patients invariably present with abdominal pain and leukocytosis; while some exhibit "pain out of proportion to examination," many do not. Importantly and unlike other vascular disorders, AMI primarily affects women; more than 70% of patients are female. Tenderness on examination suggests bowel necrosis causing peritoneal irritation. As the disease progresses and bowel ischemia sets in, lactic acidosis and signs of shock may ensue. The clinician should not wait for severe leukocytosis or lactic acidosis to intervene, as these often are markers of severe ischemia or irreversible bowel injury. A high index of suspicion is necessary with all forms of mesenteric ischemia but especially those with mesenteric venous thrombosis; lab values may be deceptively normal due to the lack of washout of the by-products of bowel ischemia secondary to a thrombosed outflow.

High-resolution computed tomographic (CT) angiography is not only diagnostic for acute mesenteric ischemia, but also helps distinguish embolic from thrombotic etiologies and aids in operative planning (Kim and Ha, 2003). In patients whom the suspicion for mesenteric venous thrombosis is high, CT angiography with a portal venous phase should be obtained. Venous filling defects or absent mesenteric flow during the venous phase are diagnostic.

Initial management includes fluid resuscitation using isotonic crystalloids, antibiotic coverage, and therapeutic anticoagulation. Visceral ischemia incites an intense inflammatory response associated with extensive third spacing and intravascular volume depletion potentially exacerbating ischemia. Prompt goal directed resuscitation is thus essential. The use of pressor therapy in the setting of shock should be a last resort. Broad spectrum antibiotics are instituted due to bacterial and toxin translocation associated with damaged intestinal epithelium. Therapeutic anticoagulation (typically unfractionated heparin) is employed to prevent further clot propagation (Klempnauer et al., 1997). Oral intake can exacerbate intestinal ischemia and patients should thus be kept NPO.

The goal of intervention is focused on expeditious restoration of visceral perfusion (Ryer et al., 2012; Corcos et al., 2013). In patients with embolism, a midline laparotomy is performed and a Fogarty embolectomy catheter is passed proximally and distally and flow is restored. This approach also allows for assessment of bowel viability. In patients with mesenteric thrombosis, thrombectomy alone is unlikely to be effective or durable. Mesenteric bypass, classically considered the "gold-standard," constructs a graft from the aorta or iliac artery to a site distal to the occlusion. It offers excellent relief and is remarkably durable, however, it can be prohibitive in patients in shock or those with extensive cardiovascular comorbidities (Johnston et al., 1995; Klempnauer et al., 1997; Björck et al., 2002; Cho et al., 2002; Roussel et al., 2015). Endovascular and hybrid approaches, typically by means of mechanical thrombectomy or angioplasty and stenting, may be as effective as traditional surgical approaches while eliminating the need for aortic cross clamping, minimizing physiologic insult (Milner et al., 2004; Wyers et al., 2007). If endovascular-only therapy is pursued, any evidence of clinical deterioration or peritonitis necessitates operative exploration (Clair and Beach, 2016). Poor-risk surgical candidates with extensive small bowel infarction may be best served by a palliative approach.

Following revascularization, the abdomen should be explored, and frankly necrotic bowel resected. Marginal appearing bowel should be observed; a second-look laparotomy in 24 to 48 hours to reevaluate the bowel is often necessary. Bowel anastomosis should not be performed in patients with questionable bowel viability or hemodynamic instability (Roussel et al., 2015; Becquemin, 2017).

Postoperatively, patients require invasive hemodynamic monitoring, end point directed resuscitation, nutritional support, and mitigation of cardiovascular risk factors. Anticoagulation should be continued postoperatively, and surveillance imaging is warranted.

In conclusion, acute mesenteric ischemia is a life-threatening disease that often presents a diagnostic challenge and requires a high index of suspicion. Prompt diagnosis and intervention is focused on expeditious restoration of visceral perfusion. Despite aggressive treatment strategies, mortality is high (Schoots et al. 2004).

ANNOTATED REFERENCES FOR MESENTERIC ISCHEMIA

Acosta S, Ögren M, Sternby N-H, Bergqvist D, Björck M. Clinical implications for the management of acute thromboembolic occlusion of the superior mesenteric artery: autopsy findings in 213 patients. *Ann Surg*. 2005;241(3):516.

A study of 213 cases of acute thromboembolic occlusion of the SMA and intestinal infarction. Clinical suspicion of intestinal ischemia was documented in about one third of patients. The embolus/thrombus ratio was 1.4 to 1. Thrombotic occlusions were located more proximally than embolic occlusions and associated with more extensive intestinal infarction.

Becquemin J. Management of the diseases of mesenteric arteries and veins: clinical practice guidelines of the European Society for Vascular Surgery (ESVS). *Eur J Vasc Endovasc Surg.* 2017;53(4):455–457.

Sixty-four recommendations from the European Society for Vascular Surgery (ESVS) guidelines committee regarding the management of acute and chronic arterial ischemia, nonocclusive mesenteric ischemia, visceral aneurysms, and dissection.

Björck M, et al. Revascularization of the superior mesenteric artery after acute thromboembolic occlusion. *Brit J Surg.* 2002;89(7):923–927.

Sixty patients with acute thromboembolic occlusion of the SMA undergoing revascularization procedures across 21 Swedish hospitals. Fifty-eight patients had an exploratory laparotomy and subsequent revascularization, and two were treated with thrombolysis alone. Mortality rates were 43% at 30 days and 67% at 5 years.

Cho J-S, et al. Long-term outcome after mesenteric artery reconstruction: a 37-year experience. *J Vasc Surg.* 2002;35(3):453–460.

A retrospective review of 48 consecutive patients who underwent revascularization for acute mesenteric ischemia (AMI) of nonembolic origin. Perioperative (<30 days) mortality rate was 52%. Major complications occurred in 60% of the cases. The late survival rates were 54% and 20% at 5 and 10 years,

Clair DG, Beach JM. Mesenteric ischemia. *N Engl J Med.* 2016;374(10):959–968.

A review article that explains the pathophysiology, diagnosis, and treatment of intestinal ischemic syndromes.

Corcos O, et al. Effects of a multimodal management strategy for acute mesenteric ischemia on survival and intestinal failure. *Clin Gastroenterol Hepatol.* 2013;11(2):158–165. e152.

A pilot study demonstrating that a multimodal management team approach of 18 consecutive patients with occlusive AMI achieved a survival rate of 95% at 30 days and 89% at 2 years.

Johnston KW, et al. Mesenteric arterial bypass grafts: early and late results and suggested surgical approach for chronic and acute mesenteric ischemia. *Surgery.* 1995;118(1):1–7.

A study of 34 patients who underwent mesenteric vascular graft placement for chronic and acute mesenteric ischemia. Of the patients who underwent only a single SMA or celiac bypass, two of five died of bowel infarction; only one of 16 patients who underwent both celiac and SMA bypass had to undergo a repeat surgical procedure because of graft occlusion. Complete revascularization of the SMA and celiac artery or pelvis or both and prograde bypass may reduce the risk of late bowel ischemia.

Kim AY, Ha HK. Evaluation of suspected mesenteric ischemia: efficacy of radiologic studies. *Radiologic Clin.* 2003;41(2):327–342.

A review article that studies the reports the utility of radiographic diagnostic studies in patients with suspected mesenteric ischemia.

Klempnauer J, et al. Long-term results after surgery for acute mesenteric ischemia. *Surgery.* 1997;121(3):239–243.

Ninety patients with acute mesenteric ischemia treated by vascular reconstruction or bowel resection, or both, between 1972 and 1993 were studied. The overall mortality was 66%. In the 31 patients who were discharged from the hospital, the 2- and 5-year survival rates were 70% and 50%.

Lim S, et al. Contemporary management of acute mesenteric ischemia in the endovascular era. *Vasc Endovasc Surg.* 2019;53(1):42–50.

A review article that supports an endovascular first approach in the management of patients with AMI, citing evidence that this strategy may have improved outcomes in the immediate postoperative period.

Mamode N, et al. Failure to improve outcome in acute mesenteric ischaemia: seven year review. *Eur J Surg.* 1999;165(3):203–208.

A study of 57 patients presenting with acute mesenteric ischemia. Only 18 (32%) patients were accurately diagnosed before operation or death. Forty-six of the 57 patients died.

Milner R, et al. Superior mesenteric artery angioplasty and stenting via a retrograde approach in a patient with bowel ischemia: a case report. *Vasc Endovasc Surg.* 2004;38(1):89–91.

This study reports a novel combination of open and endovascular techniques via a retrograde superior mesenteric artery (SMA) approach to treat acute mesenteric ischemia in the setting of an acute abdomen.

Roussel A, et al. Revascularization of acute mesenteric ischemia after creation of a dedicated multidisciplinary center. *J Vasc Surg.* 2015;62(5):1251–1256.

A study of 83 patients with AMI, 29 of whom underwent revascularization. Overall 2-year survival was 89.2%, and 30-day operative mortality was 6.9%. The 2-year primary patency rate of open revascularization was 88%.

Ryer EJ, et al. Revascularization for acute mesenteric ischemia. *J Vasc Surg.* 2012;55(6):1682–1689.

A study of 93 patients with AMI who underwent emergency arterial revascularization. Forty-five patients were treated during the 1990s and 48 during the 2000s. Patient demographics and risk factors were similar and etiology remained constant between the groups with in situ thrombosis being the most common followed by arterial embolus. Thirty-day mortality was 27% in the 1990s and 17% during the 2000s (p = 0.28). Major adverse events occurred in 47% of patients with no difference between decades. There was no significant difference in outcomes between open and endovascular revascularization.

Schoots I, et al. Systematic review of survival after acute mesenteric ischaemia according to disease aetiology. *Brit J Surg.* 2004;91(1):17–27.

A review of 45 observational studies containing 3692 patients with acute mesenteric ischemia showed that the overall survival after acute mesenteric ischemia has improved over the past four decades. Surgical treatment of arterial embolism has improved outcome whereas the mortality rate following surgery for arterial thrombosis and non-occlusive ischemia remains poor.

Wyers MC, et al. Retrograde mesenteric stenting during laparotomy for acute occlusive mesenteric ischemia. *J Vasc Surg.* 2007;45(2):269–275.

Three different revascularization methods used in 13 patients with arterial occlusive AMI. At 17%, the retrograde open stenting group had the lowest hospital mortality compared with bypass at 80% (p = 0.08) and percutaneous stent at 100% (p = 0.11).

Landmark Article of the 21st Century

SURGICAL MANAGEMENT OF THROMBOTIC ACUTE INTESTINAL ISCHEMIA

Endean et al., *Ann Surg.* 2001 June;233(6):801–808

Commentary by Eric D. Endean

Vascular causes for acute mesenteric ischemia (AMI) include arterial embolus, arterial thrombosis, and mesenteric venous thrombosis. Historically, AMI is associated with a high mortality. Many factors contribute to this poor prognosis and include the relative infrequency of mesenteric ischemia as a cause for abdominal symptoms, lack of specific physical or laboratory findings, and the fact that many patients who present with AMI are elderly with co-morbid conditions and limited physiologic reserve.

While we recognized the poor prognosis associated with AMI, we felt that the contemporary outcomes may be better than the reported 10–38% survival rate. This led us to review our experience with AMI. The study was limited to patients who had AMI either due to arterial embolus or thrombosis or mesenteric venous thrombosis.

In the entire group of patients, the survival rate was 52%, seeming to confirm our hypothesis that the survival rate was better than previously reported. However, when evaluating each cohort of patients, the survival rate for patients with arterial embolus was 41%, arterial thrombosis was 38%, and mesenteric venous thrombosis was 87%. These results, while at the high end of the reported survival rates, continued to demonstrate poor prognosis. As other authors have emphasized, we also highlighted the need for early diagnosis and intervention as a strategy to improve survival. Interestingly, in our series, 13 patients (5 embolus, 8 thrombosis) had no intervention due to the extensive bowel infarction found at laparotomy. We suggest that these patients had progressed to this point, in part because of delay in diagnosis and or intervention. If these patients were excluded from the analysis, the survival rate in those who had an intervention would have been 53% for those with an embolus and 62% for those with arterial thrombosis.

Our study again emphasizes the need for early diagnosis and intervention for patients with AMI. Since our study was done prior to the era when computed tomography was routinely utilized for patients who presented with abdominal pain, it may be that with routine CT scanning, AMI will be diagnosed earlier leading to earlier intervention and hopefully improved outcomes.

CHAPTER 19

Treatment of Variceal Bleeding in Cirrhotic Patients

Review by Robert J. Canelli

Gastroesophageal varices are present in approximately 50% of all patients with cirrhosis, with a higher percentage found in patients with Child–Turcotte–Pugh class C disease. Varices form and grow at a rate of 8% per year, with a yearly rupture rate of 5–15% [1]. Management of varices can be divided into three categories: primary prophylaxis to prevent the first episode of bleeding, emergency treatment during an acute bleeding episode, and secondary prophylaxis to prevent re-bleeding.

Acute variceal hemorrhage requires emergency treatment and is associated with a high 6-week mortality rate. Controlling hemorrhage is complex and involves a combination of urgent pharmacotherapy and procedural intervention. The immediate goals of emergency treatment are to control bleeding, prevent early re-bleeding within 5 days, and prevent 6-week mortality [2].

The first step in emergency treatment is to restore hemodynamic stability by obtaining large bore intravenous access for resuscitation. Red blood cells are administered to maintain a hemoglobin between 7 and 9 g/dL [3]. Platelet transfusion to maintain platelet count above 50,000/μL should be considered. Although hemostatic products such as fresh frozen plasma, prothrombin complex concentrate, and recombinant activated factor VII to correct coagulopathy are often considered, they have not shown clear benefit.

Airway protection including endotracheal intubation is especially important in patients presenting with hematemesis. Endotracheal intubation will also facilitate the timely performance of diagnostic and therapeutic endoscopy. Nasogastric tube placement to remove particulate matter and administration of a prokinetic agent such as erythromycin can facilitate successful endoscopic management of variceal hemorrhage. The prophylactic administration of short term antibiotics including ceftriaxone has been shown to decrease the development of infections, recurrent hemorrhage, and death [4].

Urgent pharmacologic intervention for emergency treatment includes the administration of splanchnic vasoconstrictors that will reduce blood flow through the portal venous system. Vasoactive agents such as octreotide and terlipressin are associated with lower 7-day all-cause mortality, improved control of acute hemorrhage, and lower transfusion requirements [5]. These medications should be administered as soon as

DOI: 10.1201/9781003042136-19

possible. In fact, Levacher and colleagues advocate for terlipressin administration to patients by emergency medical personnel before transfer to the hospital [6].

Temporizing measures as a bridge to definitive therapy include balloon tamponade and esophageal stent placement. Balloon tamponade is useful at controlling hemorrhage; however, severe complications such as re-bleeding upon balloon deflation and esophageal rupture can occur. Esophageal stents, self-expanding metal stents placed endoscopically, show no differences in survival when compared to balloon tamponade; however, control of bleeding was superior and side effects were significantly lower [7].

Emergent endoscopic therapy is the definitive treatment of choice for acute variceal hemorrhage and can be performed at the same time as diagnostic endoscopy. Upper endoscopy should be performed within 12 hours of presentation and when the patient is hemodynamically stable. Endoscopic variceal ligation (EVL) and endoscopic sclerotherapy are the interventional options with EVL the preferred choice [8].

Secondary prophylaxis aims to prevent re-bleeding, defined as bleeding that occurs >120 hours after the first hemorrhage provided that hemostasis was initially achieved [9]. Therapies include a combination of nonselective beta blockade and endoscopic variceal ligation [10]. If re-bleeding occurs, more definitive therapy, including transjugular intrahepatic portosystemic shunt (TIPS) or abdominal surgery, is required.

Prior to 2010, TIPS was only indicated for re-bleeding as a bridge to liver transplant. TIPS creates a low resistance channel between the hepatic vein and the portal vein. Complications of TIPS include portosystemic encephalopathy and technical complications such as cardiac arrhythmias, traversal of the liver capsule, and TIPS stenosis. TIPS is contraindicated in patients with heart failure, polycystic liver disease, severe pulmonary hypertension, uncontrolled systemic infection or sepsis, and severe tricuspid regurgitation.

In 2010, Garcia-Pagan et al. studied the early use of TIPS in patients with cirrhosis and acute esophageal variceal hemorrhage as a secondary prophylaxis therapy. The authors randomized 63 patients who had been treated with vasoactive drugs and endoscopic therapy to receive early TIPS within 72 hours or continuation of pharmacotherapy only, reserving TIPS as rescue therapy for re-bleeding. At median follow up of 16 months, 14 patients in the pharmacotherapy group met composite criteria for re-bleeding events versus one patient in the early-TIPS group (p <0.001). One year survival was 86% in the early-TIPS group as compared to 61% in the pharmacotherapy group (p <0.001) [11].

Presently, early TIPS within 72 hours of endoscopic therapy is indicated for secondary prophylaxis in patients at high risk of re-bleeding, including those with Child–Turcotte–Pugh class C cirrhosis. If early TIPS is not performed after the first bleeding episode, it is the recommended rescue therapy for patients that re-bleed despite initial secondary prophylaxis measures. TIPS is not recommended for primary prophylaxis [8].

Abdominal surgery is an alternative means to control variceal hemorrhage; however, the mortality rate is high, approaching 50% with surgery [12]. Two surgical approaches are described: a shunt operation that decompresses the portal tree or an operation involving esophageal transection or devascularization of the gastroesophageal junction. Because of the high mortality rate associated with surgery, it is usually reserved for patients who have a contraindication to TIPS.

ANNOTATED REFERENCES FOR TREATMENT OF VARICEAL BLEEDING IN CIRRHOTIC PATIENTS

1. Sass DA, Chopra KB. Portal hypertension and variceal hemorrhage. *Med Clin North Am.* 2009;93(4):837–853.

    This review article describes the classification system of portal hypertension and discusses the pathophysiology of varices and variceal hemorrhage. Authors report on the natural history of varices including the incidence of varices in patients with cirrhosis, the rate of development, and the yearly rate of variceal hemorrhage. They identify predictors of variceal hemorrhage.

2. de Franchis R; Baveno V Faculty. Expanding consensus in portal hypertension: Report of the Baveno VI Consensus Workshop: stratifying risk and individualizing care for portal hypertension. J Hepatol. 2015; 63:743–752.

    The Baveno VI faculty provides an expert consensus statement that defines key events in portal hypertension, clarifies terminology, and standardizes language regarding variceal hemorrhage. The consensus statement issues evidence-based recommendations for conducting of clinical trials, including identification of 6 week mortality as the primary endpoint that should be used for studies on acute variceal bleeding. Authors report a 6 week mortality rate of 10–20% for variceal bleeding.

3. Villanueva C, Colomo A, Bosch A, et al. Transfusion strategies for acute upper gastrointestinal bleeding. *N Engl J Med.* 2013;368:11–21.

    This randomized controlled trial enrolled 921 patients with acute upper gastrointestinal bleeding to evaluate restrictive versus liberal blood transfusion strategies. Red blood cell transfusion to a hemoglobin goal 7–9 g/dL was associated with a significant improvement in 6 week survival compared to a liberal tansfusion strategy to maintain hemoglobin of 9–11 g/dL (95% vs. 91%; p = 0.02). The subgroup analysis of patients with cirrhosis revealed significantly lower early rebleeding and mortality rates in patients randomized to restrictive PRBC transfusion.

4. Chavez-Tapia NC, Barrientos-Gutierrez T, Tellez-Avila F, et al. Meta-analysis: antibiotic prophylaxis for cirrhotic patients with upper gastrointestinal bleeding - an updated Cochrane review. *Aliment Pharmacol Ther.* 2011;34(5):509–518.

    In a meta-analysis of 12 trials including over 1200 patients with cirrhosis and GI bleeding, antibiotic prophylaxis was compared with either placebo or no intervention, and the benefit of antibiotic use was demonstrated with regard to mortality (relative risk [RR] 0.79, 95% CI 0.63–0.98), bacterial infections (RR 0.35, 95% CI 0.26–0.47), and rebleeding (RR 0.53, 95% CI 0.38–0.74).

5. Wells M, Chande N, Adams P, et al. Meta-analysis: vasoactive medications for the management of acute variceal bleeds. *Aliment Pharmacol Ther.* 2012;35:1267–1278.

    In a meta-analysis of 30 RCTs, authors report the use of vasoactive agents in acute variceal hemorrhage is associated with lower 7-day all-cause mortality (p = 0.02), improved control of acute hemorrhage (p <0.001), lower transfusion requirements (p <0.001), and shorter duration of hospitalization (p = 0.007).

6. Levacher S, Letoumelin P, Pateron D, Blaise M, Lapandry C, Pourriat JL. Early administration of terlipressin plus glyceryl trinitrate to control active upper gastrointestinal bleeding in cirrhotic patients. *Lancet.* 1995;346:865–868.

   In a prospective, randomized, double-blind trial, cirrhosis patients with upper gastrointestinal hemorrhage were randomized to receive early initiation of an infusion of terlipressin and glyceryl trinitrate at their homes prior to transport to the hospital versus placebo. Authors report improved bleeding control and improved mortality in the intervention group.

7. Escorsell A, Pavel O, Cardenas A, et al. Esophageal balloon tamponade versus esophageal stent in controlling acute refractory variceal bleeding: A multicenter randomized, controlled trial. *Hepatology.* 2016;63:1957–1967.

   A randomized, controlled trial compared esophageal stent versus balloon tamponade to control variceal hemorrhage in 28 patients with cirrhosis and variceal hemorrhage. Success of therapy was defined as survival at day 15 with control of bleeding and without serious adverse events. The esophageal stent group showed significant improvement in success of therapy (66% vs. 20%; p = 0.025) and control of bleeding (85% vs. 47%; p = 0.037), with lower rates of serious adverse events (15% vs. 47%; p = 0.077).

8. Garcia-Tsao G, Abraldes JG, Berzigotti A, Bosch J. Portal hypertensive bleeding in cirrhosis: risk stratification, diagnosis, and management: 2016 practice guidance by the American Association for the study of liver diseases. *Hepatology.* 2017;65(1):310–335.

   The American Association for the Study of Liver Diseases provides updated, evidence-based guidance on risk stratification, diagnosis, and management of portal hypertension, varices, and variceal hemorrhage.

9. Tripathi D, Stanley AJ, Hayes PC, et al; U.K. guidelines on the management of variceal haemorrhage in cirrhotic patients. *Gut.* 2015;64(11):1680–1704.

   The Clinical Services and Standards Committee of the British Society of Gastroenterology provides updated guidelines on the management of variceal hemorrhage, specifically with regards to primary prophylaxis, acute variceal hemorrhage, and secondary prophylaxis. They attempt to standardize language by defining terms such as acute variceal bleeding, variceal re-bleeding, and clinically significant bleeding.

10. Thiele M, Krag A, Rohde U, Gluud LL. Meta-analysis: banding ligation and medical interventions for the prevention of rebleeding from oesophageal varices. *Aliment Pharmacol Ther.* 2012;35(10):1155–1165.

    This meta-analysis includes 9 randomized clinical trials and 955 patients to assess the effectiveness of combination endoscopic variceal ligation and nonselective beta blockade versus monotherapy in preventing variceal rebleeding. Authors conclude that combination therapy reduces the risk of re-bleeding but not overall mortality.

11. García-Pagán JC, Caca K, Bureau C, et al. Early use of TIPS in patients with cirrhosis and variceal bleeding. *N Engl J Med.* 2010;362(25):2370–2379.

    Authors randomized 63 patients with cirrhosis and variceal bleeding who had been treated with vasoactive drugs and endoscopic therapy to receive early TIPS or continuation of pharmacotherapy only. Fourteen patients in the pharmacotherapy group met composite criteria for re-bleeding events versus 1 patient in the early-TIPS group (p <0.001). One year survival was 86% in the early-TIPS group as compared to 61% in the pharmacotherapy group (p <0.001).

12. Rikkers LF, Jin G. Emergency shunt. Role in the present management of variceal bleeding. *Arch Surg.* 1995;130(5):472–477.

This retrospective review of 42 patients treated with selective and nonselective emergency portosystemic shunt operations observed a mortality rate of 43% in patients with Child's class C cirrhosis.

Landmark Article of the 21st Century

EARLY USE OF TIPS IN PATIENTS WITH CIRRHOSIS AND VARICEAL BLEEDING

Garcia-Pagan JC et al. *N Engl J Med.* 2010;362:2370–2379

Commentary by Venkatesh A. Murugan and Hesham H. Malik

The authors sought to evaluate the role of early TIPS on re-bleeding or failure to control bleeding (composite endpoint) in Child–Pugh B and C (score <14) cirrhotics presenting with acute variceal hemorrhage. All patients (n = 63) were treated with vasoactive agents plus endoscopic therapy. Within 24 hours, patients were randomized to polytetrafluoroethylene-covered stenting (early TIPS, n = 32) to be accomplished within 72 hours or a continuation of vasoactive therapy followed by beta adrenergic blockade and long-term endoscopic band ligation (EBL, n = 31). Rescue TIPS was allowed in the control group.

Re-bleeding or failure to control bleeding was observed in 14/31 of EBL patients versus 1/32 patient in the TIPS group. Seven patients required a rescue TIPS. The probability of no re-bleeding within 1 year was significantly better for early TIPS at 97% vs. 50% for EBL. Six week and 1-year survival rates for the TIPS group was also significantly higher (97% vs. 67% and 86% vs. 61% respectively). The number of days in the ICU and percentage of time spent in the hospital were significantly lower in the TIPS group. The 1-year probability of developing hepatic encephalopathy or ascites was no different between the groups.

The study shows that in high-risk cirrhotic patients presenting with acute variceal bleeding, early TIPS is associated with significant reductions in mortality and re-bleeding, and no worsened risk of encephalopathy when compared to standard of care therapy.

This is the first randomized trial to report use of e-PTFE stents in TIPS. The study is limited by its small sample size. It was not designed to evaluate other prognostic factors influencing mortality after TIPS, such as renal function, diastolic dysfunction, and age, which limits its generalizability.

CHAPTER 20

Catheter-Related Infections

Review by Stephen Heard

Central venous catheters are essential for the care of the critically ill patient. Mechanical and infectious complications are the most common complications associated with central venous catheterization. Early efforts to reduce catheter infection included scheduled removal and reinsertion of the catheter at a different site and or scheduled exchange of the catheter by a new one over a guide wire. Although initial reports touted the efficacy of these approaches, neither strategy was found to be helpful in reducing central line associated bloodstream infections (CLABSIs). Guide wire exchange should only be performed if a catheter is malfunctioning and no infection is suspected.

The Centers for Disease Control and Prevention (CDC) define a CLABSI as a primary bloodstream infection that is not related to an infection at another and develops in a patient with a central venous catheter in place within a 48-hour period before the onset of the bloodstream infection. Because this definition does not require culturing of the catheter, CLABSIs are probably overdiagnosed. Researchers commonly culture (semi-quantitatively or quantitatively) the tip of the catheter. A catheter-related bloodstream infection (CBRBSI) is diagnosed if bacteria from the blood and catheter are the same as determined antibiograms or genomic fingerprinting. Paired blood cultures from a peripheral vein and through the catheter may be helpful in diagnosing catheter infection. If the blood obtained from a catheter grows a pathogen ≥ 120 minutes before that of peripheral blood, a CRBSI is present. Although reports suggest this method has a high sensitivity and specificity, there is the danger that a CLABSI will be diagnosed (and publicly reportable) if the blood culture from the catheter is positive while that from the peripheral blood is negative. For that reason, we do not employ this method at UMass Memorial Medical Center.

Studies in the early to mid-1990s showed that experience and education of the proceduralist was important in reducing the risk of CLABSIs. A simple educational program provided to interns was found to be effective in reducing the incidence of these infections [1]. Use of maximum barrier precautions, where the proceduralist wears a cap and mask and sterile gown and gloves, and the patient is covered with a drape that covers the entire body, reduced the incidence of CLABSIs in outpatient cancer patients [2]. Alcoholic chlorhexidine was also found to be superior to 10% povidone-iodine in preparing the patient for catheterization [3]. Advances in catheter manufacturing resulted in the development of antimicrobial and antiseptic catheters which were associated with fewer CLABSIs compared to control catheters [4, 5].

DOI: 10.1201/9781003042136-20

115

Antimicrobial catheters appear to be the most efficacious [6]. Use of a chlorhexidine impregnated dressing or sponge also reduced the incidence of high level catheter colonization. Post-hoc analyses of prospective, randomized trials studying the utility of anti-infective catheters indicated the subclavian site of insertion was associated with the lowest risk of infection, followed by the internal jugular and femoral sites. A recent large, prospective, randomized study has confirmed these findings [7].

Despite periodic publication by the CDC of evidence-based guidelines to prevent intravascular catheter infections that date back to at least 1983, the incidence of CLABSIs during the 1980s and 1990s remained stubbornly high. At the end of the 1990s, the number of CLABSIs per year in US ICUs was estimated to be 16,000, resulting in a rate of 5.3 CLABSIs per 1000 catheter-days [8]. However, it wasn't until 2004 that Berenholtz and co-workers developed a true team approach to eradicate CLABSIs. All clinicians who inserted CLABSIs had to complete an educational program. A central line cart was created where all supplies were readily available. During rounds, discussion had to occur as to whether the catheter was needed. During insertion, a checklist was utilized to ensure all evidence-based guidelines (hand hygiene, preparation of skin with chlorhexidine, use of cap, mask, sterile gloves and gown and maximum barrier precautions) followed and the nurse was impowered to stop the insertion if sterile technique was breached. The authors found that this intervention resulted in a significant and sustained reduction in CLABSIs [9]. Subsequently, larger multicenter studies have demonstrated the efficacy of this approach [10]. Studies that have incorporated a "larger" bundle (use of antibiotic impregnated catheters and chlorhexidine-impregnated dressings and tracking high risk catheters [emergency insertion and femoral catheters]), have realized a reduction in CLABSI rates to 0.3–0.8 per 1000 catheter-days that has persisted for over 8 years [11].

Use of ultrasonography has been shown to improve time to vessel cannulation and reduce mechanical complications compared to insertion by using anatomic landmarks. It would seem logical that ultrasonography would also reduce the risk of CLABSI. However, in ICUs where there is already a low CLABSI rate, use of ultrasonography has not been shown to further reduce the infection rate [12].

Catheter infection can occur by either bacterial spread via the subcutaneous wound or by the development of an intraluminal biofilm. Early infection tends to occur via the wound and most strategies of prevention focus on this route. However, several techniques have been developed to prevent infection via the catheter lumen. A meta-analysis of various lock solutions (e.g., ethanol; citrate; minocycline and EDTA; aminoglycoside and heparin) have been shown to be helpful in preventing CLABIs even in units that have a low baseline rate of infection. However, most patients in this analysis were receiving hemodialysis through a catheter. The findings may not be germane to the standard ICU patient [13]. Hubs represent another means by which bacteria can reach the catheter lumen and establish a biofilm. Several antiseptic caps are available which are applied to the hubs of the intravenous tubing and are not removed until medication is administered. Although "before and after" studies have shown a significant reduction in the rate of CLABSI, the baseline rates in these studies were higher than 1.0 per 1000 catheter-days. Consequently, if the baseline rate is low, the caps may not provide any additional benefit [14].

In summary, use of a check list and bundled approach to insertion and care of central venous catheters will result in a reduction in CLABSIs.

ANNOTATED REFERENCES FOR CATHETER-RELATED INFECTIONS

1. Sherertz RJ, Ely EW, Westbrook DM, et al. Education of physicians-in-training can decrease the risk for vascular catheter infection. *Ann Intern Med.* 2000;132(8):641–8.

   A simple education program given to interns during the first week of their residency resulted in a decrease in catheter infections compared to historical infection rates.

2. Raad II, Hohn DC, Gilbreath BJ, et al. Prevention of central venous catheter-related infections by using maximal sterile barrier precautions during insertion. *Infect Control Hosp Epidemiol.* 1994;15(4 Pt 1):231–8.

   Catheter infection rates were reduced when the proceduralist used cap, mask, sterile gloves and gown, and a sterile drape covering the entire patient when inserting a central venous catheter.

3. Maki DG, Ringer M, Alvarado CJ. Prospective randomised trial of povidone-iodine, alcohol, and chlorhexidine for prevention of infection associated with central venous and arterial catheters. *Lancet.* 1991;338(8763):339–43.

   Skin preparation with chlorhexidine was found to be superior to povidone-iodine in preventing catheter infection.

4. Raad I, Darouiche R, Dupuis J, et al. Central venous catheters coated with minocycline and rifampin for the prevention of catheter-related colonization and bloodstream infections. A randomized, double-blind trial. The Texas Medical Center Catheter Study Group. *Ann Intern Med.* 1997;127(4):267–74.

   One of two seminal investigations demonstrating the use of an antibiotic impregnated catheter reduces CLABSIs.

5. Maki DG, Stolz SM, Wheeler S, Mermel LA. Prevention of central venous catheter-related bloodstream infection by use of an antiseptic-impregnated catheter. A randomized, controlled trial. *Ann Intern Med.* 1997;127(4):257–66.

   The second of two seminal investigations demonstrating the use of antiseptic catheters reduces CLABSIs.

6. Darouiche RO, Raad II, Heard SO, et al. A comparison of two antimicrobial-impregnated central venous catheters. Catheter Study Group.
   N Engl J Med. 1999;340(1):1–8.

   Central venous catheters impregnated with minocycline and rifampin (external surface and lumen) were found to be superior in preventing CLABSIS compared to catheters impregnated with chlorhexidine and silver-sulfadiazine on the external surface.

7. Parienti JJ, Mongardon N, Megarbane B, et al. Intravascular complications of central venous catheterization by insertion site. *N Engl J Med.* 2015;373(13):1220–9.

   The subclavian insertion site was associated with the lowers risk of infection compared to internal jugular and femoral sites. However, mechanical complications were higher.

8. Mermel LA. Prevention of intravascular catheter-related infections. *Ann Intern Med.* 2000;132(5):391–402.

   A review of the state of the art in preventing catheter infections. Subsequent reviews a decade later (MMWR) demonstrated a significant decline in CLABSIs nationwide.

9. Berenholtz SM, Pronovost PJ, Lipsett PA, et al. Eliminating catheter-related bloodstream infections in the intensive care unit. *Crit Care Med.* 2004;32(10):2014–20.

   Use of a checklist and bundled approach to insertion of central venous catheters resulted in a sustained decrease in CLABSIs.

10. Pronovost P, Needham D, Berenholtz S, et al. An intervention to decrease catheter-related bloodstream infections in the ICU. *N Engl J Med.* 2006;355(26):2725–32.

    Use of the protocol outlined in reference 9 was successfully implemented in Michigan ICUs.

11. Walz JM, Ellison RT, 3rd, Mack DA, et al. The bundle "plus": the effect of a multidisciplinary team approach to eradicate central line-associated bloodstream infections. *Anesth Analg.* 2015;120(4):868–76.

    Adding antimicrobial impregnated catheters and chlorhexidine dressings to the bundle and treating very CLABSI as a sentinel event resulted in sustained reductions in CLASBIs to 0.5–0.8/1000 catheter days.

12. Cartier V, Haenny A, Inan C, Walder B, Zingg W. No association between ultrasound-guided insertion of central venous catheters and bloodstream infection: a prospective observational study. *J Hosp Infect.* 2014;87(2):103–8.

    Although use of the ultrasound during insertion of central venous catheters may prevent complications, CLABSIs do not appear to be reduced.

13. Zacharioudakis IM, Zervou FN, Arvanitis M, Ziakas PD, Mermel LA, Mylonakis E. Antimicrobial lock solutions as a method to prevent central line-associated bloodstream infections: a meta-analysis of randomized controlled trials. *Clin Infect Dis.* 2014;59(12):1741–9.

    Antimicrobial locks appear to be useful in preventing CLABSIs but the data are heavily weighted towards hemodialysis catheters.

14. Voor AF, Helder OK, Vos MC, et al. Antiseptic barrier cap effective in reducing central line-associated bloodstream infections: a systematic review and meta-analysis. *Int J Nurs Stud.* 2017;69:34–40.

    Antiseptic barrier caps may be useful in preventing CLABSIs if the baseline rate is high.

Landmark Article of the 21st Century

AN INTERVENTION TO DECREASE CATHETER-RELATED BLOODSTREAM INFECTIONS IN THE ICU

Pronovost P et al., *N Engl J Med.* 2006;355:2725–2732

Commentary by Robert C. Hyzy

I was sitting in a conference room at the headquarters of the Michigan Health and Hospitals Association in 2003 with a group of intensivists, putting the finishing touches on an ICU quality improvement toolkit, when MHA Keystone Center for

Patient Safety and Quality Executive Vice President Chris Goeshel told our group she was seeking to recruit around 20 ICUs from Michigan hospitals to participate together in a quality improvement "collaborative" along with Dr. Peter Pronovost, a physician from Johns Hopkins who had secured AHRQ funding for the project. While our toolkit seemed just another well-intentioned document destined to sit in a notebook on a shelf or languish on the MHA website, the proposed collaborative would be field work, a real world attempt to change care by implementing several evidence-based practices which had been piloted by Johns Hopkins. I immediately volunteered my ICU's participation at the University of Michigan Hospital.

Work to implement the central line insertion checklist, and other care bundles, soon commenced in my ICU, and ICUs from almost every other Michigan hospital. The entire collaborative began meeting in person, twice yearly, as Chris and Peter commanded the stage in a ballroom of more than 300 participants. Our motto was "ohana," everyone was in it together; no one gets left behind. We took that message home, having realized reducing CLABSI via a checklist really meant changing the "culture" of our respective intensive care units. When all was said and done, together we had reduced the median CLBSI rate in the state of Michigan to zero.

CHAPTER 21

Diagnosis and Prevention of Ventilator-Associated Pneumonia

Review by Kevin Dushay

Ventilator-associated pneumonia (VAP) is defined as pneumonia arising >48–72 hours following intubation. It is the most common infection in intubated patients requiring mechanical ventilation and the leading cause of death by nosocomial infections in the ICU [1, 2]. Occurring in 9–27% of intubated ICU patients, it is an expensive complication that increases ICU length of stay by 7–9 days, adding $19,000–$80,000 to the cost of stay [1, 3, 4].

Accumulation of oropharyngeal and gastric secretions above the endotracheal tube (ETT) cuff leads to micro-aspiration, and colonized biofilm inside the ETT also contributes to seeding of the lower airways, which may progress to ventilator-associated tracheobronchitis and/or pneumonia [5]. Less frequently, pathogens may reach the lungs from the bloodstream. Although viral and fungal VAP do occur, the majority of cases are due to bacteria.

The CDC definition for VAP [6] includes:

1. Two or more chest x-rays with new/progressive/persistent infiltrate, consolidation, or cavitation
2. Fever >38°, or WBC either <4000 or >12,000, or for adults over 70 years old, a change in mental status with no other recognized cause
3. At least two of the following:
   a. New onset purulent sputum, or change in sputum, or increased respiratory secretions, or increased need for suctioning
   b. Worsening gas exchange
   c. New onset or increasing cough, dyspnea, tachypnea
   d. Fine crackles or bronchial breath sounds

Other disease processes may also meet the above criteria, so their presence is not diagnostic of VAP. The clinical pulmonary infection score (CPIS) proposed by Pham et al. [7] and modified by Singh et al. is a similar tool for identifying possible VAP [8].

With suspected VAP, two sets of blood cultures and a respiratory tract culture should be obtained immediately to confirm the diagnosis and allow narrowing of antibiotic

DOI: 10.1201/9781003042136-21

coverage with their results. Samples may be obtained by suction catheter to obtain a tracheal aspirate or by protected specimen brush or balloon lavage catheter passed blindly or via bronchoscopy. Bronchoscopy also allows bronchoalveolar lavage, but with the risk of increased hypoxemia. Quantitative or semiquantitative culture should help rule out false positive diagnoses of VAP, though a false negative culture may occur in the setting of partially treated VAP. Cultures may also be positive with ventilator-associated tracheobronchitis; if this occurs in the setting of non-infectious pulmonary infiltrates, an erroneous diagnosis of VAP may delay diagnosis and treatment.

Once appropriate cultures are obtained, empiric antibiotics should be initiated immediately. A 2002 single center trial of 107 ventilated patients treated for VAP demonstrated delayed initial appropriate antibiotic therapy (DIAAT) had an adjusted odds ratio for death of 7.68 [9]. Seventy-six percent of DIAAT was due to antibiotics not being ordered promptly once patients met criteria for VAP; only 18% was due to resistant organisms. A subsequent meta-analysis in 2008 supported this conclusion but found a lower odds ratio of death of 2.33 [10]. Previously the choice of empiric antibiotics was guided by time since intubation, but more recent studies have suggested even early onset VAP may be caused by antibiotic resistant organisms such as *Pseudomonas aeruginosa*, *Acinetobacter* species, *Stenotrophomonas maltophilia*, ESBL *Klebsiella pneumoniae*, and MRSA [11, 12]. In light of these studies, initiating broad spectrum antibiotics up front followed by a more focused regimen upon identification of the causative organism(s) and sensitivity determination may be a better strategy. Since hospitals and even units within a hospital may differ in the frequency of infections by specific organisms, antibiotic therapy should be guided by hospital- or unit-specific antibiograms if possible [13, 14].

Duration of therapy may best be guided by the causative organism. Two studies have shown 8-day (short) course therapy is associated with more frequent relapses and superinfections than a 15-day regimen, but without differences in 21-day or 90-day mortality, ICU length of stay, or ventilator-days [15, 16]. Shorter course antibiotic therapy should reduce the development of antibiotic resistance and drug-related adverse events. The 2016 joint IDSA/ATS Guideline suggested using procalcitonin (PCT) levels together with clinical criteria to guide discontinuation of therapy, based on it shortening duration of therapy compared to clinical criteria alone [15]. However, this was a weak recommendation based on low quality evidence. The guideline released by the European Respiratory, Intensive Care and Infectious Disease societies opposed using PCT to reduce duration of antibiotics to less than 7–8 days. In the case of patients requiring longer courses of therapy, PCT coupled with clinical assessment was favored for stopping antimicrobial therapy [15]. A small single-center study basing antibiotic discontinuation on PCT, fever <38.5°, and WBC <15, found the group with recurrent infection was more likely to have an elevated CPIS, and/or purulent tracheal secretions [16]. Thus, efforts to minimize antibiotic resistance and adverse events by administering short-course therapy should take into account the presence of clinical indicators of infection as noted in the CPIS score or an elevated PCT or the presence of organisms prone to develop resistance such as *Pseudomonas, Acinetobacter, Stenotrophomonas*, and MRSA.

Some antibiotics only achieve a fraction of their plasma levels in alveolar and bronchial fluid. Aerosol delivery of antibiotics can achieve higher levels and reduce toxicity that systemic delivery may cause. The European Society of Clinical Microbiology and Infectious Diseases (ESCMID) 2017 meta-analysis did not find adequate support of the use of aerosolized antibiotics for treatment of ventilator-associated respiratory infections [17]. However, an international survey with most responses coming from Europe showed roughly 73% of the 410 responding units use them, the majority for the treatment of VAP and VAT, with 92% only using them in the setting of positive culture results [18]. The most frequently prescribed agents were colistin and amikacin, usually delivered by jet nebulizer.

Efforts at prevention and improving diagnosis and treatment have resulted in the development of VAP bundles. Multiple studies have now demonstrated that the development of a VAP bundle and alerting ICU staff to its existence does not result in widespread adoption of its measures. A Canadian program developed guidelines for prevention, diagnosis, and treatment of VAP and used a multifaceted approach including education of ICU physicians, nurses, respiratory therapists, and pharmacists; reminders to these groups; enlisting local opinion leaders; and using implementation teams to maintain awareness and provide compliance measurement and feedback. This program was conducted in 11 different medical, surgical, and trauma ICUs, 5 academic, 6 community. They reduced VAP rates by 38%, from 47 events/330 patients to 29/330, and demonstrated they were able to increase exposure of the staff to the bundle from 86.7% at the start of the initiative to 95.8% at the last observation period. However, despite a high degree of awareness of best practice measures, the aggregate concordance with the measures went from 50.7% at baseline to only 58.7% at the conclusion of the study [19]. However, a single shock-trauma ICU with a baseline 90th percentile rate of VAP developed a program including a VAP bundle and utilizing an infection control practitioner assigned to that unit; their VAP rates did not change after implementing their VAP bundle, but with implementation of measuring compliance daily and weekly meetings providing feedback and education, the VAP rate declined significantly and stayed low [20]. The authors emphasized the need for an implementation team that includes hospital administration, infection control, ICU medical, nursing, and RT leadership, and others that have expertise in developing a preventative program in order to succeed.

ANNOTATED ENDNOTES FOR DIAGNOSIS AND PREVENTION OF VENTILATOR-ASSOCIATED PNEUMONIA

1. Kalil AC, Metersky ML, Klompas M, et al. Management of adults with hospital-acquired and ventilator-associated pneumonia: 2016 Clinical Practice Guidelines by the Infectious Diseases Society of America and the American Thoracic Society. *Clin Infect Dis.* 2016; 63(1):e61–111.

This is the most recent guideline from the Infectious Diseases Society of America (IDSA) and the American Thoracic Society (ATS) frequently referenced in more recent literature that updates aspects of these guidelines. See also reference 15.

2. Bassi GL, Ranzini OT, Torres A. Systematic implementation of evidence-based guidelines in intensive care medicine: resistance to change is human nature. *Crit Care Med.* 2013;41(1):329–30.

This very informative editorial comments on the paper by Sinuff, Muscedere, and Cook (reference 19 below) from 2013 describing their program to implement a VAP Bundle to reduce VAP in a mix of academic and community hospital ICUs.

3. Cocanour CS, Ostrosky-Zeichner L, Peninger M, et al. Cost of a ventilator-associated pneumonia in a shock-trauma intensive care unit. Surg *Infect (Larchmt) Spring.* 2005;6(1):65–72.

Study conducted in the Shock Trauma ICU of Memorial Hermann Hospital of the University of Texas Medical School at Houston, pairing patients with VAP and those of similar age and Injury Severity Score to assess the cost difference associated with VAP.

4. Bysshe T, Gao Y, Heaney-Huls K, et al. Final Report - Estimating the additional hospital inpatient cost and mortality associated with selected hospital-acquired conditions. Agency for Healthcare Research and Quality Publication No. 18-0011-EF, November 2017.

5. Koulenti, D, Arvanitis K, Judd M, et al. Ventilator-associated tracheobronchitis: to treat or not to treat? *Antibiotics.* 2020;9(2). DOI 10.3390/antibiotics9020051

6. Horan TC, Andrus M, Dudeck MA. CDC/NHSN surveillance definition of health care-associated infection and criteria for specific types of infections in the acute care setting. *Am J Infect Control.* 2008;36(5):309–32.

7. Pham LH, Brun-Buisson C, Legrand P, et al. Diagnosis of nosocomial pneumonia in mechanically ventilated patients - Comparison of a plugged telescoping catheter with the protected specimen brush. *Am Rev Respir Dis.* 1991;143(5):1055–61.

8. Singh N, Rogers P, Atwood CW, et al. Short-course empiric antibiotic therapy for patients with pulmonary infiltrates in the intensive care unit. A proposed solution for indiscriminate antibiotic prescription. *Am J Respir Crit Care Med.* 2000;162(2):505–11.

This paper modified the CPIS (Clinical Pulmonary Infection Score) proposed in reference #7 above, making it more useful. However, the major focus of the paper is on tailoring therapy to individual patients to avoid excess antibiotic days.

9. Iregui M, Ward S, Sherman G, et al. Clinical importance of delays in the initiation of appropriate antibiotic treatment for ventilator-associated pneumonia. *Chest.* 2002;122(1):262–68.

High quality study demonstrating increased mortality attributable to VAP when appropriate antibiotics were not administered within 24 hours of patients meeting criteria for VAP.

10. Kuti EL, Patel AA, Coleman CI. Impact of inappropriate antibiotic therapy on mortality in patients with ventilator-associated pneumonia and blood stream infection: a meta-analysis. *J Crit Care.* 2008;23(1):91–100.

Meta-analysis 6 years later than Iregui et al's study (reference 9 above) confirming increased mortality with delay in administration of appropriate antibiotics for both VAP and hospital-acquired blood stream infections.

11. Gastmeier P, Sohr D, Geffers C, et al. Early- and late-onset pneumonia: is this still a useful classification? *Antimicrob Agents Chemother.* 2009;53(7):2714–18.

12. Restrepo MI, Peterson J, Fernandez J, et al. Comparison of the bacterial etiology of early-onset and late-onset ventilator-associated pneumonia in subjects enrolled in 2 large clinical studies. *Respir Care*. 2013;58(7):1220–25.
13. Namias N, Samiian L, Nino D, et al. Incidence and susceptibility of pathogenic bacteria vary between intensive care units within a single hospital: implications for empiric antibiotic strategies. *J Trauma*. 2000;49(4):638–45.

    This paper suggests optimal infection control may require monitoring pathogen frequency and susceptibility for individual units rather than just the hospital as a whole.
14. Rello J, Sa-Borges M, Correa H, et al. Variations in etiology of ventilator-associated pneumonia across four treatment sites: implications for antimicrobial prescribing practices. *Am J Respir Crit Care Med*. 1999;160(2):608–13.
15. Torres A, Niederman MS, Chastre J, et al. International ERS/ESICM/ESCMID/ALAT Guidelines for the management of hospital-acquired pneumonia and ventilator-associated pneumonia. *Eur Respir J*. 2017;50(3):17000582 doi.org/10.1183/13993003.00582-2017
16. Wang Q, Hou D, Wang J, et al. Procalcitonin-guided antibiotic discontinuation in ventilator-associated pneumonia: a prospective observational study. *Infect Drug Resist*. 2019;12:815–24.
17. Rello J, Sole-Lleonart C, Rouby JJ, et al. Use of nebulized antimicrobials for the treatment of respiratory infections in invasively mechanically ventilated adults: a position paper from the European Society of Clinical Microbiology and Infectious Diseases. *Clin Microbiol Infect*. 2017;23(9):629–39.

    Points out that limited data do not provide strong support for the use of aerosolized antibiotics as treatment for ventilator-associated tracheitis, bronchitis, or pneumonia.
18. Sole-Lleonart C, Roberts JA, Chastre J, et al. Global survey on nebulization of antimicrobial agents in mechanically ventilated patients: a call for international guidelines. *Clin Microbiol Infect*. 2016;22(4):359–64.

    Survey indicating the lack of a recommendation in favor of aerosolized antibiotics by ESCMID is not preventing a majority of surveyed intensive care units from using them to treat mostly resistant infections rather than colonization or other conditions.
19. Sinuff T, Muscedere J, Cook D, et al. Implementation of clinical practice guidelines for ventilator-associated pneumonia: a multicenter prospective study. *Crit Care Med*. 2013;41:15–23.

    Great paper describing the right way to implement a multi-institutional program to change practice in ICUs, in this case for VAP, however, the program fell short due to a failure to adequately analyze interim data and modify their program to address its failure to change behavior largely among their intensivists - see reference 20.
20. Cocanour CS, Peninger M, Domonoske BD, et al. Decreasing ventilator-associated pneumonia in a trauma ICU. *J Trauma*. 2006;61(1):122–30.

    This single ICU program performed 7 years earlier than the one noted in the reference above contained the key intervention that Sinuff et al missed - collecting and presenting data weekly to the care providers with a current graphic posted and clearly demonstrating their progress or lack thereof - these two papers provide the "How To" for any institution that needs to conquer a clinical issue requiring a change in the status quo of ICU care.

Landmark Article of the 21st Century

IMPLEMENTATION OF CLINICAL PRACTICE GUIDELINES FOR VENTILATOR-ASSOCIATED PNEUMONIA: A MULTICENTER PROSPECTIVE STUDY

Sinuff T et al., *Crit Care Med.* 2013;41:15–23

Commentary by John Muscedere

Ventilator-associated pneumonia (VAP) is a cause of morbidity and mortality in mechanically ventilated patients [1]. There is a large amount of evidence for its prevention, diagnosis, and treatment but it has not been systematically adopted into clinical practice. Although clinical practice guidelines (CPGs) synthesize evidence and can aid the delivery of evidence informed care, their uptake at the bedside is not uniform and can be poor. To improve outcomes from VAP, we first developed evidence based VAP CPGs [2, 3] and then conducted a multicenter study in which we systematically implemented the guidelines in academic and community intensive care units with a multifaceted implementation strategy including education, reminders, implementation teams and local opinion leaders to enhance guideline uptake [4]. We then measured implementation fidelity and guideline concordance [5] over the 2-year course of the study.

Our study demonstrated that the implementation strategy used resulted in a high degree of best practice awareness and increases in concordance with the recommended practices in the guidelines. In addition, it was associated with a reduction in the incidence of VAP over time. A key insight was that although our implementation strategy uniformly increased clinician awareness of guideline recommendations, the level of concordance only increased modestly suggested that there were unaddressed barriers to their adoption.

The contribution of this study to the VAP and knowledge translation literature is that the implementation of complex guidelines is feasible, must target all members of the ICU team, needs to be tailored, and can improve outcomes. However, the efficacy of education and reminder-based interventions is only modest and it is important to assess and address any barriers to behavior change in clinicians caring for critically ill patients.

REFERENCES

1. Muscedere JG, Day A, Heyland DK. Mortality, attributable mortality, and clinical events as end points for clinical trials of ventilator-associated pneumonia and hospital-acquired pneumonia. *Clin Infect Dis.* 2010; 51(Suppl 1):S120–5.
2. Muscedere J, Dodek P, Keenan S, Fowler R, Cook D, Heyland D. Comprehensive evidence-based clinical practice guidelines for ventilator-associated pneumonia: diagnosis and treatment. *J Crit Care.* 2008;23:138–47.

3. Muscedere J, Dodek P, Keenan S, Fowler R, Cook D, Heyland D. Comprehensive evidence-based clinical practice guidelines for ventilator-associated pneumonia: prevention. *J Crit Care*. 2008;23:126–37.
4. Sinuff T, Muscedere J, Cook DJ, et al.; Canadian Critical Care Trials G. Implementation of clinical practice guidelines for ventilator-associated pneumonia: a multicenter prospective study. *Crit Care Med*. 2013;41:15–23.
5. Scott IA, Harper CM. Guideline-discordant care in acute myocardial infarction: predictors and outcomes. *Med J Aust*. 2002;177:26–31.

CHAPTER 22

Treatment of Ventilator-Associated Pneumonia

Review by Gavin Tansley and Morad Hameed

Modern use of positive pressure ventilation originated in the early 1950s, when it was recognized that supportive care with endotracheal tubes and manual ventilation with an inflated rubber bag could dramatically reduce the mortality of polio-induced respiratory failure [1]. These patients were ultimately clustered together to facilitate the around-the clock ventilatory support, thus representing the birth of the intensive care unit as we know it today. Even at this time, it was acknowledged that the endotracheal tube represented a novel means of introducing potentially noxious material into the lower respiratory tract, but it wasn't until a decade later that mechanical ventilation was understood to be a substantial risk factor for hospital acquired pneumonia [2]. The following 60 years have seen a tremendous advancement in our understanding of ventilator-associated pneumonia (VAP) with the development of numerous prevention strategies and treatment guidelines. Despite this progress, the diagnosis of VAP is still imperfect and optimal treatment remains unclear, further confounding progress on this deadly infection.

VAPs complicate the ICU stays of up to 10% of mechanically ventilated patients, resulting in prolonged stays, increased mortality, as well as approximately $40,000 of added healthcare costs per patient. They are defined as any hospital associated pneumonia that develops after 48 hours of mechanical ventilation, but the diagnosis of VAP is much more challenging than this simple definition would suggest. Presently the diagnosis is dependent on a new lung infiltrate as well as a clinical suspicion that the infiltrate is infectious in origin. This can be evidenced by additional signs such as fever, leukocytosis, purulent secretions, or hypoxia [3]. As none of these signs are specific to pneumonias, the diagnosis often remains elusive. Additionally, an organism is successfully cultured from the normally sterile tracheobronchial secretions in less than half of cases, further complicating diagnosis and antibiotic selection.

An understanding of the pathophysiology of VAPs has been paramount to the development of prevention strategies. Micro-aspiration of colonized oropharyngeal secretions is felt to underlie the majority of VAPs, with the severity of disease being augmented by the number and the virulence of the aspirated organisms, in addition to host-related factors. Naturally, minimizing the duration of mechanical

DOI: 10.1201/9781003042136-22

129

ventilation will reduce the risk of VAP development, and strategies such as spontaneous breathing trials, sedation vacations, and appropriate use of non-invasive ventilation have all been shown to reduce the incidence of VAP. Reducing aspiration risk by elevating the head of the bed and minimizing the subglottic pooling of oropharyngeal secretions with specially designed endotracheal tubes have also been shown to be effective. Lastly, decontamination strategies aimed at reducing the bacterial load in the oropharynx or the GI tract using topical antiseptics or antimicrobials have demonstrated reductions in the rates of VAP in many ICUs. Supporting all of these strategies are several studies demonstrating robust reductions in VAP rates, but concomitant reductions in mortality has been a much less consistent finding.

The mutually inclusive nature of many VAP prevention strategies supports the bundling of several approaches together into quality improvement initiatives designed to reduce VAP rates further than any one intervention alone. Several of these bundles have been studied and consistently demonstrate reductions in VAP rates. Although comparison of these studies is challenged by variable interventions and VAP definitions, low rates of compliance have been consistently observed and underscore the need for continuous education and reinforcement around the importance of VAP prevention. However, despite the progress in this area, it remains unclear which components of a VAP prevention bundle are most important [4]. Furthermore, it is becoming increasingly accepted that it is infeasible to prevent all VAPs, underscoring the need for sound, evidence-based treatment strategies.

Successful VAP treatment relies on prompt diagnosis with empiric antibiotic therapy targeting the most likely pathogens, followed by appropriate tailoring of antibiotics to minimize the risk of antimicrobial resistance and antibiotic-associated complications. It has been documented that patients become colonized with hospital-acquired microbes within the first 48 hours of their stay, meaning the appropriate treatment needs to consider institutional resistance patterns. The organisms identified from patients with VAPs vary depending on if the VAP was developed within the first four days of hospitalization, or later in their course. Early VAPs are typically caused by *Staphylococcus aureus*, *Klebsiella pneumoniae*, *Haemophilus influenzae, or Pseudomonas aeruginosa*. VAPs that develop later are more likely to result from multidrug resistant organisms. Initial antibiotic selection must acknowledge these patterns, but as importantly it needs to be tailored early in situations where resistant organisms are not isolated.

One of the most important advancements in VAP treatment in recent years has been the systematic shortening of treatment durations. Guided by results from several randomized controlled trials, patients receiving shorter courses of VAP therapy have demonstrated fewer days of antibiotic therapy as well as reductions in recurrent pneumonias due to multidrug resistant organisms without adverse effects on mortality. Less drug resistance and fewer antibiotic-related complications are the obvious advantages of shorter treatment courses, but some patients may remain undertreated with the currently recommended seven days of therapy. Serum procalcitonin has been used as a biomarker to guide the discontinuation of therapy, and may be particularly useful in patients who remain clinically unwell at the end of their treatment course. Use of procalcitonin in conjunction with clinical criteria to guide antibiotic discontinuation is currently recommended. This is particularly important considering the nearly 30% failure rate of initial treatment reported by Chastre et al. in their landmark study. Deciding who to treat, and for how long is certainly one of the great challenges in VAP management. The available evidence suggests we have erred on the side of overtreatment. Identifying ways to limit antibiotic therapy and detect treatment failure early will be instrumental to ensuring we have effective drugs for our future patients [5].

ANNOTATED REFERENCES FOR TREATMENT OF VENTILATOR-ASSOCIATED PNEUMONIA

1) Lassen HCA. A preliminary report on the 1952 epidemic of poliomyelitis in Copenhagen. *Lancet.* 1953;1:37.

   This is an early description of the novel management of polio-related respiratory failure with tracheostomy and manual bag mask ventilation. The authors reported a 50% mortality reduction with this technique. This landmark finding laid the foundation for modern critical care.

2) Johanson WG, Pierce AK, Sanford JP. Changing pharyngeal bacterial flora of hospitalized patients. *N Engl J Med.* 1969;21:1137–1140.

   One of the initial pieces of work noting the changes of oropharyngeal flora in hospitalized patients and identifying the endotracheal tube as a risk factor for nosocomial pneumonia.

3) Pugin J, Auckenthaler R, Mili N, et al. Diagnosis of ventilator-associated pneumonia by bacteriologic analysis of bronchoscopic and nonbronchoscopic "blind" bronchoalveolar lavage fluid. *Am Rev Respir Dis.* 1991;143:1121–1129.

   This case series identified the clinical criteria which correlated with positive cultures obtained from tracheal secretions. They used these criteria to develop a scoring system which ultimately became known as the Clinical Pulmonary Infection Score.

4) Vazquez Guillamet C, Kollef MH. Is zero ventilator-associated pneumonia achievable?: practical approaches to ventilator-associated pneumonia prevention. *Clin Chest Med.* 2018;39:809–822.

   A systematic review of current VAP prevention strategies with a good summary of the available evidence.

5) Kalil AC, Metersky ML, Klompas M, et al. Management of adults with hospital-acquired and ventilator-associated pneumonia: 2016 Clinical Practice Guidelines by the Infectious Diseases Society of America and the American Thoracic Society. *Clin Infect Dis.* 2016;63(5):e61–e111.

   These are the most recent guidelines from the Infectious Disease Society of America on the diagnosis and treatment of VAP. These guidelines largely agree with their European equivalent.

Landmark Article of the 21st Century

COMPARISON OF 8 VS 15 DAYS OF ANTIBIOTIC THERAPY FOR VENTILATOR-ASSOCIATED PNEUMONIA IN ADULTS: A RANDOMIZED TRIAL

Chastre J et al., *JAMA*. 2003;290(19):2588-2598

Commentary by Jean Chastre

Two decades ago, most experts were recommending that treatment of ventilator-associated pneumonia (VAP) last 14 to 21 days. This recommendation was largely empirical and only justified by a higher theoretical risk of infection relapse after a short duration of antibiotic administration. However, unduly prolonging the duration of therapy may not improve the outcome and lead to the emergence of multidrug-resistant microorganisms. This is why we undertook a randomized trial in 1999 to compare the outcomes of therapy with an 8-day or 15-day antibiotic regimen in ICU patients who had developed VAP. In this study, we observed no benefit in patients randomized to the 15-day regimen. The confidence intervals for the between-group differences in mortality and pulmonary infection-recurrence rates exclude an absolute difference exceeding 10% in favor of the 15-day regimen. No differences in other outcome parameters could be established, including duration of mechanical ventilation, number of organ failure–free days, the evolution of signs and symptoms potentially linked to pulmonary infection, number of infection recurrence, or status at hospital discharge. Pertinently, multi-resistant pathogens emerged more frequently for patients with pulmonary infection recurrence who had received 15 days of antibiotics. These results are consistent with those of other studies conducted after the publication of our trial that also clearly demonstrated the possibility of safely reducing antibiotic exposure in ICU patients by shortening duration of therapy. Thus, although appropriate antibiotics may improve the survival rate of patients with VAP, their indiscriminate use after 8 days of therapy should be strongly discouraged.

CHAPTER 23

Catheter-Associated Urinary Tract Infection

Review by Emily M. Ramasra and Richard T. Ellison III

Catheterization of the bladder has been practiced for many years, with the well-known Foley catheter being developed in the 1930s. Infections and fever in the setting of indwelling urinary tract catheterization have long been recognized and are now known as catheter-associated urinary tract infections (CAUTI) which remain an ongoing challenge and concern [1].

A CAUTI is one of the most frequently encountered infections seen in hospitalized patients receiving care in both the intensive care unit and on the inpatient wards. Prolonged urinary tract catheterization is the major risk factor for urinary tract infection in hospitalized patients [2]. The strain on healthcare associated with CAUTI is significant for both increased morbidity and hospital associated costs, and based on this the Centers for Medicare and Medicaid Services has made the incidence of hospital-acquired CAUTIs a publicly reported quality measure. Additionally, patients are at risk of receiving unnecessary antibiotics which in turn can lead to antibiotic resistance [3]. It is also important to note that bacteremia due to CAUTIs is less frequent and mortality is rare.

The 2009 Infectious Disease Society of America (IDSA) guidelines define CAUTI as symptomatic bacteriuria, without another infectious source, with a single specimen urine culture growth of 1000 colony forming units of one or more bacteria, in a patient with an indwelling catheter or catheter removal within 48 hours prior to specimen collection. The guidelines further defined catheter-associated asymptomatic bacteriuria (CAASB) as 10,000 colony forming units of one or more bacteria, without symptoms of urinary tract infection, in a patient with an indwelling catheter. The constellation of symptoms that accompany CAUTI or symptomatic bacteriuria can include leukocytosis, fever, hypotension, metabolic abnormalities, suprapubic and flank pain. CAASB, where patients have bladder colonization without manifestations of clinical infection, is highly prevalent and is rarely associated with subsequent bacteremia or infectious complications. Recent single center studies have found that less than 1% of cases of catheter-associated bacteriuria were associated with bacteremia, and these did not note mortality [4, 5, 6].

The pathogenesis of CAUTI relates to colonization of the foreign catheter material and the bladder. Microorganisms form biofilms over the catheter, allowing them to

DOI: 10.1201/9781003042136-23

persist with limited susceptibility to antibiotics or host defenses. The organisms that contribute to these infections include colonizers of the genital region and gastrointestinal tract. Alternatively, they can also be introduced from within the health care setting [7]. According to the CDC, the most common pathogens involved in catheter-associated bacteriuria (combining both symptomatic and asymptomatic) in hospitals reporting to the National Healthcare Safety Network (NHSN) between 2006 and 2007 were *Escherichia coli* (21.4%), *Candida* spp (21.0%), *Enterococcus* spp (14.9%), *Pseudomonas aeruginosa* (10.0%), *Klebsiella pneumoniae* (7.7%), and *Enterobacter* spp (4.1%). Gram-negative bacteria and *Staphylococcus* spp were the infecting bacteria in a smaller percentage of cases [8].

The treatment of CAUTI depends on whether symptoms of infection are present or not. With asymptomatic bacteriuria (CAASB), it is currently recommended that antibiotic therapy not be initiated. When symptoms or signs of infection are present in a catheterized patient, 7–14 days of therapy are recommended depending on response to therapy. Notably, the optimal duration of therapy has remained unclear and the established range has largely been based on clinical response. Shorter courses are considered in certain populations. If culture results are available, empiric regimens can be narrowed to specific therapy with consideration of oral therapy again based on clinical improvement and level of antimicrobial urinary tract penetration. Where possible, removal of the urinary catheter will help to achieve source control and likely improve clinical outcome [1].

Numerous approaches to prevent CAUTIs have been studied including improving insertion technique, modifying daily catheter care, stabilizing the catheter position, varying catheter materials, behavioral changes to limit the use or decrease the duration of urethral catheterization, and assessing the need for routine diagnostic urinalysis and urine cultures in catheterized patients [9].

A key study by Mullin and colleagues, published in 2017, demonstrates the effectiveness of using a multimodal approach to limiting CAUTIs. In this study, the ICU leadership and the infection prevention department of a large academic medical center program jointly developed a CAUTI-prevention program that included assessment of the competency of catheter insertion and maintenance, maintaining a closed catheter system, starting a nurse-driven protocol for catheter removal, improving documentation on catheter usage, using preservative tubes when urine cultures were obtained, and periodically auditing catheter maintenance. They supplemented these prevention efforts with a stewardship program in accordance with national guidelines on the evaluation of fever in critically ill patients. This stewardship program considered urine cultures only in patients felt to be at high risk for systemic infection including those who were kidney transplant recipients, were neutropenic, had had recent genitourinary infection, or who had demonstrated evidence of obstruction. Over the course of 2 years, the institution's CAUTI rate progressively decreased from 3.0 per 1000 catheter days to 1.9 per 1000 catheter days and was associated with a decrease in the overall hospital-acquired bloodstream infection as well as the hospital-acquired bloodstream infection due to enteric Gram-negative bacteria. Overall, this study shows the benefits that can be achieved by an institution committing to a standardized approach to both the management of urethral catheters and the diagnostic assessment of patients who develop fever with a urethral catheter in place [6].

ANNOTATED REFERENCES FOR CATHETER-ASSOCIATED URINARY TRACT INFECTION

1. Hooton TM, Bradley SF, Cardenas DD et al. Diagnosis, prevention, and treatment of catheter-associated urinary tract infection in adults: 2009 International Clinical Practice Guidelines from the Infectious Diseases Society of America. *Clin Infect Dis.* 2010;50(5):625–663.

   The authors of this paper present the 2009 guidelines for the diagnosis, prevention, and management of catheter-associated urinary tract infections as prepared by an Expert Panel of the Infectious Diseases Society of America. The paper outlines an approach for both asymptomatic and symptomatic urinary tract infections in the inpatient and long-term care settings.

2. Nicolle LE. Urinary catheter-associated infections. *Infect Dis Clin of North Am.* 2012;26 (1):13–27.

   This paper presents a review of urinary catheter-associated infections including their epidemiology, pathophysiology, diagnosis, and treatment along with guidelines for use of catheters, maintenance, and infection-prevention strategies.

3. Gould CV, Umscheid CA, Agarwal RK, Kuntz G, Pegues DA. Healthcare Infection Control Practices Advisory Committee. Guideline for prevention of catheter-associated urinary tract infections 2009. *Infect Control Hosp Epidemiol.* 2010;31(4):319–326.

   Published in 2010, this paper proposed guideline updates and expansions on the CDC Guideline for Prevention of Catheter-Associated Urinary Tract Infections. It reviewed questions and evidence addressing patient populations who should receive urinary catheters and approaches to best practices.

4. Kizilbash QF, Petersen NJ, Chen GJ, Naik AD, Trautner BW. Bacteremia and mortality with urinary catheter-associated bacteriuria. *Infect Control Hosp Epidemiol.* 2013 Nov;34(11):1153–1159. doi: 10.1086/673456.

   The authors performed a retrospective cohort study that looked at bacteriuria, bacteremia, and associated mortality. Additionally, they looked at the effect of antimicrobial treatment of bacteriuria. Their study revealed that bacteremia due to a urinary source occurred infrequently, and that CAUTI was more associated with bacteremia than CAABU, but CAUTI and CAABU were not associated with mortality. They also found that antimicrobial therapy did not affect the outcomes.

5. Tambyah PA, Maki DG. Catheter-associated urinary tract infection is rarely symptomatic: a prospective study of 1497 catheterized patients. *Arch Intern Med.* 2000 Mar 13; 160(5):678–682. doi: 10.1001/archinte.160.5.678.

   https://www.cdc.gov/infectioncontrol/guidelines/cauti/background.html

   The authors designed a study to look at the clinical features of catheter-associated urinary tract infections with a focus on fever, symptomatic infection, and peripheral leukocytosis as measured outcomes. The study evaluated 1497 newly catheterized patients and concluded that CAUTIs are infrequently symptomatic or not a common cause of bloodstream infection. They are an important source of antibiotic-resistant organisms. Additionally, fever and leukocytosis are not good predictors in the diagnosis of CAUTI.

This CDC website outlines the definition, epidemiology, pathophysiology, and microbiology of catheter-associated urinary tract infections.

6. Mullin K, Kovacs C, Fatica C, et al. A multifaceted approach to reduction of catheter-associated urinary tract infections in the intensive care unit with an emphasis on "Stewardship of Culturing". *Infect Control Hosp Epidemiol.* 2017;38(2):186–188. doi:10.1017/ice.2016.266.

   The paper described a successful multimodal approach to limiting CAUTIs in ICUs, in a single institution, with protocols directed at placement, maintenance and removal of catheters combined with a stewardship approach to obtaining urine cultures.

7. Nicolle, LE. Catheter associated urinary tract infections. *Antimicrob Resist Infect Control.* 2014;3:23. doi: 10.1186/2047-2994-3-23.

   The author reviewed catheter-associated urinary tract infections (CAUTIs) and the related spectrum of illness and morbidity. The importance of hospital and facility infection-control programs to monitor use and maintenance of urinary tract catheterization, and treatment of infections were reviewed. The paper highlighted the need for limiting urinary tract catheterization days, and the role of catheter materials and biofilms in the disease.

8. https://www.cdc.gov/infectioncontrol/guidelines/cauti/background.html

   This CDC website outlines the definition, epidemiology, pathophysiology, and microbiology of catheter-associated urinary tract infections.

9. Pickard R, Lam T, MacLennan G, et al. Antimicrobial catheters for reduction of symptomatic urinary tract infection in adults requiring short-term catheterisation in hospital: a multicentre randomised controlled trial. *Lancet.* 2012 Dec 1;380(9857):1927–1935. doi: 10.1016/S0140-6736(12)61380-4.

   This study evaluated the use of urinary tract catheters made of various materials in relation to catheter-associated urinary tract infections. The authors concluded that routine use of antimicrobial catheters was not supported by the trial.

Landmark Article of the 21st Century

LONG-TERM PREVENTION OF CATHETER-ASSOCIATED URINARY TRACT INFECTIONS AMONG CRITICALLY ILL PATIENTS THROUGH THE IMPLEMENTATION OF AN EDUCATIONAL PROGRAM AND A DAILY CHECKLIST FOR MAINTENANCE OF INDWELLING URINARY CATHETERS: A QUASI-EXPERIMENTAL STUDY. MEDICINE (BALTIMORE)

Menegueti MG et al., *Medicine (Baltimore).* 2019 Feb;98(8):E14417

Commentary by Theofilos P. Matheos

The authors formed a multidisciplinary team to develop interventions to reduce the rate of catheter-associated urinary tract infections (CAUTIs) in the intensive care units (ICU) at the Cleveland Clinic Foundation. Protocols from the Centers for Disease Control and Prevention (CDC) for the insertion, care, and removal of the catheters were utilized. In addition, guidelines from the Infectious Disease Society of America (IDSA) and the American College of Critical Care Medicine (ACCCM) for work-up of a fever were used. Consensus on the interventions was achieved by the start of 2014.

The calendar year of 2013 was used as the baseline period and 2014 was used as the postintervention period. The device utilization ratio and the hospital-acquired bloodstream infection rates were statistically unchanged between the two periods. However, the number of urine cultures (4749 in 2013 vs. 2479 in 2014) and CAUTI rates (3.0 per 1000 catheter days in 2013 vs. 1.9 per 1000 catheter days in 2014) were statistically reduced. This study highlights that a multidisciplinary approach to care of urinary catheters and work-up of fever (notably parsimonious urine culturing) can reduce the CAUTI rates without an associated increase in hospital-acquired bloodstream infections. Weaknesses include the fact that this was a single institution study although multiple diverse ICUs were part of the study. Interventions were recommended rather than mandated and it does not appear the data were shared with each ICU on a monthly or quarterly basis.

CHAPTER 24

Fever in the ICU

Review by Juan M. Perez Velazquez and Sandeep Jubbal

Fever is common in the intensive care unit (ICU), occurring in approximately 70% of admissions. Infective and non-infective processes cause fever in approximately an equal proportion of patients [1]. An accurate and precise evaluation of body temperature is necessary to attend to ICU patients. Temperature trends provide cues regarding homeostasis, and deviation from normal parameters signal physiologic strain that may require intervention.

The hypothalamus functions as the body temperature regulatory center. Fever results from the activity of endogenous pyrogens that intensifies prostaglandin E2 production in the preoptic region of the hypothalamus [2]. Individual differences in normal body temperature vary depending on several factors, including demographics, comorbid conditions, and physiology [3]. Although arbitrary, a body temperature of 38.3°C (101°F) or higher has been the generally accepted definition of fever. A lower temperature of 38°C (100.4°F) is considered a fever in the immunocompromised or neutropenic patient, as they may have a blunted inflammatory response preventing body temperature elevation [4].

Fever in the ICU has been linked to adverse outcomes as described in a retrospective cohort study looking at 24,204 ICU admission episodes among 20,466 patients. High fever was associated with a significant increased risk for death (20.3% vs. 12%, $p < 0.0001$) [5]. Some studies support temperature lowering interventions to prevent fever complications. In a multicenter randomized controlled trial, 200 febrile patients with septic shock requiring vasopressors, mechanical ventilation, and sedation were allocated to external cooling to achieve normothermia or no external cooling. Fever control using external cooling decreased early mortality (19% vs. 34%) in septic shock [6]. Control of fever could reduce bacterial growth, promote immunomodulation, and activate white blood cells.

Several animal and human studies have suggested that suppressing infective febrile responses with antipyretic treatment might worsen outcomes for those suffering from infections [2, 7]. The possible adverse effects of fever suppression were reported in a prospective randomized controlled trial evaluating aggressive temperature control versus permissive hyperthermia in 82 ICU patients. The study was stopped after the first interim analysis due to the mortality difference identifying seven deaths in the aggressive group and only one death in the permissive group ($p = 0.06$) [9].

DOI: 10.1201/9781003042136-24

Permissive hyperthermia through avoidance of acetaminophen in known or suspected infection in the intensive care unit (HEAT) trial was a prospective, double-blind, randomized, placebo-control study conducted at 22 centers across Australia and New Zealand [10]. It was primarily designed to appraise the beneficial effects of fever, a natural or innate host defense, in patients with infection, and whether treatment with acetaminophen (or paracetamol) was associated with any adverse outcome. The study enrolled 700 ICU patients, aged 16 years or older, with a known or suspected infection and with a body (axillary) temperature ≥38°C. Eligible patients were randomly assigned to receive either scheduled 1-g intravenous acetaminophen (346/700) or scheduled 100-mL infusion of 5% dextrose in water (344/700) every 6 hours, in conjunction with the antimicrobial therapy. The acetaminophen course or the placebo were deemed complete if the study subjects reached day 28 post-randomization, the antibiotic was stopped, or the patient was discharged from the ICU. The maximum duration of study participation was 90 days. Eligible patients received the scheduled study treatment for the first 48 hours following the first elevation in fever. After that, the axillary temperatures were assessed daily in the morning, and if it measured less than 37°C for the entire past 24 hours, the study medication was withheld. However, if the body temperature rose again above 38°C within 48 hours of withholding the study drug, the 6-hourly scheduled treatment was resumed. The study groups had similar demographics, severity of illness and critical care support.

There were 53 patients in the acetaminophen and 54 patients in the placebo arm who were receiving concomitant aspirin therapy. Forty-nine out of 320 patients in the acetaminophen group, and 62 out of 327 patients in the placebo group received glucocorticoid therapy. The causative organism was identified in 217 and 214 patients in the acetaminophen and the placebo group, respectively. The number of ICU free days to day 28 (primary outcome) did not differ significantly between the acetaminophen group (median 23 days) and the placebo group (median 22 days). There was heterogeneity of response with acetaminophen treatment: the median ICU length of stay was shorter with acetaminophen therapy compared to placebo among survivors whereas the median ICU length of stay was longer among non-survivors treated with acetaminophen. No significant differences were noted for the secondary outcomes of mortality at day 28 or 90, days free from vasopressors/renal replacement therapy/mechanical ventilation, ICU/hospital length of stay, or survival time to day 90. The patients receiving acetaminophen had a lower body temperature than those who received placebo and did not have significantly more adverse events or outcomes.

The results of these studies emphasize that fever is a pathophysiological process not well understood, and while fever may be an appropriate adaptation to an infective process, it may be detrimental in other circumstances. There is a limited benefit of managing fever aggressively during an infection unless it is used for providing comfort. Scheduled antipyretics or cooling measures may also masquerade the clues to the diagnosis of certain infections presenting with a classical fever pattern or missing infection in patients presenting without localizing symptoms or signs or those with neutropenia. On the other hand, hyperthermia from non-infectious conditions or emergencies (acute brain injury or bleeding, heatstroke, malignant hyperthermia, neuroleptic malignant syndrome, etc.) necessitates rigorous control of body temperature to prevent adverse outcomes. Antipyretic treatments are mainly used in critically ill patients to provide symptomatic relief, prevent brain injury, and decrease oxygen consumption [11]. Aspirin and non-steroidal anti-inflammatory drugs (NSAIDs) are useful medications for pain and fever control; however, they can cause undesired side effects on platelets and the gastrointestinal tract. Administration of acetaminophen to lower the temperature in patients with fever and infection is broadly used in hospitalized patients, including those in the ICU where its use has been reported between 58% and 70% of patients per day [12].

Although antipyretic therapy is commonly used in ICU patients, its benefits and risks during sepsis are not well understood, and available research is conflicting. Additional randomized controlled studies assessing antipyretics use are needed to determine which temperature-lowering interventions provide the best outcomes for critically ill patients suffering from fever due to infection.

ANNOTATED REFERENCES FOR FEVER IN THE ICU

1. Circiumaru B, Baldock G, Cohen J. A prospective study of fever in the intensive care unit. *Intensive Care Med.* 1999 Jul;25(7):668–73. doi: 10.1007/s001340050928. PMID: 10470569

   This study describes fever epidemiology in a general ICU located in a tertiary care inner-city institution. It concluded that fever is a common event in the ICU, and prolonged fever is associated with poor outcomes.

2. Ryan M, Levy MM. Clinical review: fever in intensive care unit patients. *Crit Care.* 2003 Jun;7(3):221–5. doi: 10.1186/cc1879. Epub 2003 Mar 8. PMID: 12793871; PMCID: PMC270667.

   This review article evaluates the literature concerning the pathophysiology, treatment practices, potential benefits, and hemodynamic and metabolic costs of fever.

3. Obermeyer Z, Samra JK, Mullainathan S. Individual differences in normal body temperature: longitudinal big data analysis of patient records. *BMJ.* 2017 Dec 13;359:j5468. doi: 10.1136/bmj.j5468. PMID: 29237616; PMCID: PMC5727437.

   This study evaluates individual-level body temperature and correlates it with other physiological and health measures in patients without infection. It concluded that baseline temperatures correlated with demographics, comorbid conditions, and physiology, but these factors explained only a small part of individual temperature variation and that unexplained variation in baseline temperature strongly predicted mortality.

4. O'Grady NP, Barie PS, Bartlett JG, et al.; American College of Critical Care Medicine; Infectious Diseases Society of America. Guidelines for evaluation of new fever in critically ill adult patients: 2008 update from the American College of Critical Care Medicine and the Infectious Diseases Society of America. *Crit Care Med.* 2008 Apr;36(4):1330–49. doi: 10.1097/CCM.0b013e318169eda9. Erratum in: Crit Care Med. 2008 Jun;36(6):1992. PMID: 18379262.

This article presents clinical practice guidelines for adult patients who develop a new fever in the intensive care unit.

5. Laupland KB, Shahpori R, Kirkpatrick AW, Ross T, Gregson DB, Stelfox HT. Occurrence and outcome of fever in critically ill adults. *Crit Care Med.* 2008 May;36(5):1531–5. doi: 10.1097/CCM.0b013e318170efd3. PMID: 18434882.

This study evaluates the occurrence of fever defined by temperature > or = 38.3°C and high fever > or = 39.5°C in the critically ill and assesses its effect on ICU outcomes. It concluded that fever was not associated with increased ICU mortality, and high fever was associated with a significantly increased risk for death.

6. Schortgen F, Clabault K, Katsahian S, et al. Fever control using external cooling in septic shock: a randomized controlled trial. *Am J Respir Crit Care Med.* 2012 May 15;185(10):1088–95. doi: 10.1164/rccm.201110-1820OC. Epub 2012 Feb 23. PMID: 22366046.

This study evaluates the effect of fever control by external cooling on vasopressor requirements in patients with septic shock. It concluded that fever control using external cooling was safe and decreased vasopressor requirements and early mortality in septic shock.

7. Kluger MJ, Kozak W, Conn CA, Leon LR, Soszynski D. The adaptive value of fever. *Infect Dis Clin North Am.* 1996 Mar;10(1):1-20. doi: 10.1016/s0891-5520(05)70282-8. PMID: 8698984.

This article evaluates the literature concerning the survival value of fever in animal and human models. It concludes that a rise in body temperature following infection is overall beneficial and decreases morbidity and mortality.

8. Lee BH, Inui D, Suh GY. et al; Fever and Antipyretic in Critically ill patients Evaluation (FACE) Study Group. Association of body temperature and antipyretic treatments with mortality of critically ill patients with and without sepsis: multi-centered prospective observational study. *Crit Care.* 2012 Feb 28;16(1):R33. doi: 10.1186/cc11211. Erratum in: *Crit Care.* 2012;16(1):450. PMID: 22373120; PMCID: PMC3396278.

This study examines the association of fever and antipyretic (acetaminophen and NSAIDs) treatments with mortality in critically ill patients with and without sepsis. It concluded that in non-septic patients, high fever (≥39.5°C) was independently associated with mortality and that in septic patients, antipyretic administration was independently associated with mortality, without association of fever with mortality.

9. Schulman CI, Namias N, Doherty J, et al. The effect of antipyretic therapy upon outcomes in critically ill patients: a randomized, prospective study. *Surg Infect (Larchmt).* 2005 Winter;6(4):369–75. doi: 10.1089/sur.2005.6.369. Erratum in: *Surg Infect (Larchmt).* 2010 Oct;11(5):495. PMID: 16433601.

This study evaluates the impact of antipyretic therapy strategies on patients admitted to the trauma intensive care unit, excluding those with traumatic brain injury. Patients were randomized into aggressive or permissive groups. The aggressive group received acetaminophen for a temperature of >38.5°C, and a cooling blanket was added for a temperature of >39.5°C. The permissive group received no treatment for a temperature of >38.5°C but instead had treatment initiated at a temperature of >40°C, at which time acetaminophen and cooling blankets were used until the temperature was <40°C. The study was stopped after the first interim analysis due to significantly higher mortality in the aggressive group.

10. Young P, Saxena M, Bellomo R, et al.; HEAT Investigators; Australian and New Zealand Intensive Care Society Clinical Trials Group. Acetaminophen for fever in critically ill

patients with suspected infection. *N Engl J Med.* 2015 Dec 3;373(23):2215–24. doi: 10.1056/NEJMoa1508375. Epub 2015 Oct 5. PMID: 26436473.

This study evaluated acetaminophen use in the ICU for patients with a temperature ≥38°C who have suspected infection. The primary outcome was ICU-free days (days alive and free from the need for intensive care) from randomization to day 28. The study concluded that administration of acetaminophen to treat fever due to probable infection did not affect the number of ICU-free days.

11. Egi M, Morita K. Fever in non-neurological critically ill patients: a systematic review of observational studies. *J Crit Care.* 2012 Oct;27(5):428–33. doi: 10.1016/j.jcrc.2011.11.016. Epub 2012 Jan 9. PMID: 22227089.

This systematic review of observational studies assesses the association of fever with mortality in non-neurological critically ill patients. It concluded that limited evidence suggests that the recommended definition of fever (38.3°C) might be too low to predict increased mortality.

12. Young P, Saxena M, Eastwood GM, Bellomo R, Beasley R. Fever and fever management among intensive care patients with known or suspected infection: a multicentre prospective cohort study. *Crit Care Resusc.* 2011 Jun;13(2):97–102. PMID: 21627577.

This study describes the duration of fever, fever management, and outcomes among intensive care patients with fever of ≥38.0°C and known or suspected infection, excluding those with neurological injury or elective surgery. It reported the typical time course of fever in patients with known or suspected infection and concluded that these patients have more than double the mortality rate of ineligible patients.

Landmark Article of the 21st Century

ACETAMINOPHEN FOR FEVER IN CRITICALLY ILL PATIENTS WITH SUSPECTED INFECTION

Young P et al., *N Engl J Med.* 2015;373:2215–2224

Commentary by Paul J. Young

We conducted the HEAT trial because we were concerned that the antipyretic effect of acetaminophen might result in harm in febrile intensive care unit (ICU) patients with infections. The reason for this concern was that fever, a metabolically costly response, is conserved broadly across many animal species. We considered that such a broadly conserved response was likely to confer a survival advantage and that suppressing it with medication might be harmful. We also noted that there were many interesting historical examples of induction of fever or hyperthermia being used to treat infectious diseases, including the example of patients being infected with malaria to successfully treat neuro-syphilis which led to the Nobel Prize for Physiology or Medicine being awarded to Julius Wagner-Jauregg in 1927.

At the time that the HEAT trial was conceived, I was a novice researcher. I had conducted one small, single-center pilot RCT working in isolation. Realizing that I had no future in research without support and mentorship, I sought help from someone with the knowledge and experience. I looked through the list of clinical studies funded by the Health Research Council of New Zealand (New Zealand's peak health research funding body) and found one clinician researcher in my hospital, Professor Richard Beasley. Professor Beasley had a funded community-based clinical trial evaluating the use of acetaminophen to treat fever in patients with influenza. I approached him and asked if he would be interested in collaborating on a similar trial in patients with fever and suspected infection in the ICU. He agreed. I wrote a funding application with his name on it. The study was funded and the HEAT study, my second RCT, ended up published in the *New England Journal of Medicine*. I think that this highimpact publication was a result of the fact we investigated a ubiquitous therapy and that what we studied was of interest to many clinicians.

Ultimately, the findings from the HEAT trial were reassuring. Although acetaminophen did reduce body temperature, it neither increased nor decreased ICU-free survival days or mortality. These findings suggest that when ICU clinicians chose to administer acetaminophen to treat fever or to treat pain in patients who happen to be febrile, this practice is unlikely to result in demonstrable harm.

CHAPTER 25

Fulminant Colitis

Review by Michael F. Musso and Adrian W. Ong

In a patient with colitis, the term "fulminant" denotes a rapidly deteriorating condition with systemic toxicity and progression to multiorgan failure and, possibly, death if not managed aggressively. Although general treatment principles are the same, the lack of standardized criteria for defining what constitutes fulminant colitis (FC) makes it difficult to compare outcomes from different studies and across disease processes. From the provider's standpoint, the lack of a standardized definition of FC might result in uncertainty as to how, and when, treatments should be initiated or escalated.

While colitis can stem from a number of inciting processes, the most common etiologies of FC are ulcerative colitis (UC) and *Clostridioides difficile* (*C. difficile*) colitis. Other less common causes are ischemic colitis (IC), Crohn's disease, bacterial, viral, and parasitic organisms such as *Salmonella, Shigella, Cytomegalovirus,* and *Entamoeba histolytica.* It is important to determine the etiology of FC expeditiously, as treatment varies considerably. The intensivist is likely to encounter FC due to *C. difficile,* UC, or colon ischemia.

Originally identified as the cause of pseudomembranous colitis in 1978, *C. difficile* has emerged as a major cause of nosocomial infections [1]. A 2017 clinical practice guideline defines FC due to *C. difficile* as severe infection (white blood count [WBC] >15,000/μL or serum creatinine of >1.5 mg/dL) with hypotension or shock, ileus, or megacolon [2]. While oral vancomycin 125 mg four times a day is recommended for severe colitis, treatment for FC consists of oral vancomycin 500 mg four times a day with intravenous metronidazole 500 mg every 8 hours, especially with concomitant ileus. It is also prudent to administer vancomycin as an enema if ileus is present due to inhibited motility. The addition of intravenous metronidazole was associated with decreased mortality when compared to vancomycin monotherapy in a retrospective study [3].

Criteria for operative intervention in *C. difficile* FC have not been well defined. Peritonitis, perforation, toxic megacolon, and hypotension are clear indicators, but these may not be present in many patients. A retrospective study found that age ≥70 years, WBC of >35,000 or <4,000/μL or bandemia, and need for intubation or vasopressors predicted mortality in FC [4]. When all three criteria were present, mortality was 57% vs. 0% when all three were absent. Lamontagne et al. [5] reviewed 165 patients with *C. difficile* colitis requiring intensive care unit admission.

DOI: 10.1201/9781003042136-25

Risk factors for mortality were age ≥75 years, WBC of ≥50,000 µL, immunosuppression, need for vasopressors, and a lactate level of ≥5 mmol/L. Colectomy reduced adjusted odds of death by 78%. Subgroup analyses showed that colectomy was of mortality benefit in those aged ≥75 years, WBC >20,000 µL, and lactate of >2.2 and <5 mmol/L. They and others found that 75–80% of patients with a lactate of >5 mmol/L died whether or not there was operative intervention. These studies suggest that certain clinical criteria may signal the need for expeditious operation.

Total abdominal colectomy (TAC) is the operation of choice for FC. An acceptable alternative, loop ileostomy with antegrade colonic lavage has been used in a minority of patients. Neal et al. [6] compared 42 matched historical controls undergoing TAC to patients who underwent loop ileostomy, intraoperative antegrade polyethylene glycol colonic lavage, and postoperative antegrade vancomycin enemas and found lower mortality (19% vs. 50%) in the latter group. In a multicenter study by Ferrada et al., loop ileostomy was associated with a lower adjusted mortality (17% vs. 39%). Other larger studies have not shown mortality benefit for loop ileostomy. It remains debatable if the type of operation is associated with improved outcomes.

In patients with inflammatory bowel disease, FC is seen more often with UC than Crohn's colitis. Severity of UC has been commonly classified according to the criteria by Truelove and Witts as mild or severe depending on the number of daily bowel movements, temperature, heart rate, anemia, and erythrocyte sedimentation rate [7]. Since then, several scoring systems have been developed to quantify disease severity. The 2019 American College of Gastroenterology clinical guidelines propose four categories (remission, mild, moderate-severe, fulminant) based on laboratory values, patient reported outcomes, and endoscopic disease severity [8].

For patients with active severe UC, it is important to rule out *C. difficile* disease and *Cytomegalovirus* infection. Flexible sigmoidoscopy with biopsies is therefore recommended early during treatment of UC [8]. Intravenous steroid therapy should be initiated, as approximately 60–70% will respond positively. The use of empiric broad spectrum antibiotics is controversial. Surgical intervention should be considered in cases of massive hemorrhage, perforation, or toxic megacolon. For the remainder who are refractory to steroids after 3–5 days, options include rescue therapy with cyclosporine A (CSA) or infliximab, or colectomy. CSA was demonstrated to be efficacious in a small, randomized trial versus placebo (9 of 11 patients vs. 0 of 9 patients) [9]. Another study randomizing patients with steroid-refractory UC to either infliximab or placebo on day 4 of therapy found that infliximab was associated with a lower 90-day colectomy rate (7 of 24) than placebo (14 of 21) [10]. While rescue therapy with CSA or infliximab is appropriate in steroid-refractory UC, clinical deterioration should prompt total colectomy. For patients with a long disease duration or known colonic dysplasia, colectomy should also be considered.

Causes of ischemic colitis are generally divided into occlusive disease (e.g., surgery, thromboemboli, vasculitides) and non-occlusive disease (e.g., various shock etiologies, drugs). Segmental involvement of the colon is typical, with the left colon being most commonly affected. Pancolonic involvement is unusual, occurring in 13% in one study [11]. While 50–60% have non-gangrenous IC that resolves with resuscitation and empiric antibiotics, the remainder will develop irreversible colonic damage manifested by gangrene, stricture, or, rarely, a fulminant course characterized by a toxic, rapidly progressing course with colectomy being necessary [12].

FC is an emergency requiring prompt diagnosis and treatment. Clinicians should be cognizant of common causes of FC and maintain a heightened awareness of the need for operative intervention. A multidisciplinary approach to management including critical care practitioners, gastroenterologists, and surgeons is necessary to optimize outcomes.

ANNOTATED REFERENCES FOR FULMINANT COLITIS

1. Bartlett JG, Chang TW, Gurwith M, Gorbach SL, Onderdonk AB. Antibiotic-associated pseudomembranous colitis due to toxin-producing clostridia. *N Engl J Med.* 1978;298:531–534.

   This is the first paper to correctly identify Clostridium difficile as the pathogen responsible for pseudomembranous colitis.

2. McDonald LC, Gerding DN, Johnson S, et al. Clinical practice guidelines for *Clostridium difficile* infection in adults and children: 2017 update by the Infectious Diseases Society of America (IDSA) and Society for Healthcare Epidemiology of America (SHEA). *Clinical Infect Dis.* 2018;66:e1–e48.

   Comprehensive guidelines for the diagnosis, management, and prevention of C. difficile infection. Metronidazole, a long-time recommended first-line agent, was replaced in favor of vancomycin and fidaxomicin. Nucleic acid amplification testing was also recommended as a stand-alone or confirmatory test.

3. Rokas KE, Johnson JW, Beardsley JR, Ohl CA, Luther VP, Williamson JC. The addition of intravenous metronidazole to oral vancomycin is associated with improved mortality in critically ill patients with *Clostridium difficile* infection. *Clin Infect Dis.* 2015;61:934–941.

   While metronidazole is no longer recommended as a first line therapy for Clostridium difficile infections, this study examined its use in combination with oral vancomycin for patients with fulminant colitis.

4. Sailhamer EA, Carson, K, Chang Y, et al. Fulminant *Clostridium difficile* colitis. Patterns of care and predictors of mortality. *Arch Surg.* 2009;144(5):433–439.

   Four percent of 4796 patients had fulminant C. difficile colitis with a 35% mortality. Three independent risk factors for mortality were found.

5. *Lamontagne F, Labbé A, Haeck O, et al. Impact of emergency colectomy on survival of patients with fulminant *Clostridium difficile* colitis during an epidemic caused by a hyper-virulent strain. *Ann Surg.* 2007;245:267–272.

   This is a retrospective study of 165 cases of fulminant C. difficile colitis with 23% undergoing colectomy and 53% overall 30-day mortality. Outcomes of patients undergoing colectomy were compared to those who did not, analyzed for each of several risk factors.

Benefit of colectomy was demonstrated for age ≥75 years, lactic acid of >2.2 and <5 mmol/L, immunocompetent patients, and a white blood cell count of >20,000/μL.

6. Neal MD, Alverdy JC, Hall DE, Simmons RL, Zuckerbraun BS. Diverting loop ileostomy and colonic lavage: an alternative to total abdominal colectomy for the treatment of severe, complicated *Clostridium difficile* associated disease. *Ann Surg.* 2011;254:423–427.

This study compared 42 cases of fulminant C. difficile infection managed by diverting ileostomy, antegrade polyethylene glycol lavage, and vancomycin flushes via ileostomy compared to historical matched controls undergoing total colectomy. Ileostomy with antegrade lavage was a safe alternative surgical option which preserved the colon.

7. Truelove SC, Witts LJ. Cortisone in ulcerative colitis; final report on a therapeutic trial. *BMJ* 1955;2:1041–1048.

This paper provides details of a controlled study of cortisone versus placebo in ulcerative colitis classified by disease severity in 210 patients.

8. Rubin DT, Ananthakrishnan AN, Siegel CA, Sauer BG, Long MD. ACG clinical guideline: ulcerative colitis in adults. *Am J Gastroenterol.* 2019;114: 384–413.

This provides comprehensive clinical practice guidelines on ulcerative colitis.

9. Lichtiger S, Present DH, Kornbluth A, et al. Cyclosporine in severe ulcerative colitis refractory to steroid therapy. *N Engl J Med.* 1994;330:1841–1845.

This paper describes a randomized trial showing efficacy of Cyclosporine A as rescue therapy for severe ulcerative colitis refractory to steroids.

10. Jarnerot G, Hertervig E, Friis–Liby I, et al. Infliximab as rescue therapy in severe to moderately severe ulcerative colitis: a randomized, placebo-controlled study. *Gastroenterology.* 2005;128:1805–1811.

This is the first randomized placebo-controlled study to show benefit of infliximab as rescue therapy in steroid-refractory ulcerative colitis patients.

11. Scharff JR, Longo WE, Vartanian SM, Jacobs DL, Bahadursingh AN, Kaminski DL. Ischemic colitis: spectrum of disease and outcome. *Surgery.* 2003;134:624–630.

Large series of patients with ischemic colitis discussing patient characteristics, clinical presentation, extent of colonic disease and outcome.

12. Brandt LJ, Boley SJ. Colonic ischemia. *Surg Clin North Am.* 1992;72:203–229.

This paper discusses the pathophysiology, clinical presentation, and management of ischemic colitis.

Landmark Article of the 21st Century

DONOR FECES INFUSION IN THE DUODENUM FOR RECURRENT *CLOSTRIDIUM DIFFICILE* INFECTIONS

Van Nood E et al., *New Engl J Med.* 2013;368:407–415

Commentary by Josbert Keller and Els van Nood

In 2006, an epidemic of *Clostridium difficile* infection (CDI) stimulated an interest in investigation of more effective treatment strategies. We were trainees in the Departments of Internal Medicine and Gastroenterology at the Academic Medical Centre in Amsterdam when a patient was scheduled for colectomy because of persistent recurrence of CDI. Fortunately, visiting gastroenterologists from Scandinavia mentioned the possibility of FMT (feces microbiota transplantation). It was not performed in the Netherlands before. However, our supervisor Joep Bartelsman became suddenly enthused by this idea, and this patient was cured by the first FMT performed in The Netherlands. Everybody was astonished by the prompt effects of this unconventional therapy. Word of this novel treatment spread quickly through the Netherlands, and together with the ongoing *C. difficile* outbreak, more patients were referred to us for curative FMT. In those "early days", FMT was considered both non-appealing and peculiar by colleagues but provided salvation for desperate patients after months of chronic diarrhea caused by recurrent CDI. Our mentor and professor, Peter Speelman, a distinguished infectious disease specialist, was surprised that, at the end of his career, he had to change his mind about the effects of bacteria on human health. Still, skeptics persisted because of the lack of evidence.

To overcome the skepticism toward FMT and driven by the unexpected high cure rate in patients for whom no other rescue treatment was available, we decided to initiate a randomized controlled trial. The trial was supervised by a gastroenterology fellow (Josbert Keller) and run by an internal medicine fellow (Els van Nood). We must mention Marcel Levi, Peter Speelman, and Marcel Dijkgraaf for their support, and the Netherlands Organization for Health Research and Development for funding this study. The evidence of the beneficial effect of FMT was overwhelming, and our DSMB advised early termination of the trial to prevent further allocation to the vancomycin treatment arm. Fortunately, early termination of the trial did not prevent our study from publication in the *New England Journal of Medicine*, which led to a change in the management of recurrent CDI worldwide. However, the most valuable result of our efforts was the cure of the large majority of our patients with recurrence of CDI.

CHAPTER 26

Necrotizing Soft Tissue Infections

Review by Mark D. Sawyer

INTRODUCTION

...when the exciting cause was a trivial accident or a very small wound...the erysipelas would quickly spread widely in all directions. Flesh, sinews, and bones fell away in large quantities...there were many deaths

—Hippocrates

Necrotizing soft tissue infections (NTSIs) remain a highly lethal disease process. There has been a gradual improvement in survival over the decades from 40% or so down to around 20% currently. This is mostly likely due to multifactorial advances in critical care medicine, antibiotics, prompt recognition, and expeditious and complete surgical debridement. By nature, the patients are usually critically ill at the time of presentation, and rapid institution of resuscitative and supportive intensive care is vitally important for survival. Cases are rare, about a thousand or so per year in the United States.

CLASSIFICATION

NSTIs are most usefully classified by virtue of their microbial makeup. Type I NSTIs are the most common, and are polymicrobial infections which consist of Gram-negative, anaerobic, streptococcal and sometimes fungal organisms. They are typically in the perineal area and account for 70–80% of cases with a preponderance in diabetic patients. Type II infections are primarily Group A streptococcus and while often referred to in the literature as "monomicrobial" they are frequently accompanied by MRSA and may have toxic shock syndrome as an accompaniment. These are often rapidly lethal—sometimes within 24 hours—and may require a rapid decision for radical treatment such as amputation of the affected extremity. Type III infections are the least common, are more accurately described as monomicrobial, and are due to organisms such as *Clostridial* species (*perfringens* and *septicum*, the latter usually from perforated colon cancers), *Vibrio vulnificans*, and *Aeromonas* species.

DIAGNOSIS

Often the diagnosis is strongly suggested by clinical presentation, and imaging studies can provide additional evidence. With the rapid advances in scan resolution, CT imaging has become increasingly useful and can help guide operative therapy as well as

DOI: 10.1201/9781003042136-26

diagnostic evidence. While initially promising, the LRINEC (laboratory risk indicator for necrotizing fasciitis) score has not been confirmed in subsequent studies as useful in ruling out NSTIs; however, it may have some benefit in prognosticating outcome. Frozen section biopsy was touted as the gold standard for diagnosis in the past, but has largely been supplanted by bringing the patient to the operating room to perform an open biopsy with visual confirmation to make certain of the diagnosis and proceeding with debridement as soon as possible. High levels of clinical suspicion, surgical consultation, and early biopsy remain the vanguards of early diagnosis.

TREATMENT

The definitive treatment of NSTIs includes source control (radical and complete surgical debridement), tissue and blood cultures, broad spectrum antibiotics, and resuscitative and supportive critical care. The effectiveness of adjunctive strategies is often difficult to ascertain due to the rarity of the disease.

These patients are usually critically ill and require ICU admission. They often present in septic shock aggravated by dehydration, with renal failure, and sometimes may suffer toxic shock syndrome as well. The usual measures of aggressive crystalloid resuscitation, early culture and empiric antibiotics, and source control by aggressive operative debridement are paramount. While a complete initial debridement is the desired goal, the patient may not tolerate this and require second and additional returns to the operating room once they are hopefully more stable. However, if the patient fails to stabilize in the initial postoperative period, requiring ongoing resuscitation and pressors, the assumption should be made that there is progression of disease, and early return to the OR for more aggressive debridement is critically important. Even in the cases where the initial debridement is thought to be complete, the necrosis may continue to spread beyond the boundaries of the resection postoperatively, and a second look should be mandatory. Debridements should continue on a daily basis until the surgeon is satisfied that there is no further necrotic progression. Once the tissues are clean without further evidence of disease, vacuum wound dressings may be placed to minimize wound size and facilitate wound healing and closure. If renal failure or dysfunction result, continuous renal replacement therapy may be required early in the course; patients are often too labile to tolerate hemodialysis. Pressors may be required to maintain blood pressure and perfusion in accordance with the latest SCCM guidelines. The 2018 update to the 2016 Surviving Sepsis guidelines advocates even earlier establishment of the previous bundles to a 1-hour time frame: measurement of lactate, blood cultures, broad spectrum antibiotics, crystalloid infusion, and vasopressors to restore blood pressure and perfusion. Nutritional support is key to recovery, with caloric and protein requirements that can be similar to those of burn patients in severe cases. IVIG may be of value as an adjunctive measure in patients with Type II (Group A Streptococcal) NSTIs and concomitant toxic shock syndrome. The evidence for this is not strong, but there are some indications it may be beneficial in these patients. Hyperbaric oxygen therapy remains unproven and incurs significant additional burdens on the patient and care teams, and its use should not delay the mainstays of treatment.

After initial resuscitative care and source control, supportive critical care is necessary as patients undergo multiple debridements and recover from their septic insult. While most aspects of the management of these patients is according to general critical care support, they may have very substantial surface area wounds, with extensive evaporative losses of fluid from their wounds and increased fluid requirements, and concomitant electrolyte fluctuations requiring close attention. Once the wounds are satisfactorily clean enough to allow its use, negative pressure wound therapy may be helpful to limit wound size, accelerate healing, contract wounds, and aid in tracking the amount of insensible losses.

An element of critical care that has deservedly received more attention in recent years is preparing for the longer term recovery these patients will endure. Early multidisciplinary care involving physical and occupational therapy, plastic surgery, and close attention to long-term nutrition and psychological care should begin in the intensive care unit as soon as practicable once they patient has moved into a more stable phase of their illness.

SUMMARY

Intensive care of the NSTI patient remains daunting, with high morbidity and mortality. For survivors, long term recovery will pose additional challenges. The principles for successful treatment have not changed appreciably in recent years: early, aggressive resuscitation and debridement, broad-spectrum antimicrobial therapy as per IDSA guidelines, and adherence to the critical care principles delineated in the Surviving Sepsis guidelines. Adjunctive therapies remain of questionable efficacy and should not interfere with the pillars of treatment.

ANNOTATED REFERENCES FOR NECROTIZING SOFT TISSUE INFECTIONS

Cocanour CS, Chang P, Huston JM, et al. Management and novel adjuncts of necrotizing soft tissue infections. *Surg Infect (Larchmt)*. 2017;18(3):250–272. doi: 10.1089/sur.2016.200

An evidence-based, GRADE-recommendation review of 64 manuscripts addressing novel and adjunctive therapies in detail, including hyperbaric oxygen, IVIG, LRINEC score, antibiotics, toxic shock syndrome, and other elements.

de Prost N, Sbidian E, Chosidow O, Brun-Buisson C, Amathieu R. Management of necrotizing soft tissue infections in the intensive care unit: results of an international survey. *Intensive Care Med*. 2015;41:1506–1508. doi: 10.1007/s00134-015-3916-9

A letter to the editor describing an international survey the authors performed with regards to NSTI management. Their survey of NSTIs in 100 ICUs showed significant heterogeneity in most aspects of care including adherence to the latest guidelines. They identified two major and modifiable prognostic factors—delayed diagnosis of NSTI and lack of priority access to the operating room—as being of significant concern and causing delays in definitive treatment.

Fernando SM, Tran A, Cheng W, et al. Necrotizing soft tissue infection: diagnostic accuracy of physical examination, imaging, and LRINEC score. A systematic review and meta-analysis. *Ann Surg.* 2019;269:58–65.

Thorough, very recent review of the current state of diagnostic modalities in NSTIs, with conclusions on the utility of the various measures. Twenty-three studies were analyzed for physical examination, imaging, and Laboratory Risk Indicator for Necrotizing Fasciitis (LRINEC) score in diagnosis of necrotizing soft tissue infection (NSTI) in adults with a soft tissue infection clinically concerning for NSTI. Findings included: absence of any single feature of the physical examination feature was found to be insufficient to rule-out NSTI, CT is superior to plain radiography, and LRINEC had poor sensitivity, ruling it out as a test to exclude the diagnosis of NSTI. The authors felt that given the poor sensitivity of these diagnostic modalities, high clinical suspicion and early surgical consultation remain the most important factors in early diagnosis.

Jeffrey S, Ustin JS, Malangoni MA. Necrotizing soft-tissue infections. *Crit Care Med.* 2011;39:2156–2162.

In this clear, succinct paper by Drs. Ustin and Malangoni, all the key elements of NSTIs are covered with a solid evidence-based approach to the literature, and with explicit recommendations regarding diagnosis, critical care, antimicrobials, source control, and adjunctive treatments. An excellent first-line reference to utilize when treating these diseases. The sometimes confusing issue of microbiologic classification is clear and reflects the latest understanding and impact of individual microorganisms.

Lauerman MH, Scalea TM, Eglseder WA, Pensy R, Stein DM, Henry S. Physiology, not modern operative approach, predicts mortality in extremity necrotizing soft tissue infections at a high-volume center. *Surgery.* 2018;164:105–109.

This review looks at mortality in patients with NSTIs at a large referral center with aggressive attempts to preserve limbs. Their results suggest that the aggressive limb salvage approach as opposed to early amputation did not adversely affect mortality at their center, and that patient outcome with regards to mortality was instead related to the physiology of the patient and their response.

Levy MM, Evans LE, Rhodes A. The surviving sepsis campaign bundle: 2018 update. *Intensive Care Med.* 2018;44:925–928.

Central to any discussion of the intensive care of critically ill patients suffering from sepsis are the Surviving Sepsis guidelines. The two references above are the 2016 Surviving Sepsis guidelines, and a 2018 update urging that previous 3- and 6-hour bundles be moved to a more aggressive timeline of a 1-hour bundle, including measurement of lactate, blood cultures, broad spectrum antibiotics, crystalloid infusion, and vasopressors to restore blood pressure and perfusion.

Parks T, Wilson C, Curtis N, Norrby-Teglund A, Sriskandan S. Polyspecific intravenous immunoglobulin in clindamycin-treated patients with streptococcal toxic shock syndrome: a systematic review and meta-analysis. *Clin Infect Dis.* 2018;67:1434–1436.

The authors performed a small meta-analysis of five studies to evaluate the effect of intravenous immunoglobulin (IVIG) on mortality in clindamycin-treated NSTIs with streptococcal toxic shock syndrome. Mortality fell from 33.7% to 15.7% in the pooled data with a p value of 0.01. While encouraging, the results certainly should be viewed with caution; only one of the five studies was randomized and none of the studies achieved a significantly decreased mortality on their own, and clindamycin is not the antimicrobial of choice in Group A streptococcal NSTIs.

Peetermans M, de Prost N, Eckmann C, Norrby-Teglund A, Skrede S, De Waele JJ. Necrotizing skin and soft-tissue infections in the intensive care unit. *Clin Microbiol Infect.* 2020;26:8.

A meta-analysis of NSTIs using PubMed and Cochrane. From an initial search result of 435 papers, it was narrowed down to 222 manuscripts. Some additional granularity was deduced by analysis of the data; overall, a good summary of a large amount of recent clinical data.

Rhodes A, Evans LE, Alhazzani W, et al. Surviving sepsis campaign: international guidelines for management of sepsis and septic shock. *Intensive Care Med.* 2017 Mar;43(3):304–377. doi: 10.1007/s00134-017-4683-6. Epub 2017 Jan 18.

Stevens DL, Bisno AL, Chambers HF, et al. Practice guidelines for the diagnosis and management of skin and soft tissue infections: 2014 update by the Infectious Diseases Society of America. *Clin Infect Dis.* 2014;59(2):e10–52.

A panel of national experts was convened by the Infectious Diseases Society of America (IDSA) to update the 2005 guidelines for the treatment of skin and soft tissue infections (SSTIs). This is an antimicrobial-centered review which covers the gamut of skin and soft tissue infections, and is an evidence-based, expert consensus guideline that could reasonably be considered to be the most definitive guide on the most appropriate antibiotics for these infections. It covers other elements of treatment as well and is an excellent overall resource.

Landmark Article of the 21st Century

IMPACT AND PROGRESSION OF ORGAN DYSFUNCTION IN PATIENTS WITH NECROTIZING SOFT TISSUE INFECTIONS: A MULTICENTER STUDY

Bulger et al., *Surg Infect.* 2015;16(6):694–701

Commentary by Eileen M. Bulger

This paper represents an important piece of a journey to better understand the trajectory of systemic illness in the setting of NSTI in order to define meaningful clinical endpoints for subsequent clinical trials. Due in part to our role as a major referral center for burns, trauma, and complex critical illness, my home, Harborview Medical Center in Seattle, has become a regional referral center for NSTI patients across the Pacific Northwest. We currently manage approximately 150 cases per year. Our experience in caring for these critically ill patients has driven us to study novel interventions to improve the outcome. One such intervention is a novel immune modulator known as Reltecimod or AB103 which binds to the CD28 receptor on T cells resulting in transient inhibition of the response to superantigens. In 2014 we published a Phase 2a RCT for patients with NSTI demonstrating the safety and optimal dose of AB103. While not powered for efficacy, there was evidence of improved resolution of organ dysfunction in the treatment arm [1]. As a result, in this study we sought to evaluate the pattern of organ dysfunction in a larger cohort (n = 198) of patients who would be representative of a cohort that would be eligible for a subsequent Phase 3 trial. This study laid the ground work for the development of a composite endpoint known as the NICCE [2] (necrotizing infection clinical composite endpoint) which was developed, validated, and then used as the primary endpoint in our recently completed Phase 3 RCT involving 65 clinical enrolling sites in the United States and France [3]. Reltecimod is now under review at the US FDA. This 10-year journey illustrates the challenges of studying a rare disease which requires time sensitive surgical intervention and the importance of taking a methodical approach to understanding the trajectory of the disease process in order to develop meaningful clinical trial endpoints.

REFERENCES

1. Bulger EM, Maier RV, Sperry J, et al. A novel drug for treatment of necrotizing soft-tissue infections. *JAMA Surg.* 2014 Jun 1;149(6):528–529.
2. Bulger EM, May A, Dankner W, Maislin G, Robinson B, Shirvan A. Validation of a clinical trial composite endpoint for patients with necrotizing soft tissue infections. *J Trauma Acute Care Surg.* 2017 May 22;83(4):622–627.
3. Bulger EM, May AK, Robinson BRH, et al. A novel immune modulator for patients with necrotizing soft tissue infections (NSTI): results of a multicenter, phase 3 randomized controlled trial of Reltecimod (AB 103). *Ann Surg.* 2020 Jul 8;272(3):469–478.

CHAPTER 27

Sepsis I: Antibiotic Therapy

Review by Catherine Kuza

One of the major causes of intensive care unit (ICU) admission is sepsis. Annually, in the United States (US), there are over 970,000 septic patients admitted to the hospital, and the incidence increases each year. Sepsis places a heavy burden on hospital resources in addition to hospital costs. Sepsis management costs the highest of all diseases in the US, and accounts for more than $24 billion in hospital expenses annually. Approximately 50% of patients with sepsis will develop severe sepsis and 25% will develop septic shock. Sepsis may result in multi-organ system failure and acute respiratory distress syndrome in ICU patients. These complications result in a longer length of stay and a need for hospital resources. Over 50% of hospital deaths are attributed to sepsis, and the mortality rate increases with disease severity [1].

It is crucial that sepsis is diagnosed and treated as soon as possible. Sepsis may present with nonspecific signs and symptoms, resulting in delayed recognition and management. Delayed diagnosis and management of sepsis results in increased patient mortality. Previous studies have demonstrated that the median time to the administration of appropriate antimicrobial therapy in patients with septic shock after the initial onset of persistent hypotension was 6 hours. The survival to hospital discharge rate of patients who receive empiric broad-spectrum antibiotics within an hour of sepsis-related hypotension was 79.9%. The survival decreases approximately 7.6% with each additional 1-hour delay from hypotension onset [2]. These findings prompted updates in initiatives such as the "Surviving Sepsis Campaign (SSC)" (latest edition in 2016) which provided education for healthcare workers on sepsis awareness and management, which includes prompt recognition, early ICU supportive care, early goal-directed therapy (EGDT) resuscitation protocol, and early initiation of empiric antibiotics [3, 4].

It is recommended that hospitals have quality improvement efforts for sepsis, which entail screening for early diagnosis in high-risk patients [4]. This has led to the development of the "sepsis bundle," which has been instrumental in implementing the guidelines of the SSC. The most recent edition of the SSC emphasizes the importance of immediate diagnosis, resuscitation, and treatment of sepsis. Two preexisting bundles, the 3-hour and 6-hour bundles, were combined into the "1-hour bundle." The bundle, which should ideally be performed within one hour of presentation, includes: measuring a lactate level, obtaining blood cultures prior to initiating antibiotics, administering broad-spectrum antibiotics, delivering crystalloid fluids at a rate of 30 mL/kg for hypotension or lactate ≥4 mmol/L, and administering vasopressors if the patient remains hypotensive during or after fluid administration with the goal of

DOI: 10.1201/9781003042136-27

maintaining the mean arterial pressure (MAP) at ≥65 mmHg [5]. The implementation of and compliance with the sepsis bundles is associated with improved survival rates in patients with sepsis and septic shock [6].

Serum lactate is a good surrogate marker for measuring tissue perfusion, and lactate-guided resuscitation has demonstrated a substantial reduction in mortality rates in patients with sepsis. Serum lactates should be trended approximately every 4 hours if the initial lactate level is elevated (>2 mmol/L), to measure the response to resuscitation [7].

It is imperative to obtain microbiological cultures, including at least two sets of blood cultures, prior to the initiation of antibiotics, as culture sterilization can occur within minutes after antibiotic administration. Antibiotic administration should not be delayed if obtaining the cultures is time consuming or there is difficulty in obtaining the culture specimens. The culture results help identify the underlying organism responsible for the sepsis, and help guide antibiotic therapy. Antibiotic therapy should be narrowed as soon as the cultures have resulted, the sensitivities are available, or there is clinical improvement noted. It is recommended that empiric IV broad-spectrum antibiotics be administered within one hour of sepsis presentation, and the antibiotics should provide coverage against all suspected pathogens, which may include bacterial, viral, and fungal coverage. Daily assessment of antibiotic de-escalation should be performed [4].

The antibiotic choice is patient-specific, and should take into account patient comorbidities, previous infections or antibiotics received, the underlying signs and symptoms of clinical presentation, surgical history, and local antibiotic susceptibility patterns and recommendations from the antibiotic stewardship committee. Gram-positive cocci are the most common pathogen associated with sepsis, followed by gram-negative bacilli [8]. It is important to cover all suspected pathogens, as there is an increase in mortality rates in patients who received inappropriate initial antibiotic therapy. At least one antibiotic agent must have in vitro activity against the underlying pathogen in order to accomplish appropriate antibiotic therapy. Empiric coverage against gram-negative bacteria should be considered as this antibiotic regimen resulted in increased rates of appropriate initial antibiotic therapy when compared with monotherapy [9]. Combining an aminoglycoside to a beta-lactam antibiotic could result in superior coverage and more effective treatment against an underlying infection in a patient with septic shock. However, a recent meta-analysis did not report a difference in outcomes when comparing combination therapy to beta-lactam therapy alone, and the combination of these two agents should be discouraged as there is no difference in mortality rates and it results in an increased incidence of nephrotoxicity [10]. The recommended duration of antimicrobial therapy per the SSC is 7–10 days for most serious infections; however, the duration may be shorter or longer depending on the pathogen, infection source, and overall clinical pictures [4].

Finally, in addition to antibiotic management, the anatomic source of the infection should be identified as soon as possible. If there is an infectious source which is amenable to intervention, then source control should occur as soon as possible, once the patient has been stabilized and resuscitated. Source control may entail open surgical intervention or percutaneous intervention. Ideally, source control should be achieved within 6–12 hours after diagnosis; after this window of time, the survival rate decreases [4, 11, 12]. Additionally, any intravascular devices or foreign bodies which are contributing to sepsis, should be removed, if possible [4].

ANNOTATED REFERENCES FOR SEPSIS I: ANTIBIOTIC THERAPY

1. Paoli CJ, Reynolds MA, Sinha M, et al. Epidemiology and costs of sepsis in the United States—An analysis based on timing of diagnosis and severity level. *Crit Care Med*. 2018; 46(12):1889–1897.

   This was a retrospective observational study. There were 2,566,689 adult patients with sepsis. The overall mortality was 12.5%, but it increased with increasing disease severity (5.6% for sepsis without organ dysfunction, 14.9% for severe sepsis, and 34.2% for septic shock). Similarly, the hospital cost of the admission increased with increasing disease severity. Sepsis which was not diagnosed until after the admission, and more severe disease had higher economic burden and mortality.

2. Kumar A, Roberts D, Wood KE, et al. Duration of hypotension before initiation of effective antimicrobial therapy is the critical determinant of survival in human septic shock. *Crit Care Med*. 2006;34(6):1589–1596.

   This is a retrospective cohort study which evaluated 2731 patients with septic shock from 14 ICUs and 10 hospitals. The median time to effective antimicrobial therapy was 6 hours. Among patients who received antimicrobial therapy within the first hour of hypotension, there was a survival rate of 79.9%. There was an approximate decrease in survival of 7.6% with each hour that antibiotic administration was delayed. The time to initiation of antimicrobial therapy was the strongest predictor of outcome.

3. Herran-Monge R, Muriel-Bombin A, Garcia-Garcia MM, et al. Epidemiology and changes in mortality of sepsis after the implementation of Surviving Sepsis Campaign guidelines. *J Intensive Care Med*. 2019;34(9):740–750.

   This was a prospective, multicenter, observational study comparing 262 patients with severe sepsis or septic shock to a historical cohort of 324 patients from 2002. The incidence of sepsis/septic shock did not change over the 10-year period, however, the implementation of the Surviving Sepsis Campaign guidelines resulted in a decrease in overall mortality. There was a lower severity of patients on ICU admission which suggests earlier diagnosis and management.

4. Rhodes A, Evans LE, Alhazzani W, et al. Surviving Sepsis Campaign: International guidelines for management of sepsis and septic shock: 2016. *Intensive Care Med*. 2017;43:304–377.

   These are the most recent Surviving Sepsis Campaign guidelines which provide evidence-based recommendations on early management and resuscitation of patients with sepsis or septic shock. There were recommendation provided based on graded evidence for the screening for sepsis, initial resuscitation, diagnosis, and antimicrobial therapy.

5. Levy MM, Evans LE, Rhodes A. The Surviving Sepsis Campaign bundle: 2018 update. *Crit Care Med*. 2018;46:997–1000.

   The authors review the elements of the 1-hour bundle in the treatment of sepsis.

6. Seymour CW, Gesten F, Prescott H, et al. Time to treatment and mortality during man-dated emergency care for sepsis. *N Engl J Med*. 2017;376:2235–2244.

There were 49,331 patients with sepsis or septic shock who were studied. Of these patients, 83% had the 3-hour sepsis bundle. The median time to completing the bundle was 1.3 hours, and the median time to administering antibiotics was 0.95 hours. The patients who received the antibiotics earlier on in their course and had the bundle completed more rapidly, had a lower risk-adjusted in-hospital mortality.

7. Jansen TC, van Bommel J, Schoonderbeek FJ, et al. Early lactate-guided therapy in inten-sive care unit patients: a multicenter, open-label, randomized controlled trial. *Am J Respir Crit Care Med*. 2010;182:752–761.

There were 348 ICU patients with a lactate level >3 mmol/L who were randomized to receive lactate-guided resuscitation or be managed without monitoring the lactate levels (control group). Patients in the lactate group had reduced hospital mortality rates compared to the control group.

8. Leibovici L, Shraga I, Drucker M, et al. The benefit of appropriate empirical antibiotic treatment in patients with bloodstream infection. *J Intern Med*. 1998;244(5):379–386.

This was a prospective observational cohort study evaluating the in-hospital mortal-ity rates and length of hospital stay in patients with bloodstream infections who either received appropriate empirical antibiotic therapy or inappropriate antibiotic therapy (the antibiotic regimen did not match the in vitro susceptibility of the pathogen). Of 3440 patients with bloodstream infections, 2158 received appropriate antibiotic therapy. The inappropriate antibiotic therapy group was associated with higher mortality rates.

9. Micek ST, Welch EC, Khan J, et al. Empiric combination antibiotic therapy is associated with improved outcome against sepsis due to Gram-negative bacteria: a retrospective analysis. *Antimicrob Agents Chemother*. 2010;54(5):1742–1748.

Seven-hundred-sixty ICU patients with severe sepsis or septic shock from gram-negative bacteremia were evaluated. Patients who received antibiotic regiments directed against gram-negative bacteria were less likely to receive inappropriate initial antimicrobial therapy compared to patients receiving antibiotic monotherapy.

10. Paul M, Lador A, Grozinsky-Glasberg S, et al. Beta lactam antibiotic monotherapy versus beta lactam-aminoglycoside antibiotic combination therapy for sepsis. *Cochrane Database Syst Rev*. 2014.

This was a systematic review of randomized controlled trials that compared patients with sepsis who received beta lactam monotherapy as their initial antibiotic therapy to those who received both beta lactam and an aminoglycoside. There were 69 studies with 7863 patients included in the analysis. There was no decrease in mortality and an increased risk of nephrotoxicity in the beta lactam and aminoglycoside group compared to the monotherapy group.

11. Jimenez MF, Marshall JC. Source control in the management of sepsis. *Intensive Care Med*. 2001;27:S49–S62.

There were evidence-based recommendations based on graded evidence provided on source control in the management of sepsis. There are recommendations provided as answers to common questions for source control management of sepsis.

12. Azuhata T, Kinoshita K, Kawano D, et al. Time from admission to initiation of surgery for source control is a critical determinant of survival in patients with gastrointestinal perfora-tion with associated septic shock. *Crit Care*. 2014;18(3):R87.

This was a prospective observational study evaluating 154 patients with GI perforation with septic shock. The time from admission to initiation of surgery for source control that was associated with more favorable outcomes was within 6 hours of admission.

Landmark Article of the 21st Century

DURATION OF HYPOTENSION BEFORE INITIATION OF EFFECTIVE ANTIMICROBIAL THERAPY IS THE CRITICAL DETERMINANT OF SURVIVAL IN HUMAN SEPTIC SHOCK

Kumar A et al., *Crit Care Med.* 2006;34:1589–1596

Commentary by Anand Kumar

Through the 1980s to the early 2000s, the landscape of septic shock therapy centered on the concept that septic shock was the consequence of an inflammatory mediator cascade initiated by, but ultimately divorced from, the triggering infection. As a consequence, fluid and vasopressor resuscitation was the priority with antimicrobial therapy a secondary concern. Because of the lack of benefit found with the many anti-mediator and immunomodulatory randomized controlled trials done to that point, we thought that the persistence of infection may play a more substantial role in driving the aberrant inflammatory response driving septic shock. Based on promising work in a murine animal model, we decided we'd look at this question in humans. Since a randomized controlled trial was not an ethical option, we decided to do a retrospective analysis of a comprehensive cohort of >2000 septic shock patients from 10 hospitals and 14 ICUs in Canada and the United States. This study showed that every hour delay in initiation of microbially appropriate antimicrobial therapy after documentation of hypotension results in an absolute decrease in survival of 7–8% per hour over the first 6 hours. Multiple high quality observational studies since that time have reinforced the observation. Other studies have consistently shown that the most impactful element in septic shock bundles is rapid administration of antimicrobials. The Surviving Sepsis Campaign guidelines from 2006 onward have consistently recommended antimicrobial initiation within the first hour of septic shock. Although the question of the need for similarly rapid antimicrobials for sepsis without shock remains uncertain, a broad consensus in favor of early initiation of antimicrobials in septic shock is now well established.

CHAPTER 28

Sepsis II: Monitoring and Resuscitation

Review by Shahla Siddiqui

The word sepsis is derived from the Greek word for "decomposition" or "decay," and its first documented use was about 2700 years ago in Homer's poems. Sepsis and septic shock have remained a persistent and recurrent source of mortality in surgical ICU patients. Sepsis and infections have been recognized as a perplexing cause of mortality since at least 1000 BC. In early Muslim, Roman, and European literature, scientists and scholars and then physicians have struggled with the pathophysiology and treatment of sepsis. Currently more than 33 million cases occur yearly with roughly 5 million annual deaths. These are simply very rough estimates from mostly Western countries as the true estimates remain uncertain [1]. During the current COVID-19 pandemic these rates have risen exponentially. Despite a dramatic increase in our understanding of sepsis, its origins, progression and resolution, our ability to treat and diagnose the disease has been only partially successful. The mortality from sepsis still remains close to 50%. Although in-hospital mortality from sepsis has declined over the past decade, this improvement is the result of the advances made for early diagnosis and treatment of underlying causes of sepsis, as well as better compliance with best-practice supportive therapies.

The manifestations of sepsis and evolution of septic shock can no longer be attributed only to the infectious agent and the immune response it creates, but also to significant alterations in coagulation, immunosuppression, and organ dysfunction. Many sepsis patients develop profound hypotension and can quickly have multi-organ failure including acute kidney injury, acute respiratory distress syndrome, and liver failure. They may also have dysregulated coagulation [2].

The first modern definition was given by Hugo Schottmüller in 1914 who wrote that "sepsis is present if a focus has developed from which pathogenic bacteria, constantly or periodically, invade the blood stream in such a way that this causes subjective and objective symptoms." Over the century, numerous trials were able to demonstrate the importance of the host immune response and its suppression to the clinical manifestations of sepsis. However, due to the vast heterogeneity of the disease process, it posed serious challenges in diagnosing, managing and treating sepsis. Finally, at a SCCM-ACCP conference in 1991, Roger Bone and his colleagues laid the foundation for the first consensus definition of sepsis [3]. There have been significant advances in the pathobiology of sepsis in the last two decades. We have a better understanding of cell biology, biochemistry, immunology, and morphology, as well as changes in circulation and organ function. This understanding has led to the changes in the definition of sepsis.

DOI: 10.1201/9781003042136-28

Development of scores such as the APACHE-II and sequential organ failure assessment (SOFA) have provided simple but useful clinical tools in the assessment and prognostication of sepsis [4].

The third international consensus definition developed by a task force is that "Sepsis is a life-threatening organ dysfunction caused by dysregulated host response to infection." Suspected or documented infection and an acute increase of ≥2 SOFA points. The task force considered that positive qSOFA (quick SOFA) criteria should also prompt consideration of possible infection in patients not previously recognized as infected [5].

A revolutionary change in the way we manage sepsis has been the adoption of early goal-directed therapy (EGDT). A concept introduced by Rivers and colleagues in 2001. This involves the early identification of at-risk patients and prompt treatment with antibiotics, hemodynamic optimization, and appropriate supportive care. Although early recognition and treatment remains the cornerstone of sepsis management, further well-designed trials have shown that there was no difference in mortality between EGDT and standard management. This finding was confirmed in the 2014 ARISE and 2015 ProMISe trials. Other criticisms of the Rivers trial was that it was single center and the ED staff were not blinded to the treatment arms [6].

Surviving Sepsis Campaign guidelines from 2004, have incorporated the EGDT into the first 6-hour sepsis resuscitation bundle, although it has been found to increase resource demand unnecessarily without reducing mortality, length of stay, or organ dysfunction. However, this initial trial by Rivers changed how we manage sepsis and septic shock care. Timed and urgent fluid and antibiotic initiation, and setting short and long term goals in the initial and 24-hour management of patients were introduced, and was subsequently incorporated in the SSC guidelines [7]. The 2019 updated SSC guidelines have combined the 3-hour and 6-hour bundle into the 1-hour bundle which includes: 1) measure lactate level, 2) obtain blood cultures before administering antibiotics, 3) administer broad spectrum antibiotics, 4) begin rapid administration of crystalloid at 30 mL/kg for hypotension (MAP <65) or lactate >4 mmol/L, 5) apply vasopressors (with noradrenaline being the optimal choice) if hypotension before or during fluid resuscitation to maintain MAP. Remeasure lactate if >2 mmol/L [8]. Also, an integral part of sepsis treatment remains early source control and identification. This could include surgical management, such as drainage of an abscess, removal of the offending viscera such as inflamed appendix, or gallbladder, or a gangrenous extremity.

Sepsis and septic shock remain a major source of morbidity and mortality in the surgical ICU. Early recognition and treatment have improved outcomes dramatically over the past century; however, implementation of the guidelines, bundles, and standards of care remain an uphill struggle, especially in the third world. COVID-19 sepsis and shock present a myriad new complications such as severe hypoxemia with normal lung compliance and generalized micro-clots in the circulation resulting in pulmonary emboli or strokes in addition to the inflammatory storm seen with other types of sepsis and septic shock states. Profound and long lasting myocarditis has also been described. Whilst sepsis remains a significant burden on health systems worldwide, the advances made in understanding its pathogenesis and the extensive efforts at providing guidelines for its effective management in the past 20 years exceed anything that has been done before. Early recognition and targeted management remain the pillars of treatment goals for sepsis and septic shock [9].

ANNOTATED REFERENCES FOR SEPSIS II: MONITORING AND RESUSCITATION

1. Funk DJ, Parrillo JE, Kumar A. Sepsis and septic shock: a history. *Crit Care Clin.* 2009; 125(1):83–101.

   The authors provide a historical perspective of the name and understanding of sepsis.

2. Beal AL, Cerra FB. Multiple organ failure syndrome in the 1990s: systemic inflammatory response and organ dysfunction. *JAMA.* 1994;271(3):226–233.

   The authors review the pathophysiology of SIRS and MODS, and emphasize definitions, common clinical patterns, metabolic responses, and pathophysiological changes. A brief discussion of treatment concepts is also included.

3. Bone RC, Balk RA, Cerra FB, et al. Definitions for sepsis and organ failure and guidelines for the use of innovative therapies in sepsis: the ACCP/SCCM consensus conference committee. American College of Chest Physicians/Society of Critical Care Medicine. *Chest.* 1992;101(6):1644–1655.

   The first consensus definition of sepsis with collaboration from the American College of Critical Care Medicine and the Society of Critical Care Medicine.

4. Vincent JL, Moreno R, Takala J, et al. Working group on sepsis-related problems of the European Society of Intensive Care Medicine: the SOFA (Sepsis-related Organ Failure Assessment) score to describe organ dysfunction/failure. *Intensive Care Med.* 1996;22(7):707–710.

   The authors provide a validated use of the SOFA score to assess the incidence of organ dysfunction/failure in intensive care units: results of a multicenter, prospective study. This was a working group on "sepsis- related problems" of the European Society of Intensive Care Medicine.

5. Singer M, Deutschman CS, Seymour CW, et al. The third international consensus definitions for sepsis and septic shock (Sepsis-3). *JAMA.* 2016;315(8):801–810.

   The third and latest iteration of the definition based on further understanding of the disease pathogenesis and etiology.

6. Nguyen HB, Jaehne AK, Jayaprakash N, et al. Early goal-directed therapy in severe sepsis and septic shock: insights and comparisons to ProCESS, ProMISe, and ARISE. *Crit Care.* 2016;20(1):160.

   The authors compare three large RCTs comparing EGDT and standard care and found no significant difference between them. While reporting an all-time low sepsis mortality, the authors question the continued need for all of the elements of early goal-directed therapy or the need for protocolized care for patients with severe and septic shock.

7. Rhodes A, Evans LE, Alhazzani W, et al. Surviving Sepsis Campaign: International guidelines for management of sepsis and septic shock: 2016. *Intensive Care Med.* 2017 Mar;43(3):304–377. doi: 10.1007/s00134-017-4683-6. Epub 2017 Jan 18.

   The authors present the international consensus guidelines for management of sepsis and the recent inclusion of the new sepsis definition. Here the 3- and 6-hour bundles are combined into the 1-hour bundle.

8. Levy MM, Evans LE, Rhodes A. The Surviving Sepsis Campaign bundle: 2018 update. *Intensive Care Med.* 2018 Jun;44(6):925–928. doi: 10.1007/s00134-018-5085-0. Epub 2018 Apr 19.

   Here the 3- and 6-hour sepsis bundles are combined into the 1-hour bundle.

9. Rivers E, Nguyen B, Havstad S, et al. Early goal-directed therapy in the treatment of severe sepsis and septic shock. *N Engl J Med.* 2001;345(19):1368–1377.

Landmark Article of the 21st Century

EARLY GOAL-DIRECTED THERAPY IN THE TREATMENT OF SEVERE SEPSIS AND SEPTIC SHOCK

Rivers E et al., *N Engl J Med.* 2001 NOV 8;345(19):1368–1377

Commentary by Emanuel P. Rivers

Almost 20 years ago, early goal directed therapy (EGDT) challenged the existing paradigm of sepsis care by expanding the landscape to the most proximal aspect of hospital presentation. At that time sepsis was considered an "intensive care unit (ICU) disease." The reality was that the majority of patients admitted to the ICU were from the emergency department (ED) after experiencing long durations of stay. The principles of EGDT was developed from prior work of numerous pioneers in sepsis, critical care, and shock resuscitation. These principles included early identification using the systemic inflammatory response syndrome (SIRS), risk stratification (lactate), antibiotics, source control, and hemodynamic optimization. There was no standard for early sepsis care at that time [1]. The study of EGDT simply compared a systems based approach using these principles (similar to acute myocardial infarction, stroke and trauma) to existing standard care [1]. The outcome benefit was a reduction in mortality from 46.5% to 30.5%, never seen in previous sepsis trials. Since the publication of the EGDT trial, the external validity, reliability, and feasibility of this approach to sepsis care have been replicated in both the clinical and public health circles [2, 3]. Significant scientific interest was generated to question the outcome benefit of EGDT as a whole and its individual components (systemic inflammatory response syndrome [SIRS], antibiotics, lactate, fluids, vasopressors, central venous pressure, and central venous oxygen saturation). All have been shown to contribute in the mortality reduction of sepsis in part or as a whole when accompanied by a continuous quality improvement initiative [3]. Two decades later, a systems based approach to early sepsis care or EGDT has been shown to decrease sepsis mortality internationally. As a result, EGDT has been shown to be a verb—series of actions—and not a noun.

REFERENCES

1. Rivers E, Nguyen B, Havstad S, et al. Early goal-directed therapy in the treatment of severe sepsis and septic shock. *N Engl J Med.* 2001;345(19):1368–1377.
2. Nguyen HB, Jaehne AK, Jayaprakash N, et al. Early goal-directed therapy in severe sepsis and septic shock: insights and comparisons to ProCESS, ProMISe, and ARISE. *Crit Care.* 2016;20(1):1–16.
3. Levy MM, Gesten FC, Phillips GS, et al. Mortality changes associated with mandated public reporting for sepsis: the results of the New York State initiative. *Am J Respir Crit Care Med.* 2018;198(11):1406–1412.

CHAPTER 29

Steroids in Septic Shock

Review by Philip Chan and Somnath Bose

INTRODUCTION

Septic shock is a state of dysregulated response to an infection, resulting in circulatory, cellular and metabolic abnormalities associated with life-threatening organ dysfunction. Corticosteroids may dampen pro-inflammatory over-activity, improve cardiovascular function and response to catecholamines [1]. Early studies on high dose steroids demonstrated a reduction in mortality by 25–30% (2); however, follow-up studies found no difference possibly attributable to secondary infections [3, 4]. Subsequently, lower doses have been suggested to be beneficial in treating a presumed critical illness-related corticosteroid deficiency (CIRCI), but it remains unclear whether steroids improve patient-centered outcomes in septic shock.

EVIDENCE

In 2002, Annane et al. found that among septic shock patients refractory to vasopressors and with CIRCI, steroids prolonged the median time to death from 12 to 24 days [5]. Corticosteroids also accelerated the time to vasopressor weaning from 10 to 7 days in non-responders of corticotropin test. Though commonly referenced, 28-day mortality in non-responders was only significant after an adjusted mortality analysis, despite baseline characteristics being similar between two groups (53% vs. 63%, RR 0.83, 95%CI 0.66–1.04. Adjusted OR 0.54, 95%CI 0.31–0.91, $p = 0.04$).

Despite the stated intention to study all patients regardless of corticotropin response, the CORTICUS trial was powered to detect a mortality difference among non-responders [6]. There was no difference in 28-day mortality in the hydrocortisone group among non-responders or responders, but median time to shock reversal was shorter by 2.5 days in all patients with steroids. Of note, this trial was underpowered because actual mortality was lower than estimated, and enrollment did not achieve the initial target recruitment of 800 participants.

Since the two largest trials to date diverged in survival benefits, Annane et al. randomized 1241 septic shock patients requiring ≥0.25 mcg/kg/min of norepinephrine to either hydrocortisone plus fludrocortisone or placebo in the APROCCHSS trial [7]. The authors found a significant reduction in 90-day mortality in the steroid group (43.0% vs. 49.1%), but with a fragility index of just 3. Multiple secondary outcomes, including vasopressor-free days, organ-failure-free days, ICU and hospital mortality, were also in favor of the intervention group.

The ADRENAL trial randomized 3800 participants who required vasopressors for at least 4 hours to either hydrocortisone infusion or placebo [8]. There was no difference in either primary outcome of 90-day mortality or secondary 28-day mortality. However, steroids reduced time to shock resolution by 1 day, time of initial ventilation by 1 day, and time to ICU discharge by 2 days. The steroid group had more adverse events (1.1% vs. 0.3%, $p = 0.009$; 4 of 6 serious events).

A Cochrane review was updated in 2019 and summarized 61 trials involving 12,192 total participants and concluded that corticosteroids probably slightly reduced 28-day mortality, ICU stay (by 1 day), and hospital stay (by 1.5 days), and increased the rate of shock reversal at day seven [9]. Two other meta-analyses in 2018 also concluded that corticosteroids may achieve a small reduction in short-term mortality and time to resolution of shock [10, 11].

COMPARISON OF TRIALS

Severity of Illness: It is important to realize the patient populations of these four major trials were not identical. The initial Annane trial enrolled patients who had persistent hypotension despite vasopressors, requiring about 1.0 mcg/kg/min of norepinephrine, and with SAPS II scores of 60. Similarly, the patient cohort in APROCCHSS was required to have ≥0.25 mcg/kg/min of norepinephrine for 6 hours (91% received about 1.08 mcg/kg/min) and SAPS II scores were around 56.

In comparison, CORTICUS enrolled patients on any amount of vasopressor, requiring about a maximum of 0.5 mcg/kg/min norepinephrine and with SAPS II scores of 50. Similarly, the participants in ADRENAL required on average 30 mcg/min of norepinephrine on day one. The hydrocortisone group in the >15 mcg/min subgroup (45.7% of total patients) trended toward improved mortality (33.1% vs. 36.1%).

Mortality at 28 days in placebo groups appear to be consistent with the observation that the study populations were dissimilar in severity of illness (61% in Annane, 38.9% in APROCCHSS, 31.5% in CORTICUS, and 24.3% in ADRENAL). In a post-hoc analysis of ADRENAL participants who fulfilled either Sepsis-3 definition or APROCCHSS inclusion criteria, there was no effect of hydrocortisone despite overall 90-day mortality being higher [12].

Timing: Proponents of corticosteroid therapy emphasize that the timing of treatment is crucial. Inclusion criteria in the original Annane study required participants to be within 8 hours of shock onset. In contrast, the CORTICUS study included patients up to 72 hours of shock onset, but 77% of participants received the study drug within 12 hours and authors reported no between-group difference among this subgroup.

Both APROCCHSS and ADRENAL excluded patients outside 24 hours of shock onset. In ADRENAL, the median time from shock onset to randomization was 21 hours, and from randomization to starting study drug was 0.8 hours. There was an improvement in 90-day mortality with hydrocortisone in the subgroup that was randomized within 6–12 hours from shock onset, but there were no differences in the <6-hour group. Timing of steroid therapy continues to be a potential confounder and source of heterogeneity in trials.

Identifying CIRCI: The Annane trial's positive outcomes were among those identified to have CIRCI. Despite mortality being higher among non-responders in CORTICUS and APROCCHSS, there were no between-group differences among responders or non-responders in either trial. ADRENAL did not utilize the corticotropin test. In the Cochrane meta-analysis, the subgroup of CIRCI did not have an improvement in mortality with corticosteroids. Corticotropin response has not been found to reliably diagnose CIRCI or consistently reflect severity of illness, likely due to multiple confounders and variability in methodology and interpretation [13].

CONCLUSION

The use of corticosteroids in septic shock continues to be a controversial issue with inconsistent data on short and long-term mortality. Steroids appear to benefit patients with high vasopressor requirements and higher illness severity scores regardless of response to corticotropin test. Given its safety at low dosages, early administration of corticosteroids may be a reasonable strategy in septic shock to accelerate weaning off vasopressors, reducing ICU days, and potentially reduce short-term mortality.

ANNOTATED REFERENCES FOR STEROIDS IN SEPTIC SHOCK

1. Annane D. The role of ACTH and corticosteroids for sepsis and septic shock: an update. *Front Endocrinol.* 2016;7.

   Review of rationale behind mechanism of disrupted HPA axis, corticosteroids effect on cardiovascular and organ function, and potential complications.

2. Schumer W. Steroids in the treatment of clinical septic shock. *Ann Surg.* 1979;184(3):333–9.

   Early double-blinded, placebo-controlled, three-arm trial over a 9 year period (1967–1976) of short-course high-dose 30 mg/kg methylprednisolone, 6 mg/kg dexamethasone, and placebo, which demonstrated a 25–30% improvement in mortality among 172 septic VA patients and a subsequent retrospective review of 328 patients.

3. Sprung CL, Caralis PV, Marcial EH, et al. The effects of high-dose corticosteroids in patients with septic shock. *N Engl J Med.* 1984;311(18):1137–43.

   Double-blinded, placebo-controlled, three-arm trial at Miami hospitals in 1979–1982 found that methylprednisolone and dexamethasone improved shock reversal at 24 hours and mortality at 133 hours but subsequently disappeared around 200 hours. Dexamethasone significantly increased rate of superinfections.

4. Bone RC, Fisher CJ, Clemmer TP, Slotman GJ, Metz CA, Balk RA. A controlled clinical trial of high-dose methylprednisolone in the treatment of severe sepsis and septic shock. *N Engl J Med*. 1987;317(11):653–8.

Double-blinded, placebo-controlled, multi-center randomized trial in the US from 1982–1985, found that high-dose methylprednisolone did not improve shock prevention, shock reversal, and overall mortality. Steroids increased mortality in subgroup of kidney failure and increased mortality related to secondary infections.

5. Annane D, Sébille V, Charpentier C, et al. Effect of treatment with low doses of hydrocortisone and fludrocortisone on mortality in patients with septic shock. *JAMA*. 2002;288(7):862–71.

A multi-center, double-blinded, parallel group randomized trial in France found that hydrocortisone and fludrocortisone prolonged the median time to death in participants with relative adrenal insufficiency, and hypotension despite fluids and vasopressors, within 8 hours of septic shock onset. This trial was powered in a 1-sided test to detect a 20% reduction in mortality with corticosteroids in non-responders, assuming a baseline mortality rate of 95% in the placebo group. Steroids prolonged primary outcome of median time to death from 12 to 24 days (HR 0.67, 95%CI 0.47–0.95, p = 0.02) and reduced median time to vasopressor withdrawal in non-responders (7 vs. 10 days, HR 1.91, 95%CI 1.29–2.84, p = 0.001) and all patients (7 vs. 9 days, HR 1.54, 95%CI 1.10–2.16, p = 0.01).

6. Sprung CL, Annane D, Keh D, et al. Hydrocortisone therapy for patients with septic shock. *N Engl J Med*. 2008;358(2):111–24.

The Corticosteroid Therapy for Septic Shock (CORTICUS) trial was an international, double-blinded, randomized, placebo-controlled study that found hydrocortisone 50 mg every 6 hours for 5 days tapered to day 12 in septic shock requiring vasopressors did not have an effect on 28-day mortality (non-responders 39.2% vs. 36.1%, p = 0.69), but was likely underpowered. The median time until shock reversal was shorter in the hydrocortisone group for all patients (3.3 vs. 5.8 days, p <0.001). Separate outcomes of new sepsis or septic shock were combined post-hoc and found to be increased in the intervention group (OR 1.37, 95%CI 1.05–1.79).

7. Annane D, Renault A, Brun-Buisson C, et al. Hydrocortisone plus fludrocortisone for adults with septic shock. *N Engl J Med*. 2018;378(9):809–18.

The Activated Protein C and Corticosteroids for Human Septic Shock (APROCCHSS) trial was a multi-center, double-blinded, randomized, placebo-controlled study that found steroids reduced 90-day mortality (43.0% vs. 49.1%, RR 0.88, 95%CI 0.78-0.99, p = 0.03), but fragility index of 3. It was initially designed to evaluate hydrocortisone plus fludrocortisone and drotrecogin alfa in a 2-by-2 factorial design, but continued with two parallel groups when drotrecogin alfa was withdrawn.

8. Venkatesh B, Finfer S, Cohen J, et al. Adjunctive glucocorticoid therapy in patients with septic shock. *N Engl J Med*. 2018;378(9):797–808.

The Adjunctive Corticosteroid Treatment in Critically Ill Patients with Septic Shock (ADRENAL) trial was an international, double-blinded, randomized, placebo-controlled, parallel-group study with enough patients to provide 90% power to detect a 5% absolute risk reduction, from a baseline mortality rate of 33%. The intervention was hydrocortisone infusion 200 mg per day for 7 days without fludrocortisone. Time to randomization was 21 hours on average (19.1% <6 hours, 27.4% 6–12 hours, 23.6% 12–18 hours, 29.9%

>18 hours). There were no differences in 90-day (27.9% vs. 28.8%, p = 0.50), or 28-day mortality but steroids improved median days to shock resolution (3 vs. 4 days, HR 1.32; 95%CI 1.23–1.41, P ≤0.001), time to cessation of initial ventilation (6 vs. 7 days, HR 1.13; 95%CI 1.05–1.22, P ≤0.001), time to discharge from ICU (10 vs. 12 days, HR 1.14, 95%CI 1.06–1.23, P ≤0.001) and number of transfusions (37.0% vs. 41.7%, OR 0.82; 95%CI 0.72–0.94, P = 0.004). Four of six serious adverse events were in steroid group (two myopathy, one ischemic bowel and one circulatory shock). Long-term neuromuscular weakness was not assessed. Interestingly, only Australia out of all other regions had an improvement in 28-day mortality (19.9% vs. 23.3%, OR 0.82, 95%CI 0.68–0.98) and trended towards improvement in 90-day mortality with steroids.

9. Annane D, Bellissant E, Bollaert PE, et al. Corticosteroids for treating sepsis in children and adults. *Cochrane Database Syst Rev.* 2019.

   Cochrane review updated in 2019 and summarized the effects of 61 trials in sepsis involving 12,192 total participants and concluded that corticosteroids probably slightly reduce 28-day mortality (RR 0.91, 95%CI 0.84–0.99, p = 0.04; 11,233 participants; 50 studies; moderate certainty), reduced ICU and hospital length of stay, with a mean difference of about 1 day and 1.5 days, and increased the number of participants with shock reversal at day 7. The subgroup of CIRCI did not have an improvement in mortality with corticosteroids (RR 0.92, 95%CI 0.82–1.03, p = 0.16; 1079 participants; 12 studies; I² = 0%). There was an increased the risk of muscle weakness, hypernatremia, and hyperglycemia.

10. Fang F, Zhang Y, Tang J, et al. Association of corticosteroid treatment with outcomes in adult patients with sepsis. *JAMA Intern Med.* 2019;179(2):213.

    Recent systematic review and meta-analysis of corticosteroid therapy in patients with sepsis is associated with reduction in 28-day mortality (RR 0.90, 95%CI 0.82–0.98; I² = 27%), ICU and in-hospital mortality, ICU length of stay, SOFA at day 7 and time to resolution of shock.

11. Rochwerg B, Oczkowski SJ, Siemieniuk RAC, et al. Corticosteroids in sepsis. *Crit Care Med.* 2018;46(9):1411–20.

    Recent systematic review and meta-analysis found that corticosteroids may achieve a small reduction or no reduction in short-term mortality (RR 0.93, 95%CI 0.84–1.03; 1.8% absolute risk reduction), small effect on long-term mortality (RR 0.94, 95%CI 0.89–1.00; 2.2% absolute risk reduction), small reductions in length of stay in ICU and hospital, higher rates of shock reversal at day 7, lower SOFA scores at day 7, and higher risk of hypernatremia, hyperglycemia, and neuromuscular weakness.

12. Venkatesh B, Finfer S, Cohen J, et al. Hydrocortisone compared with placebo in patients with septic shock satisfying the sepsis-3 diagnostic criteria and APROCCHSS study inclusion criteria. *Anesthesiology.* 2019;131(6):1292–300.

    In a post-hoc analysis of ADRENAL participants who fulfilled either sepsis-3 definition or APROCCHSS inclusion criteria, overall mortality rates at 90 days were higher, but there was no effect of hydrocortisone regardless of analysis with either odds ratio or rate ratio.

13. Venkatesh B, Cohen J. The utility of the corticotropin test to diagnose adrenal insufficiency in critical illness: an update. *Clin Endocrinol.* 2015;83(3):289–97.

    Review of evidence concluding that the use of corticotropin test in assessing adrenocortical function and guiding steroid therapy in critically ill patients is limited due to several confounding variables, methodology differences, and lack of relationship between the test and severity of illness.

Landmark Article of the 21st Century

ADJUNCTIVE GLUCOCORTICOID THERAPY IN PATIENTS WITH SEPTIC SHOCK

Venkatesh B et al., *N Engl J Med*. 2018 MAR 1;378(9):797–808

Commentary by Stephen Heard

The ADRENAL study was an investigator initiated, prospective, multicenter, randomized study of patients with septic shock (n = 3800) to determine if administration of 200 mg of hydrocortisone per day as a continuous infusion for 7 days or to death or discharge from the ICU would result in a lower 90-day mortality rate compared to placebo. Although resolution from shock was faster in the steroid treated group, there was no difference in either 28-day or 90-day mortality. Duration of mechanical ventilation was lower and time to ICU discharge was shorter in the steroid treated group. Need for transfusion was lower in the steroid group. More adverse events were observed in the study group. The findings from this study support those from previous studies and are in line with international guidelines for the use of steroids in septic shock.

However, in the same issue of the *New England Journal of Medicine* was another study (APROCCHSS) where patients (n = 1241) with septic shock were treated with either placebo or hydrocortisone plus fludrocortisone. (Drotrecogin alfa was initially included in the 2 × 2 study design but was dropped when the drug was removed from the market.) The investigators found that treatment with 50 mg of IV hydrocortisone every 6 hours and 50 mg of fludrocortisone via nasogastric tube every day resulted in lower 90-day mortality. In addition, vasopressor-free and organ-failure-free days were significantly higher in the steroid group.

Differences in patient populations and severity of illness may explain some of the differences in results between the two studies. However, at a minimum, the findings from these studies support the use of hydrocortisone in patients with septic shock. The use of a mineralocorticoid may be an important adjunct to reduce mortality.

CHAPTER 30

Treatment of Abdominal Sepsis

Review by Addison K. May

Abdominal sepsis is a common clinical condition requiring management in the intensive care unit (ICU) and may present significant diagnostic and management challenges. The core principles of therapy include appropriate and timely resuscitation, antimicrobial therapy, and source control; each impacting the outcome of critically ill patients with abdominal sepsis. Recognition by the intensivist and surgeon that critically ill patients with intraabdominal infections have significant risk of failure of source control and anastomotic disruption despite achieving these core principles is critical to successful management [1].

For ICU patients with sepsis and septic shock, the abdomen is a common source of infection, ranking second behind pulmonary sources [2, 3]. Although a variety of etiologies can cause intraabdominal infections, secondary peritonitis from bowel perforation and bowel ischemia/infarction together causes nearly 50% cases of abdominal sepsis [2]. Other causes include spontaneous bacterial peritonitis, *Clostridium difficile* colitis, intraabdominal abscess, hepatobiliary sources such as cholangitis, cholecystitis, and hepatic abscess, and infected necrotizing pancreatitis. As with other causes of sepsis and septic shock, time to appropriate resuscitation and appropriate empiric antibiotic therapy significantly alters the outcome. In large observational studies, each 30 minute delay in antibiotic therapy for patients with abdominal sepsis and shock is associated with a 12% increase in mortality and adequate empiric antibiotic therapy independently associated with survival (odds ratio ~9) [2, 3].

Appropriate selection of empiric antibiotics requires an understanding of likely pathogens involved and the implications if some pathogens remain uncovered. Most intraabdominal infections are due to enteric bacteria. Community acquired secondary peritonitis is typically polymicrobial with facultative and aerobic gram-negative, gram-positive, and anaerobic organisms. *Escherichia coli* is most common, isolated in nearly three quarters of cases. *Klebsiella* spp. and *Pseudomonas aeruginosa* are isolated in 10–20% of cases with other gram-negative bacteria isolated less frequently. Even in community acquired infections, extended spectrum beta-lactamase positive enteric pathogens are present roughly 10% of cases. Species of *Bacteroides* are involved in greater than three quarters of cases and *Streptococcus* spp. in over one third. For critically ill patients, empiric therapy should be directed to include all these pathogens with either single agent or combination therapy. Single agent recommendations include imipenem/cilastatin, doripenem, meropenem, or piperacillin/tazobactam. Combination regimens include cefepime or ceftazidime in combination with metronidazole. A fluoroquinolone in combination with metronidazole had been recommended in the past, but increasing resistance among *E. coli* requires that local sensitivity should be considered in choosing these agents. Patient severity of illness increases the importance of covering microorganisms with less virulence and pathogenic potential increases. *Enterococcus* spp. and yeast can be isolated with relative frequency in secondary peritonitis. While in non-critically ill patients, antimicrobial coverage of these pathogens does not alter outcome, doing so in critically ill patients does and coverage of both microbes should be considered.

Prior antibiotic exposure greatly increases the likelihood of resistant pathogens, particularly to the previous agents used and antibiotic history should be considered. Patients with recurrent or persistent peritonitis (tertiary peritonitis) and with nosocomial infections have an increased prevalence of resistant gram-negative pathogens, *Enterococcus* spp., methicillin resistant *Staphylococcus aureus* (MRSA), and yeast typically requiring three agents to achieve appropriate coverage of pathogens.

In addition to appropriate and timely resuscitation and antimicrobial therapy, time to source control has a very significant association with outcome. Definitive source control includes three components: 1) elimination of infectious foci and reduction of bacterial burden 2) the removal of diseased or non-viable material and control/closure of enterostomies, and 3) correct or control anatomic derangements to restore normal physiologic function.

While significant organ dysfunction or septic shock is present in the minority of cases of peritonitis (5% of patients with peritonitis), those with organ dysfunction and/or septic shock are at significantly greater risk of both failure of source control and mortality (relative risk—19) [1, 4]. For this summary, failure of source control is defined as persistent or recurrent intraabdominal infection and/or anastomotic failure in the setting of technically appropriate source control procedures. Failure of source control in this setting represents an altered ability to clear pathogens and heal anastomoses. Several patient factors present on ICU admission are independently associated with subsequent failure of source control following treatment of peritonitis, most of which reflect severity of illness, including high APACHE score, low serum albumin, need for vasoactive/inotropic support, degree of peritoneal inflammation/contamination, and age. An analysis of a randomized trial of antibiotic therapy treating peritonitis demonstrated that an APACHE II score of ≥15 was associated with a 50% rate of failed source control [5]. While no prediction tools for failure of source control have been validated for clinical practice, recognizing that patients requiring vasoactive support and with significant organ dysfunction in the perioperative period may have source control failure rates exceeding 50% is critical for appropriate management.

Critically ill abdominal sepsis patients with failure of source control present significant diagnostic challenges. Timely recognition of failed source control and intervention are associated with improved outcomes [6]. Fever and leukocytosis add minimally to the diagnosis, both common in the post-operative period, yet roughly 40% of post-operative patients with infectious complications do not have an elevated white blood cell count and greater than 50% will not manifest a fever [7]. Several clinical features present in post-operative period are associated with the existence of failed source control including persistence or progression of organ dysfunction, post-operative tachycardia, fever, persistence of ileus, and elevation of C-reactive protein beyond post-operative day 2. Their presence in high-risk patients requires evaluation for failed source control.

While timely initiation of empiric antibiotics is associated with improved outcomes, extending the length of antibiotic therapy does not improve outcomes and delays recognition of failed source control. In a landmark study, Sawyer and colleagues demonstrated that a fixed course of 4–5 days of antibiotic therapy had a similar outcome to longer antibiotic therapeutic courses even with persistent signs of inflammation [8]. These findings occurred in both low and high severity of illness groups and have been confirmed in subsequent studies.

ANNOTATED REFERENCES FOR TREATMENT OF ABDOMINAL SEPSIS

1. Mazuski JE, Tessier JM, May AK, et al. The Surgical Infection Society revised guidelines on the management of intra-abdominal infection. *Surg Infect (Larchmt).* 2017;18(1):1–76.

   The most recent revision of the Surgical Infection Society's Guidelines on the management of intraabdominal infections. Reviews and provides a reference for the diagnosis, treatment, and management including critically ill patients with abdominal sepsis and risk factors for mortality and failure of source control.

2. Kumar A, Roberts D, Wood KE, et al. Duration of hypotension before initiation of effective antimicrobial therapy is the critical determinant of survival in human septic shock. *Crit Care Med.* 2006;34(6):1589–96.

   A retrospective cohort study performed in 14 ICUs in Canada and the United States of 2731 patients with septic shock. Includes a significant portion of patients with abdominal sepsis and demonstrates a pronounced association of time to initiation of antimicrobial therapy with survival.

3. Kumar A, Ellis P, Arabi Y, et al. Initiation of inappropriate antimicrobial therapy results in a five-fold reduction of survival in human septic shock. *Chest.* 2009;136(5):1237–48.

   A 10 year retrospective analysis of 5715 patients with septic shock admitted to 22 medical centers in Canada, the United States, and Saudi Arabia, examining the impact of inappropriate empiric antimicrobial therapy on outcome. Includes a large cohort of abdominal sepsis patients and demonstrates a very strong association of inappropriate therapy with survival.

4. Anaya DA, Nathens AB. Risk factors for severe sepsis in secondary peritonitis. *Surg Infect (Larchmt).* 2003;4(4):355–62.

   A retrospective analysis of 11,202 patients with peritonitis from a statewide dataset to determine the incidence of and risk factors for severe sepsis in abdominal sepsis. Multivariate analysis was performed to estimate the impact of sepsis on outcome.

5. Barie PS, Vogel SB, Dellinger EP, et al. A randomized, double-blind clinical trial comparing cefepime plus metronidazole with imipenem-cilastatin in the treatment of complicated intra-abdominal infections. Cefepime Intra-abdominal Infection Study Group. *Arch Surg.* 1997;132(12):1294–302.

In an analysis of a randomized, double-blind trial examining 2 antibiotic regimens including 350 patients from 17 centers in the US and Canada, APACHE II and prolonged pre-study length of hospitalization as the only two independent risk factors for treatment failure. Demonstrates the high rate of failure of source control when patients have high APACHE II scores.

6. Koperna T, Schulz F. Relaparotomy in peritonitis: prognosis and treatment of patients with persisting intraabdominal infection. *World J Surg.* 2000;24(1):32–7.

Retrospective case-control study including 105 patients who required relaparotomy for failed source control. The authors identify risk factors for failure of source control and that delay in relaparotomy beyond 48 hours in patients with failed source control was associated with increased mortality.

7. Crabtree TD, Pelletier SJ, Antevil JL, Gleason TG, Pruett TL, Sawyer RG. Cohort study of fever and leukocytosis as diagnostic and prognostic indicators in infected surgical patients. *World J Surg.* 2001;25(6):739–44.

Prospective, 1-year, single center observational study of all surgical patients suspected of having an infectious complication to examine the incidence of fever and leukocytosis and their diagnostic and prognostic value.

8. Sawyer RG, Claridge JA, Nathens AB, et al. Trial of short-course antimicrobial therapy for intraabdominal infection. *N Engl J Med.* 2015;372(21):1996–2005.

Landmark Surgical Infection Society sponsored randomized trial examining two different periods of antibiotic therapy following source control in complicated intra-abdominal infections; a fixed duration of antibiotic therapy (4+/- 1 calendar days) versus duration 2 days beyond resolution of fever, leukocytosis, and ileus for a maximum of 10 days.

Landmark Article of the 21st Century

TRIAL OF SHORT-COURSE ANTIMICROBIAL THERAPY FOR INTRAABDOMINAL INFECTION

Sawyer RG et al., *N Engl J Med.* 2015 MAY 21;372(21):1996–2005

Commentary by Robert Sawyer

The 1990s saw the acknowledgment of the importance of two significant concepts in surgical infection: The primacy of source control and the realization that the host inflammatory response could still be severe even after the causative organisms had been killed by antimicrobial agents. A logical consequence of this thought process was the questioning of how long it took for bacteria to be adequately diminished to the point where the host response itself could eradicate the residual infection without any more antibiotics.

Intraabdominal infections are the most important infections treated by surgeons. As such, the Surgical Infection Society worked to develop a study with a unique design, comparing a fixed duration of antibiotic therapy (4 days) versus what was felt to be the standard of care at that time, continuing antibiotics until fever, leukocytosis, and ileus had resolved. Ultimately, this idea evolved into the STOP-IT trial, which resulted in two important findings. The first was using 4 days of antibiotics versus continuing antibiotics until resolution of inflammatory markers resulted in equivalent outcomes in terms of death, recurrent intra-abdominal infection, and surgical site infection. The mean duration of therapy was 4 days in the experimental group and 8 days in the control group. The second was that even under ideal circumstances the complication rate following intraabdominal infection remains painfully high at 23%, regardless of antimicrobial management. Further improvements in outcomes will depend on a better understanding of the pathophysiology of the disease and novel technologies.

CHAPTER 31

Diabetic Ketoacidosis

Review by Rae M. Allain

Diabetic ketoacidosis (DKA) is a medical emergency of hyperglycemia, metabolic acidosis, and hyperketonemia. It occurs most commonly in patients with Type 1 diabetes mellitus (T1DM) but is possible in patients with T2DM who are under extreme stress or who are "ketosis prone." American Diabetes Association (ADA) criteria for DKA are glucose >250 mg/dL, acidemia (pH <7.3, bicarbonate <18 mEq/L, anion gap >10), and ketosis [1]. The pathophysiology involves insulin deficiency and increased counterregulatory hormones (catecholamines, cortisol, glucagon) which further impair insulin's effects. The result is gluconeogenesis, impaired peripheral insulin utilization, hyperglycemia, and lipolysis-induced free fatty acid conversion to ketone bodies. Both hyperglycemia and hyperketonemia contribute to an osmotic diuresis with resultant severe hypovolemia. As strong acids, ketone bodies contribute to the anion-gap metabolic acidosis of DKA.

CDC data show a rising US hospitalization rate for DKA, particularly in the age group <45 years; overall hospital mortality is 0.4% but 2.6% for age ≥75 and >5% for those with concomitant critical illness [2, 3]. Wide variability in practice patterns of ICU admission for DKA exists, largely determined by institutional practices.

Laboratory assessment of DKA includes testing for increased production of ketone bodies: ß-hydroxybutyric acid, acetoacetic acid, and acetone. The latter two are detectable in blood or urine by the semiquantitative nitroprusside test. This test fails to detect ß-hydroxybutyric acid, which is important because it is the predominant ketone in DKA, produced more than acetoacetic acid by a factor of 7–10. For this reason, the direct assay for ß-hydroxybutyric acid is preferred.

Management of DKA consists of identification and treatment of precipitating cause, of which infection and insulin noncompliance are most common. Other causes include MI, stroke, pancreatitis, gastrointestinal disorders, and medications (atypical antipsychotics, sodium-glucose co-transporter 2 [SGLT2] inhibitors). Infection without fever is typical and may require procedural or surgical intervention for source control while simultaneous medical treatment of DKA proceeds.

Volume resuscitation is a mainstay of therapy. Recommendations include 15–20 mL/kg intravenous bolus of isotonic crystalloid in first hour followed by 250 mL/h, but the appropriate resuscitation should be guided by the hemodynamic

DOI: 10.1201/9781003042136-31

status of the patient, other significant compromising conditions (e.g., renal or conges-tive heart failure), and frequent bedside assessment of response. Fluid resuscitation alone improves hyperglycemia and acidosis via decreased plasma osmolality, dimin-ished counterregulatory hormones, and enhanced renal perfusion promoting glucose and acid excretion. The optimal resuscitation fluid is controversial; most guidelines recommend initial 0.9% sodium chloride followed by 0.45% sodium chloride when corrected sodium is normal or high (see equation below). When hyperchloremic nonanion gap metabolic acidosis is a concern, a balanced electrolyte solution may be administered instead of 0.9% sodium chloride. Findings from small studies indicate that as compared to 0.9% sodium chloride, Plasma-Lyte showed less hyperchloremia, higher bicarbonate, and more rapid acidosis resolution [3, 4]. Lactated Ringer's (LR) compared to 0.9% sodium chloride showed non-significant trends in improved pH and sodium bicarbonate levels in the LR group [5]. Definitive evidence for superior performance of balanced electrolyte solutions in clinically important outcomes is lacking such that the decision of which resuscitation fluid to use should be guided by individual patient characteristics, institutional formulary, and clinician familiarity.

DKA treatment requires close monitoring with every 1-hour glucose measurement and every 2-hour electrolytes, including measurement of anion gap (AG). Blood gas mea-surement is not essential but may be preferred in special circumstances (e.g., mechani-cal ventilation) or if easily obtained; venous blood gases are just as useful as arterial for treatment.

Insulin initiation should be delayed if hypokalemia (K^+ <3.3 mEq/L) is present because DKA produces a total body potassium deficit. Insulin administration and acidemia correction induce an intracellular potassium shift, causing worsened hypo-kalemia with risk of life-threatening dysrhythmias. Goal potassium is 4.0–5.0 mEq/L during treatment, replenished intravenously and concurrently with insulin while labo-ratory values are closely followed. Only if the potassium is >5.0 mEq/L may insulin be initiated without potassium supplementation (and while following every 2-hour measurement).

When hypokalemia is corrected, insulin infusion at 0.14 units/kg body weight/h is started. Alternatively, a bolus of IV insulin, 0.1 units/kg, followed by infusion at 0.1 units/kg/h, may be substituted, but comparisons of the two regimens show that bolusing insulin does not improve outcomes (time to DKA resolution, length of stay) but does increase incidence of hypoglycemia [6, 7]. The goal of insulin infusion is to reduce serum glucose by 50–75 mg/dL/h [1]. If inadequate response, the infusion dose may be doubled every hour (up to ~ 0.3 units/kg/h), with or without bolus of 0.1 units/kg. Once serum glucose is reduced to 200 mg/dL, the insulin infusion is titrated down (as low as 0.05 units/kg/h), and supplemental dextrose (D5 or 10%) is added to intravenous fluids to prevent hypoglycemia, targeting glucose 150–200 mg/dL. Insulin infusion should be continued until resolution of ketoacidosis/normalization of the AG. Intensivists should adjust for hypoalbuminemia's effect on AG, utilizing the following equation, which may be easily accessed in a medical app.

$$Corrected\ AG\left(\frac{mEq}{L}\right) = AG + \left\{2.5 \times \left[4 - albumin\left(\frac{g}{dL}\right)\right]\right\}$$

Hyponatremia is common in DKA, due to a shift of water from the intracellular to the extracellular space triggered by hyperglycemia and insulin deficiency. Calculating the corrected sodium is important for assessment and management; it is determined by the following equation, also available in a medical app.

$$Corrected\ Na\left(\frac{mEq}{L}\right) = Measured\ Na\left(\frac{mEq}{L}\right) + .024 \times \left[serum\ glucose\left(\frac{mg}{dL}\right) - 100\right]$$

Routine sodium bicarbonate administration for DKA is not recommended for venous pH $\geq$6.9 since no benefit in DKA reversal or outcomes has been demonstrated [1, 8–10]. This point is controversial, however, and conditions of diminished cardiac contractility, impaired catecholamine response, dysrhythmias, or severe renal dysfunction may support its use. Some advocate that if, following DKA resolution, a hyperchloremic, non-anion gap metabolic acidosis exists, then sodium bicarbonate infusion should be instituted to hasten replenishment of serum bicarbonate and restore acid-base homeostasis. When implemented, recommendations are for an isotonic solution of 100 mEq sodium bicarbonate (2 ampules 8.4%) in 400 mL sterile water [1], administered over 1–2 hours. Potassium chloride should be added or supplemented when potassium is $\leq$5.3 mEq/L.

DKA resolution is marked by hyperglycemic control with glucose <250 mg/dL and absence of ketoacidosis, with serum bicarbonate >18 mEq/L, pH >7.3, and a normal AG. At this point, a basal long-acting insulin may be administered subcutaneously (SQ) with overlapping insulin infusion for 2–4 hours [9]. In some cases of uncomplicated DKA, a patient's usual once-daily insulin may even be administered early in the course, simultaneously with IV insulin infusion; this strategy can provide a smoother transition to SQ therapy with less rebound hyperglycemia. Preferred SQ regimens are glargine or detemir as once-daily basal insulin combined with a rapid-acting insulin analog (lispro, aspart, or glulisine) immediately pre-meals. A higher incidence of hypoglycemia is seen when basal insulin is NPH (which peaks 4–6 hours following administration) [11].

Patients who are unable to eat (postsurgical, GI contraindications) should be continued on insulin infusion until oral intake is tolerated or an alternate nutritional source (e.g., enteral feeding tube, TPN) is secured.

Children undergoing treatment for DKA are at elevated risk for cerebral edema with high mortality. Pathophysiology likely involves ischemia/reperfusion injury and inflammation. Risk for cerebral edema in children has been associated with sodium bicarbonate treatment such that it is not recommended in treatment of pediatric DKA. The child's clinical neurologic exam should be closely monitored with rapid implementation of hyperosmolar therapy if cerebral edema occurs [12].

Abdominal pain, nausea, and vomiting are common complaints on presentation with DKA, and ≥25% of patients will have amylase and lipase elevations [1, 8, 9]. These findings are not necessarily due to pancreatitis, which requires confirmation by clinical and imaging examination.

ANNOTATED REFERENCES FOR DIABETIC KETOACIDOSIS

1. Kitabchi AE, Umpierrez GE, Miles JM, Fisher JN. Hyperglycemic crises in adult patients with diabetes. *Diabetes Care.* 2009;32(7):1335–1343. doi:10.2337/dc09-9032

    Consensus statement from the ADA describing features and treatment of DKA and hyperosmolar hyperglycemic state (HHS).

2. Benoit SR, Zhang Y, Geiss LS, Gregg EW, Albright A. Trends in diabetic ketoacidosis hospitalizations and in-hospital mortality—United States, 2000–2014. *MMWR Morb Mortal Wkly Rep.* 2018;67(12):362–365. doi:10.15585/mmwr.mm6712a3

    Data analysis from the CDC US Diabetes Surveillance System showing rising rates of DKA hospitalizations, particularly in younger people with postulated causes.

3. Chua HR, Venkatesh B, Stachowski E, et al. Plasma-Lyte 148 vs. 0.9% saline for fluid resuscitation in diabetic ketoacidosis. *J Crit Care.* 2012;27(2):138–145. doi:10.1016/j.jcrc.2012.01.007

    Small, retrospective study comparing laboratory and clinical outcomes of Plasma-Lyte versus normal saline in DKA. Patients receiving Plasma-Lyte had faster resolution of acidemia in first 12 hours and less hyperchloremia.

4. Mahler SA, Conrad SA, Wang H, Arnold TC. Resuscitation with balanced electrolyte solution prevents hyperchloremic metabolic acidosis in patients with diabetic ketoacidosis. *Am J Emerg Med.* 2011;29(6):670–674. doi:10.1016/j.ajem.2010.02.004

    Small, prospective, randomized study of Plasma-Lyte versus normal saline resuscitation in DKA via monitoring of serum chloride, bicarbonate, and calculated anion gap. The study achieved statistical significance showing Plasma-Lyte as opposed to normal saline prevented hyperchloremic metabolic acidosis.

5. van Zyl DG, Rheeder P, Delport E. Fluid management in diabetic-acidosis Ringer's lactate versus normal saline: a randomized controlled trial. *QJM.* 2012;105(4):337–343. doi:10.1093/qjmed/hcr226

    Small, randomized trial of normal saline versus Lactated Ringer's in DKA showing nonsignificant trends toward faster resolution of acidemia; results may have been affected by premature study cessation due to inability to obtain intended sample size.

6. Kitabchi AE, Murphy MB, Spencer J, Matteri R, Karas J. Is a priming dose of insulin necessary in a low-dose insulin protocol for the treatment of diabetic ketoacidosis? *Diabetes Care.* 2008;31(11):2081–2085. doi:10.2337/dc08-0509

    Small, randomized trial of insulin regimens in DKA, one with a bolus and two without, showing no difference in time to DKA resolution with bolus.

7. Goyal N, Miller JB, Sankey SS, Mossallam U. Utility of initial bolus insulin in the treatment of diabetic ketoacidosis. *J Emerg Med.* 2010;38(4):422–427. doi:10.1016/j.jemermed.2007.11.033

Prospective, observational chart review of ~150 DKA presentations which showed no clinically relevant superiority to an insulin bolus plus infusion regimen compared to infusion without bolus; there was a trend toward higher incidence of hypoglycemia in the bolus group.

8. Umpierrez G, Korytkowski M. Diabetic emergencies-ketoacidosis, hyperglycaemic hyperosmolar state and hypoglycaemia. *Nat Rev Endocrinol.* 2016;12(4):222–232. doi:10.1038/nrendo.2016.15

Thorough and well-referenced review of the epidemiology, pathophysiology, and management of DKA and HHS, including risk of DKA from SGLT2 inhibitors. Excellent graphics, including management flowcharts and highlighted treatment protocols. Detailed discussion of presentation and management of hypoglycemia is also helpful to the intensivist.

9. Long B, Willis GC, Lentz S, Koyfman A, Gottlieb M. Evaluation and management of the critically ill adult with diabetic ketoacidosis. *J Emerg Med.* 2020;59(3):371–383. doi:10.1016/j.jemermed.2020.06.059

Best review of DKA from a critical care perspective; references ADA definitions and guidelines, discusses controversies in management. Offers clinically useful, practical recommendations with a comprehensive list of references.

10. Kamel KS, Halperin ML. Acid–base problems in diabetic ketoacidosis. *N Engl J Med.* 2015;372(6):546–554. doi:10.1056/nejmra1207788

A review of the biochemical basis of DKA, emphasizing chemical formulae. Good discussion of the pathophysiology of cerebral edema and controversies of its management.

11. Umpierrez GE, Jones S, Smiley D, et al. Insulin analogs versus human insulin in the treatment of patients with diabetic ketoacidosis: a randomized controlled trial. *Diabetes Care.* 2009;32(7):1164–1169. doi:10.2337/dc09-0169

Small, randomized controlled trial important for showing that in DKA, treatment transition from IV infusion insulin to NPH insulin resulted in a higher incidence of hypoglycemia as compared to transition to glargine or glulisine insulin.

12. Glaser, N. Diabetic ketoacidosis in children: cerebral injury (cerebral edema). In: Wolfsdorf J, Randolph A, eds. UpToDate. Waltham, MA: *UpToDate;* 2020. https://www.uptodate.com/contents/diabetic-ketoacidosis-in-children-cerebral-injury-cerebral-edema; last updated November 12, 2020

The author, a lead researcher in studying pediatric neurologic injury associated with DKA, provides a comprehensive review of the most recent studies and hypotheses about the pathophysiology and causative factors of cerebral edema in children with DKA.

Landmark Article of the 21st Century

EFFICACY OF SUBCUTANEOUS INSULIN LISPRO VERSUS CONTINUOUS INTRAVENOUS REGULAR INSULIN FOR THE TREATMENT OF PATIENTS WITH DIABETIC KETOACIDOSIS

Umpierrez GE et al., *Amj Med.* 2004;117:291–296

Commentary by Stephen M. Cohn

Assessment: This is was a prospective randomized trial of 40 patients with diabetic ketoacidosis (DKA) randomized to hourly subcutaneous lispro versus continuous intravenous regular insulin. The subcutaneous intermittent injections of lispro were shown to be equal to the continuous regular insulin in terms of glucose control and resolution of acidosis, potentially permitting administration in a non-intensive care setting.

Limitations: This was a small study of patients with uncomplicated DKA (exclusions were hypovolemic shock, comatose state, acute myocardial ischemia, heart failure, end-stage renal disease, anasarca, or pregnancy). It is uncertain what proportion of DKA in the general population is uncomplicated versus complicated. It is also unclear what percentage of the overall diabetic population develops DKA due to failure of adherence to their glucose control program (as were most of the patients) versus other etiologies. There is a potential for inadequate absorption of subcutaneous medication if the patient requires significant fluid resuscitation. The nursing ratio required to achieve the reported 100% compliance is not stated, and likely not achievable at most institutions outside of an investigational protocol. A large proportion of patients with DKA may have other reasons for admission to an intensive care setting (such as sepsis as an etiology of the DKA), which might negate any perceived cost effectiveness benefit. On an ethical note, it is unclear how the patient (or surrogate) research-informed consent was obtained in these typically very ill patients that required immediate therapy upon hospital arrival.

Conclusions: The authors concluded that intermittent subcutaneous insulin was safe for management of DKA and was more cost effective than insulin drips. This somewhat limited paper represents the best recent paper the editors could identify focusing upon DKA, reflecting the paucity of quality investigations on this subject.

CHAPTER 32

Glucose Management in the ICU

Review by Jan Gunst and Greet Van den Berghe

Evoked by the severe physical stress induced by a major trauma, surgery, or medical illness, critically ill patients usually develop hyperglycemia. This response was traditionally considered to be adaptive, to temporarily increase non-insulin mediated glucose uptake in vital organs and immune cells at a time when food intake is scarce. Illness severity is intrinsically linked to more severe insulin resistance, and numerous observational studies have found a U-shaped association between spontaneous blood glucose concentrations and outcome of critically ill patients, whereby the lowest mortality risk associates with blood glucose concentrations in the normal fasting range. Since the metabolic response was considered to be adaptive, hyperglycemia used to be treated only when it exceeded the renal threshold, in which case it induces obvious complications including osmotic diuresis and fluid shifts. Nevertheless, severe hyperglycemia may induce metabolic stress, and apart from being an illness severity marker, the association between more severe hyperglycemia and adverse outcome could point to a detrimental role of elevated blood glucose.

A landmark RCT performed in an adult, surgical intensive care unit (ICU) in 2001 in Leuven, Belgium, found that lowering blood glucose to the healthy fasting range (80–110 mg/dL for adults) with insulin significantly reduced morbidity and mortality as compared to tolerating hyperglycemia up to the renal threshold (215 mg/dL) [1]. Subsequently, the same research group confirmed clinical benefit in medical ICU patients [2] and in critically ill children [3]. In the three RCTs, often referred to as the Leuven studies, tight glucose control inherently increased the risk of hypoglycemia, especially in critically ill children, in whom the blood glucose target was age-adjusted to account for the lower reference range in children (50–80 mg/dL for infants, 70–100 mg/dL for children older than 1 year). Importantly, a 4–year neurocognitive follow-up of children included in the pediatric RCT revealed no long-term harm associated with hypoglycemia, and children randomized to tight glucose control even performed better on certain neurocognitive tasks [4]. After the Leuven studies, numerous centers adopted tight glucose control as part of routine care, and several large observational studies confirmed clinical benefit after implementation of this treatment strategy (reviewed in 5). Subsequent mechanistic studies attributed the benefit of the intervention to avoidance of cellular glucose overload and associated metabolic stress rather than to glycemia-independent effects of insulin [6, 7].

DOI: 10.1201/9781003042136-32

Nevertheless, the efficacy and safety of tight glucose control remains debated, since the benefit has not been confirmed by large multicenter RCTs. The largest multicenter RCT, the NICE-SUGAR study, even found harm by the intervention [8]. Indeed, in NICE-SUGAR, tight glucose control increased mortality, which was attributed to the increased incidence of hypoglycemia [9]. The discrepant results between the pioneer Leuven RCTs showing benefit and the multicenter RCTs showing no benefit or even harm could be explained by the substantial methodological differences between the RCTs. Two crucial differences emerge: differences in the accuracy and safety of the glucose control protocol, and differences in feeding strategy [7]. The NICE-SUGAR RCT has been criticized for potentially hazardous aspects in the glucose control protocol, whereas the practice of early parenteral nutrition is a weakness of the Leuven studies. Indeed, patients in the Leuven RCTs received early parenteral nutrition as part of standard treatment at that time, which increases the severity of hyperglycemia and which was subsequently found to be harmful when feeding-induced hyperglycemia is treated. On the other hand, in contrast to NICE-SUGAR, the glucose control protocol in Leuven was standardized and reliable, by including accurate glucose measurements (arterial sampling, blood gas analyzer measurement) and preventing large swings in blood glucose through avoiding insulin boluses (only continuous infusion of insulin). In NICE-SUGAR, the protocol was not standardized and allowed potentially unreliable measurements by inaccurate glucometers as well as capillary and venous measurements that are potentially unreliable through poor capillary perfusion and intravenous infusion of glucose, respectively. The combination of potentially inaccurate measurements and insulin boluses (also allowed in NICE-SUGAR) may have provoked considerable blood glucose variability, and episodes of prolonged and undetected hypoglycemia. In the absence of a large RCT investigating the impact of tight glucose control with a validated protocol in the context of withholding early parenteral nutrition, the ideal glucose target for critically ill patients remains unclear. The TGC-fast multicenter RCT is currently addressing this important knowledge gap (clinicaltrials.gov NCT03665207).

In the past two decades, several strategies to improve the quality of blood glucose control in critically ill patients have been developed [5]. These include the use of software algorithms that advise insulin/glucose doses and the time of consecutive glucose measurements, as well as continuous glucose monitoring systems and closed-loop glucose control. Use of validated decision-support software was found to result in a high time in target range, with a very low risk of hypoglycemia (reviewed in 5). However, in view of the ongoing debate on the optimal glucose target, use of these algorithms and of continuous glucose monitoring is mainly restricted to centers performing research on the topic.

Some evidence suggests that the glucose target may need to be individualized according to the level of pre-admission glucose control [10]. Indeed, observational studies have shown that the ideal target may be higher in patients with pre-existing diabetes, especially in patients with poor antecedent glucose control; but, conclusive RCT evidence is lacking. The CONTROLING RCT, which randomized patients to individualized glucose control versus standard care was stopped prematurely by the data safety monitoring board (latest announcement on clinicaltrials.gov in 2018; NCT02244073). The study results have not been published yet.

In conclusion, the ideal blood glucose target for critically ill patients remains unclear. In the absence of new evidence, it seems prudent to avoid both severe hyperglycemia and hypoglycemia in critically ill patients. The efficacy and safety of tight glucose control, performed with a validated protocol in the absence of early parenteral nutrition, is currently being investigated.

ANNOTATED REFERENCES FOR GLUCOSE MANAGEMENT IN THE ICU

1. Van den Berghe G, Wouters P, Weekers F, et al. Intensive insulin therapy in critically ill patients. *N Engl J Med*. 2001;345(19):1359–1367.

   Landmark RCT including adult critically ill patients admitted to the surgical ICU (n =1548). The RCT showed a reduction in morbidity and mortality by tight glucose control, provided with a standardized protocol (arterial blood glucose measurements by blood gas analyzer, avoidance of insulin boluses). According to feeding guidelines at that time, all patients received early parenteral nutrition. This feeding practice was subsequently shown to be detrimental, also when feeding-induced hyperglycemia is treated.

2. Van den Berghe G, Wilmer A, Hermans G, et al. Intensive insulin therapy in the medical ICU. *N Engl J Med*. 2006;354(5):449–461.

   First RCT in adult critically ill patients admitted the medical ICU (n = 1200). The RCT confirmed a beneficial impact of tight glucose control, provided with a standardized protocol (predominantly arterial blood glucose measurements by blood gas analyzer, avoidance of insulin boluses). According to feeding guidelines at that time, all patients received early parenteral nutrition. This feeding practice was subsequently shown to be detrimental, also when feeding-induced hyperglycemia is treated.

3. Vlasselaers D, Milants I, Desmet L, et al. Intensive insulin therapy for patients in paediatric intensive care: a prospective, randomised controlled study. *Lancet*. 2009;373(9663):547–556.

   This pioneer RCT in critically ill children (n = 700) demonstrated that tight glucose control significantly decreased morbidity and mortality as compared to tolerating stress hyperglycemia, while increasing the risk of hypoglycemia. In the intervention group, continuous intravenous insulin was titrated to maintain blood glucose within the normal age-adjusted fasting range for blood glucose (50–80 mg/dL for infants, 70–100 mg/dL for children older than 1 year). The glucose control protocol was well standardized. All patients received early parenteral nutrition.

4. Mesotten D, Gielen M, Sterken C, et al. Neurocognitive development of children 4 years after critical illness and treatment with tight glucose control: a randomized controlled trial. *JAMA*. 2012;308(16):1641–1650.

   Prospective follow-up study of critically ill children randomized to tight versus liberal glucose control, including 569 (84%) patients enrolled in the parent RCT (Vlasselaers et al. Lancet 2009). The study showed that clinical benefit was maintained on the long-term. Indeed, full neurodevelopmental testing 4 years after randomization revealed that children randomized to tight glucose control behaved similar or better on selected neurocognitive tasks. A short episode of hypoglycemia was not associated with long-term neurocognitive harm.

5. Gunst J, De Bruyn A, Van den Berghe G. Glucose control in the ICU. *Curr Opin Anaesthesiol.* 2019;32(2):156–162.

Recent review summarizing the clinical evidence on tight glucose control, as well as the open questions and recent areas of improvement (software-guided glucose control, continuous glucose monitoring, closed-loop blood glucose control).

6. Ellger B, Debaveye Y, Vanhorebeek I, et al. Survival benefits of intensive insulin therapy in critical illness: impact of maintaining normoglycemia versus glycemia-independent actions of insulin. *Diabetes.* 2006;55(4):1096–1105.

Detailed animal study elucidating the impact of glucose lowering versus increasing insulin availability on outcome of critically ill animals. The study showed that maintenance of normoglycemia rather than high insulin levels improved morbidity and mortality.

7. Gunst J, Van den Berghe G. Blood glucose control in the ICU: don't throw out the baby with the bathwater! *Intensive Care Med.* 2016;42(9):1478–1481.

Recent opinion article as part of series of opinion papers on tight glucose control in the ICU. Apart from providing a brief overview of clinical evidence, the article summarizes animal evidence and mechanistic studies on how preventing hyperglycemia with insulin therapy may be beneficial.

8. NICE-SUGAR Study Investigators; Finfer S, Chittock DR, Su SY, et al. Intensive versus conventional glucose control in critically ill patients. *N Engl J Med.* 2009;360(13):1283–1297.

The largest multicenter RCT on tight versus liberal blood glucose control in adult critically ill patients (n = 6104). The RCT reported increased mortality by tight glucose control, fueling a vivid debate on the topic. The RCT has been criticized for the use of potentially inaccurate metrics to perform tight glucose control.

9. NICE-SUGAR Study Investigators; Finfer S, Liu B, Chittock DR, et al. Hypoglycemia and risk of death in critically ill patients. *N Engl J Med.* 2012;367(12):1108–1118.

This secondary analysis of the NICE-SUGAR RCT attributed the clinical harm of tight glucose control to the increased incidence of severe hypoglycemia.

10. Van den Berghe G, Wilmer A, Milants I, et al. Intensive insulin therapy in mixed medical/surgical intensive care units: benefit versus harm. *Diabetes.* 2006;55(11):3151–3159.

This secondary analysis of the adult Leuven RCTs on tight versus liberal glucose control (n = 2748) addressed important questions raised by the first adult RCTs. The study showed that tight glucose control decreased mortality in all subgroups of critically ill patients, except in patients with pre-admission diabetes mellitus. Also, benefit was present regardless of the parenteral glucose load. Thirdly, the study could not attribute short-term harm to a brief episode of iatrogenic hypoglycemia. Finally, the study suggested a dose-response relationship between blood glucose lowering and outcome. Indeed, patients with intermediate blood glucose control (110–150 mg/dL) had better survival than patients with blood glucose above 150 mg/dL, but worse outcome as compared to patients with blood glucose between 80 and 110 mg/dL.

Landmark Article of the 21st Century

INTENSIVE INSULIN THERAPY IN CRITICALLY ILL PATIENTS

Van den Berghe G et al., *N Engl J Med*. 2001;345(19):1359–1367

Commentary by Jan Gunst and Greet Van den Berghe

Critically ill patients usually develop hyperglycemia, which has been associated with poor outcome. In 2001, a potentially causal link was confirmed, since a landmark randomized controlled trial (RCT) in adult surgical critically ill patients demonstrated significantly reduced morbidity and mortality in patients randomized to strict control of blood glucose concentrations with insulin therapy [1]. The RCT has had major impact worldwide, with many centers adopting tight glucose control as standard practice, a seemingly simple intervention with potentially great outcome benefit. Although different implementation studies and single-center RCTs confirmed benefit by tight glucose control, multicenter RCTs were neutral and the largest RCT demonstrated potential harm, fueling a vivid, ongoing debate on the ideal blood glucose target in critically ill patients [2–4]. The outcome differences between the pioneer RCT and largest multicenter RCT are likely explained by important methodological differences, including differences in blood glucose target, feeding strategies, glucose measurement technology, and insulin administration protocol [5]. Tight glucose control has been shown to be effective and safe in critically ill patients receiving early parenteral nutrition, provided that glucose is measured with accurate devices and insulin titrated with a validated protocol that minimizes the incidence of hypoglycemia. The efficacy and safety of the intervention with a validated protocol in the context of withholding early parenteral nutrition—the current feeding standard—is currently being investigated.

REFERENCES

1. Van den Berghe G, Wouters P, Weekers F, et al. Intensive insulin therapy in critically ill patients. *N Engl J Med*. 2001;345(19):1359–1367.
2. Van den Berghe G, Wilmer A, Hermans G, et al. Intensive insulin therapy in the medical ICU. *N Engl J Med*. 2006;354(5):449–461.
3. Vlasselaers D, Milants I, Desmet L, et al. Intensive insulin therapy for patients in paediatric intensive care: a prospective, randomised controlled study. *Lancet*. 2009;373(9663):547–556.
4. NICE-SUGAR Study Investigators; Finfer S, Chittock DR, Su SY, et al. Intensive versus conventional glucose control in critically ill patients. *N Engl J Med*. 2009;360(13):1283–1297.
5. Gunst J, De Bruyn A, Van den Berghe G. Glucose control in the ICU. *Curr Opin Anaesthesiol*. 2019;32(2):156–162.

CHAPTER 33

Acute Stroke

Review by Magdy Selim

In 1996, the US Food and Drug Administration approved the use of intravenous (IV) recombinant tissue-plasminogen activator (rt-PA) for the treatment for acute ischemic stroke (AIS) based on the results of the National Institute of Neurological Disorders and Stroke (NINDS) IV rt-PA Stroke Study. Patients treated with IV rt-PA within 3 hours of stroke symptom-onset were at least 30% more likely to have minimal or no disability at 3 months compared to placebo. Intravenous thrombolysis was a major breakthrough for the treatment of AIS. In practice, the narrow treatment window and eligibility for IV rt-PA coupled with its marginal efficacy in achieving reperfusion in patients with large vessel occlusion (LVO) limited its use and benefit to only a small number of patients with AIS. This led to multiple attempts to find new ways to expand the treatment window and improve recanalization of LVO. Endovascular thrombectomy (EVT) appeared to be an appealing and logical therapeutic strategy to achieve reperfusion after AIS due to LVO. However, the results from the interventional management of stroke (IMS)-III [1], magnetic resonance and recanalization of stroke clots using embolectomy (MR-RESCUE) [2], and intra-arterial versus systemic thrombolysis for acute ischemic stroke (SYNTHESIS EXP) [3] trials, which were published in 2013, were disappointing. They showed that the EVT did not have additive benefits compared to IV rt-PA or standard care for AIS.

The stroke community learned valuable lessons from IMS-III, MR-RESCUE, and SYNTHESIS EXP trials, and was relentless in its efforts to expand treatment for AIS beyond IV rt-PA. Only 2 years later, the results of five thrombectomy trials; MR CLEAN, ESCAPE, SWIFT PRIME, EXTEND-IA, and REVASCAT were simultaneously published in the *New England Journal of Medicine* [4–8]. Doubts about the utility of EVT as an effective treatment for AIS due to LVO were replaced by euphoria and optimism for a brighter future. These trials were conducted within various health care systems in different countries. Yet they all showed that mechanical thrombectomy with or without IV rt-PA is effective in improving the outcomes of patients with AIS due to LVO compared to IV rt-PA or usual care alone. The absolute difference in the proportion of patients achieving functional independence at 3 months varied from 13.5% to 31.4% in favor of EVT, and the numbers needed to treat to benefit from EVT varied from 3 to 7. These trials confirmed the efficacy of EVT when performed within 6 hours from stroke onset in AIS due to LVO. Increased emphasis on the use of vascular and advanced brain imaging to select patients with confirmed LVO and to exclude those with large infarcted brain tissue, coupled with the development of easy-to-use

DOI: 10.1201/9781003042136-33

and more effective clot retrieval devices, such as stent retriever was instrumental to the successful results of MR CLEAN, ESCAPE, SWIFT PRIME, EXTEND-IA, and REVASCAT. All these trials implemented imaging-based criteria to select patients with proximal intracranial LVO and to exclude patients with a large infarct core. They also emphasized speed and achieved a median imaging-to-groin-puncture time of less than 60 minutes, and imaging-to-reperfusion time of less than 90 minutes. These trials were "a first step in the right direction," but there was still a need to further expand the treatment time window.

The DAWN trial (DWI or CTP assessment with clinical mismatch in the triage of wake up and late presenting strokes undergoing neurointervention with trevo) [9] examined the safety and efficacy of EVT performed within 6–24 hours of stroke onset in patients with LVO based on pre-specified perfusion imaging-based criteria. This was an international, multicenter, prospective, randomized, open-label trial with a Bayesian adaptive–enrichment design and with blinded assessment of end points. Two-hundred-six patients with occlusion of the intracranial internal carotid artery or proximal middle cerebral artery who had last been known to be well 6 to 24 hours earlier and who had a mismatch between the penumbral ischemic tissue and the infarct volume on perfusion MRI or CTP were randomly assigned to EVT plus standard care or to standard care alone. More than 60% of patients in this trial woke from sleep with stroke symptoms, i.e., the exact time of stroke onset was unknown. In essence, the investigators replaced the traditional clock-based therapeutic window with a tissue-based window using perfusion imaging. The results of DAWN were similar to its predecessors. The rate of functional independence at 3 months was 49% in the EVT group as compared with 13% in the standard care group (adjusted difference, 33 percentage points; 95% credible interval, 24–44; posterior probability of superiority >0.999). The rate of symptomatic intracranial hemorrhage and/or 3-month mortality did not differ significantly between the two groups. The concept and results of DAWN were validated in the subsequent Endovascular Therapy Following Imaging Evaluation for Ischemic Stroke 3 (DEFUSE 3) trial, which showed that endovascular thrombectomy for AIS 6–16 hours after a patient was last known to be well, plus standard medical therapy, resulted in better functional outcomes than standard medical therapy alone among patients with LVO and an initial infarct size of less than 70 mL, and a ratio of the volume of ischemic tissue on perfusion imaging to infarct volume of 1.8 or more [10].

The DAWN trial represented a new dawn for a conceptual and paradigm shift in stroke care from clock-based to tissue-based selection of patients with AIS who are likely to benefit from reperfusion therapy far beyond the first few hours from stroke onset. Treatment decisions can now be based on individualized imaging-based analyses. These studies and DAWN only mark the beginning of a new era for stroke care, and the 2020s promise to be exciting times for the stroke field. Innovations in device technology and imaging, new opportunities to deliver neuroprotective therapies, and a rejuvenated stroke community will undoubtedly continue to advance stroke care to minimize the morbidity and mortality of this devastating disease.

ANNOTATED REFERENCES FOR ACUTE STROKE

1. Broderick JP, Palesch YY, Demchuk AM, et al. Endovascular therapy after intravenous tPA versus tPA alone for stroke. *N Engl J Med.* 2013;68:893–903.

   In this randomized controlled trial (RCT) in 656 patients with AIS who received IV rt-PA within 3 hours of stroke onset, additional EVT did not result in improved functional outcomes.

2. Ciccone A, Valvassori L, Nichelatti M, et al. Endovascular treatment for acute ischemic stroke. *N Engl J Med.* 2013;368:904–913.

   In this RCT in 362 patients with AIS who were randomized to IV rt-PA or EVT within 4.5 hours of stroke onset, EVT was not superior to treatment with IV rt-PA.

3. Kidwell CS, Jahan R, Gornbein J, et al. A trial of imaging selection and endovascular treatment for ischemic stroke. *N Engl J Med.* 2013;368:914–923.

   In this trial, 118 patients with AIS due to LVO were randomized within 8 hours of stroke onset to EVT vs. standard care. EVT was not superior to standard care.

4. Berkhemer OA, Fransen PSS, Beumer D, et al. A randomized trial of intraarterial treatment for acute ischemic stroke. *N Engl J Med.* 2015;372:11–20.

   In this trial, 500 patients with AIS due to LVO were randomized within 6 hours of stroke onset to either EVT plus standard care or standard care alone. EVT improved functional outcomes at 90 days and was safe.

5. Campbell BCV, Mitchell PJ, Kleinig TJ, et al. Endovascular therapy for ischemic stroke with perfusion imaging selection. *N Engl J Med.* 2015;372:1009–1018.

   In this trial, 70 AIS patients with LVO and evidence of salvageable brain tissue and ischemic core <70 mL on perfusion CT were randomized within 4.5 hours of stroke onset to either EVT or IV rt-PA. EVT, compared with alteplase alone, improved reperfusion, early neurologic recovery at day 3, and functional outcome at 90 days.

6. Goyal M, Demchuk AM, Menon BK, et al. Randomized assessment of rapid endovascular treatment of ischemic stroke. *N Engl J Med.* 2015;372:1019–1030.

   In this trial, 316 patients with AIS due to LVO who had a small infarct and good collateral circulation were randomized within 12 hours of stroke onset to either EVT plus standard care or standard care alone. EVT improved functional outcomes at 90 days and reduced mortality.

7. Jovin TG, Chamorro A, Cobo E, et al. Thrombectomy within 8 hours after symptom onset in ischemic stroke. *N Engl J Med.* 2015;372:2296–2306.

   In this trial, 206 patients with AIS due to LVO were randomized within 8 hours of stroke onset to either medical therapy including IV rt-PA or medical therapy including IV rt-PA and EVT. EVT increased the rate of functional independence at 90 days.

8. Saver JL, Goyal M, Bonafe A, et al. Stent retriever thrombectomy after intravenous tPA vs. tPA alone in stroke. *N Engl J Med.* 2015;372:2285–2295.

   In this RCT trial, 196 patients with AIS due to LVO were randomized to within 6 hours of stroke onset to IV rt-PA alone or IV rt-PA and EVT. EVT improved functional outcomes at 90 days.

9. Nogueira RG, Jadhav AP, Haussen DC, et al. Thrombectomy 6 to 24 hours after stroke with a mismatch between deficit and infarct. *N Engl J Med.* 2018;378:11–21.

10. Albers GW, Marks MP, Kemp S, et al. Thrombectomy for stroke at 6 to 16 hours with selection by perfusion imaging. *N Engl J Med.* 2018;378:708–718.

In this RCT trial, 182 AIS patients with LVO, initial infarct volume <70 mL and a ratio of the volume of ischemic tissue on perfusion MRI or CT to infarct volume of 1.8 or more were randomized within 6–16 hours of stroke onset to EVT plus medical therapy vs. medical therapy alone. EVT resulted in better functional outcomes at 90 days.

Landmark Article of the 21st Century

THROMBECTOMY 6 TO 24 HOURS AFTER STROKE WITH A MISMATCH BETWEEN DEFICIT AND INFARCT

Nogueira RG et al., *N Engl J Med.* 2018;378:11–21

Commentary by Stephen M. Cohn

Prior studies had demonstrated the benefit of endovascular thrombectomy if performed within 6 hours of an ischemic stroke. Nonrandomized studies suggested that patients who had mismatch between the volume of brain tissue that might be salvaged and the volume of the infarcted tissue could benefit from reperfusion of the occluded proximal cerebral vessels. Essentially, those patients with a significant diminution of neurologic examination, but a relatively limited amount of infarcted brain were considered candidates for reperfusion, despite the delay in presentation.

Assessment: The role of endovascular thrombectomy more than 6 hours after onset of ischemic stroke was studied. Two-hundred-six patients were randomized in this multicenter prospective trial, if they were known to have been well 6–24 hours prior to admission and had a mismatch between the severity of the clinical deficit and the infarct volume, to standard care alone (control group) or thrombectomy with standard care. The study population represents approximately one third of patients presenting with ischemic stroke who present in a delayed fashion. The trial was multicenter at 26 institutions worldwide and all had significant experience with thrombectomy (>40 procedures per year). Functional independence and disability scores were determined by individuals blinded to study group. The study was stopped early at interim analysis due to the superiority of the thrombectomy group over the control group (49% vs. 13% achieved functional independence). No difference was noted in intracranial hemorrhage or mortality. Infarct volume at 24 hours was 8 mL in the study group and 22 mL in the control group.

Limitations: The trial was unblinded to the clinicians. There were some subtle differences of uncertain importance between the two patient groups: more of the super elderly (>80 years) in the control group (29% vs. 23%); infarct volume was larger in the controls (8.9 mL vs. 7.6 mL); and more controls had an unwitnessed stroke (38% vs. 27%). The primary endpoint for the study was altered during the trial with functional independence changed from secondary to co-primary endpoint.

Conclusions: Disability outcomes were significantly improved following thrombectomy in addition to standard care when compared to standard care alone in patients with ischemic stroke presenting 6–24 hours after being known to be well. This important study established to beneficial effect of aggressive endovascular management in stroke patients who have a mismatch between their neurologic exam and their infarct volume, even when they present late to the hospital.

CHAPTER 34

Subarachnoid Hemorrhage

Review by Dominic A. Harris and Ajith J. Thomas

Intracranial aneurysms typically occur in 1–2% of the population and aneurysmal subarachnoid hemorrhage (aSAH) remains a morbid and lethal condition [1]. Atraumatic subarachnoid hemorrhage is caused by the rupture of an intracranial aneurysm in 80% of cases. Other causes include vascular malformations such as arteriovenous malformations and vasculopathies including vasculitis. Even though the earliest description of subarachnoid hemorrhage dates back over 2400 years, successful treatment and management of these patients were not achieved until the advances in neurosurgery significantly improved morbidity and mortality throughout the 20th century [2].

HISTORY

The term "aneurysm" was first coined by the Greek physician Galen (*anu*: across and *eurys*: broad, forming aneurysma: a widening) [2]. During the Middle Ages, the management of peripheral aneurysms became standard practice, but intracranial aneurysms were not described until the 18th century [2]. Italian anatomist, Morgagni of Padua, described an unruptured dilatation of the carotid arteries on autopsy in 1761. The link between subarachnoid hemorrhage and ruptured intracranial aneurysms were more explicitly made by John Blackall in 1810, when he attributed the sudden death of the Swedish crown prince Charles August to a ruptured basilar artery aneurysm [2]. Subsequent autopsy studies further characterized the features of ruptured intracranial aneurysms, and the term spontaneous subarachnoid hemorrhage was finally coined in a postmortem case series published in 1859 [2].

The treatment of an intracranial aneurysm was first documented by Victor Horsley in 1885 when he discovered a large aneurysm in the middle cranial fossa while operating on a patient with suspected tumor. This was successfully treated with ligation of the cervical carotid artery, which the patient tolerated due to collateral circulation [2]. Carotid ligation became the standard treatment of cerebral aneurysms in the 1930s, but it was recognized that this treatment strategy was less than ideal given the high incidence of postoperative hemiparesis. Advances in the direct treatment of cerebral aneurysms occurred after Harvey Cushing's resident, Norman Dott, was the first to successfully treat a ruptured intracranial aneurysm by wrapping the aneurysm with muscle as well as developing the technique of suture ligation of the aneurysm neck [2].

DOI: 10.1201/9781003042136-34

Suture ligation, however, was technically challenging given the friable wall of the aneurysm. It wasn't until Walter Dandy performed the first clipping of an intracranial aneurysm in 1937 that modern vascular neurosurgery was born [2]. Clipping became the mainstay of treatment, turning ruptured aneurysms into a treatable condition. Surgical clipping involves placing a titanium clip across the neck of the aneurysm while preserving blood flow through the parent artery and adjacent vessels [3]. This is done with the use of the operating microscope to open the subarachnoid space around the cerebral arteries and carefully mobilize the brain parenchymal without causing injury [3].

The next paradigm shift occurred in the 1990s with the introduction of endovascular coiling for cerebral aneurysms. Guido Guglielmi developed the detachable coil using electrolysis and successfully treated his first patient in 1990 [2]. Endovascular treatment is performed under fluoroscopic guidance where a catheter is navigated to the parent artery of the aneurysm. A microcatheter is then advanced into the aneurysm sac where metal coils are deployed into the aneurysm. This causes thrombus formation inside the aneurysm sac, and thus occludes the aneurysm and eliminates risk of rerupture [3].

Currently, endovascular coiling is preferred compared to neurosurgical clipping in aneurysmal subarachnoid hemorrhage patients who are considered equally suitable for both treatment options. This shift has been largely influenced by the findings from the International Subarachnoid Aneurysm Trial (ISAT) [4] which is one of the landmark papers that has dramatically changed the field of vascular neurosurgery.

CLINICAL PRESENTATION

Aneurysmal subarachnoid hemorrhage classically presents with a severe, acute onset headache, often described as "the worst headache of life" [3]. In some patients, this headache is preceded by an aneurysm leak or "sentinel" headache, which may occur weeks prior to overt subarachnoid hemorrhage [5]. Associated symptoms include nausea, vomiting, photophobia, neck stiffness, focal neurologic deficits, and a brief loss of consciousness [5, 6]. In more severe cases, patient may present with altered mental status ranging from mild lethargy to profound coma.

The initial management of the aneurysmal subarachnoid hemorrhage is directed at reversing or stabilizing acute life-threatening sequelae, particularly in the case of comatose patients. Establishing a secure airway, normalizing cardiovascular function, treating seizures, and treating acute hydrocephalus with an external ventricular drain are common first steps.

There are two main grading systems that are used to correlate the clinical status of the patient at the time of presentation with the long-term neurologic outcome: the Hunt–Hess classification [7] and the World Federation of Neurosurgical Societies classification [8]. In both scales, the severity of encephalopathy is the major determinant of poor outcomes. Aneurysm rupture produces widespread brain dysfunction including both immediate and "late" events such as cerebral vasospasm and delayed cerebral ischemia.

Rebleeding of ruptured aneurysms is associated with a much higher risk of death and neurologic injury. The risk of rerupture is highest in the first 24 hours after aneurysmal subarachnoid hemorrhage but remains elevated for 30 days after the initial rupture if the aneurysm is not treated [3, 9].

TREATMENT OF RUPTURED CEREBRAL ANEURYSMS

Treatment of ruptured aneurysms through either surgical clipping or endovascular options have become a safe and effective way to eliminate the immediate risk of aneurysm rerupture [4, 10].

Two randomized trials have compared endovascular treatment with open-surgical treatment for ruptured intracranial aneurysms: the International Subarachnoid Aneurysm Trial (ISAT) [4] and the Barrow Ruptured Aneurysm Trial (BRAT) [10]. ISAT was a landmark multicenter, randomized controlled trial that enrolled 2143 patients with subarachnoid hemorrhage across 43 centers and randomized them to either surgical clipping or endovascular coiling [4]. In patients where both treatments were deemed suitable, a survival benefit was found in those treated with endovascular coiling compared to surgical clipping at 1-year follow-up. BRAT, a single-center trial, showed a similar benefit of endovascular treatment compared to open-surgical treatment at 1-year follow-up [10]. However, the differences between the two groups were no longer significant at year 3 or year 6 [11].

The results of these randomized controlled trials have led to a dramatic shift towards endovascular treatment of ruptured aneurysms [12]. Furthermore, treatment paradigms for unruptured intracranial aneurysms have shifted with the development of new endovascular devices, particularly flow diverting technology. Flow diverters are stents that redirect blood flow inside the parent vessel, allowing aneurysms to thrombose over time and causing remodeling of the parent artery. The caveat to this treatment is the requirement of dual antiplatelet therapy to prevent in-stent stenosis or thromboembolic events causing ischemic stroke in the first several months after placement. Up until recent years, the need for dual-antiplatelet therapy has previously precluded the use of flow diverters in the setting of ruptured aneurysms. However, this may change in the near future as endovascular technology continues to develop.

ANNOTATED REFERENCES FOR SUBARACHNOID HEMORRHAGE

1. Wiebers DO, Whisnant JP, Huston J, 3rd, et al. Unruptured intracranial aneurysms: natural history, clinical outcome, and risks of surgical and endovascular treatment. *Lancet.* 2003;362:103–110.

This was a landmark multicenter prospective study that aimed to assess the natural history of unruptured aneurysms and determine the risk associated with treatment versus observation.

2. Milinis K, Thapar A, O'Neill K, Davies AH. History of aneurysmal spontaneous subarachnoid hemorrhage. *Stroke.* 2017;48:e280–e283.

   This is a thorough overview of the history of aneurysmal subarachnoid hemorrhage. It provides an excellent historical perspective on the development of our understanding intracranial aneurysms and the advances in our treatment of them.

3. Lawton MT, Vates GE. Subarachnoid hemorrhage. *N Engl J Med.* 2017;377:257–266.

   A thorough overview of aneurysmal subarachnoid hemorrhage including a comprehensive literature review and description of epidemiology, clinical presentation, treatment, and current controversies.

4. Molyneux A, Kerr R, Stratton I, et al. International Subarachnoid Aneurysm Trial (ISAT) of neurosurgical clipping versus endovascular coiling in 2143 patients with ruptured intracranial aneurysms: a randomised trial. *Lancet.* 2002;360:1267–1274.

   This is a randomized, multicenter trial comparing clipping and endovascular treatment in 2143 patients presenting with ruptured intracranial aneurysms. In patients where both treatments were suitable, a survival benefit was found in those treated with endovascular coiling compared to surgical clipping.

5. Connolly ES, Jr., Rabinstein AA, Carhuapoma JR, et al. Guidelines for the management of aneurysmal subarachnoid hemorrhage: a guideline for healthcare professionals from the American Heart Association/American Stroke Association. *Stroke.* 2012;43:1711–1737.

   This is a literature review that summarizes the literature and guidelines on the epidemiology, clinical presentation, and management of aneurysmal subarachnoid hemorrhage.

6. Perry JJ, Stiell IG, Sivilotti ML, et al. Clinical decision rules to rule out subarachnoid hemorrhage for acute headache. *JAMA.* 2013;310:1248–1255.

   This is large prospective multicenter study evaluating clinical risk factors that predict the presence of subarachnoid hemorrhage in patients presenting with headache.

7. Hunt WE, Hess RM. Surgical risk as related to time of intervention in the repair of intracranial aneurysms. *J Neurosurg.* 1968;28:14–20.

   This is a landmark paper that summarizes the risk of mortality of aneurysmal subarachnoid hemorrhage patients based on clinical presentation on admission. The results of this study formed the basis for the widely used Hunt–Hess grading scale in describing the severity of clinical presentation.

8. Hijdra A, van Gijn J, Nagelkerke NJ, Vermeulen M, van Crevel H. Prediction of delayed cerebral ischemia, rebleeding, and outcome after aneurysmal subarachnoid hemorrhage. *Stroke.* 1988;19:1250–1256.

   This study analyzes variables associated with delayed cerebral ischemia, rebleeding, and poor outcomes in patients with aneurysmal subarachnoid hemorrhage. The authors found that death or severe disability after 3 months was best predicted by amount of subarachnoid hemorrhage and grade on the Glasgow Coma Scale. The results of this study provides the basis for the World Federation of Neurological Surgeons (WFNS) grading scale.

9. Hillman J, Fridriksson S, Nilsson O, Yu Z, Saveland H, Jakobsson KE. Immediate administration of tranexamic acid and reduced incidence of early rebleeding after aneurysmal subarachnoid hemorrhage: a prospective randomized study. *J Neurosurg.* 2002;97:771–778.

This prospective study found that an early and short course of antifibrinolytics reduced the risk of early rebleeding in subarachnoid hemorrhage. This provides a medical alternative in cases where early treatment of ruptured aneurysms cannot be achieved.

10. McDougall CG, Spetzler RF, Zabramski JM, et al. The Barrow Ruptured Aneurysm Trial. *J Neurosurg.* 2012;116:135–144.

    This is a prospective, randomized single-center trial comparing clipping versus coil embolization in the treatment of intracranial aneurysms. There were no differences in morbidity between the surgical and endovascular group, but rates of retreatment and complete obliteration favored patients who underwent clipping compared to coiling.

11. Spetzler RF, McDougall CG, Zabramski JM, et al. Ten-year analysis of saccular aneurysms in the Barrow Ruptured Aneurysm Trial. *J Neurosurg.* 2019;132:771–776.

    This study presents the 10-year results of the Barrow Ruptured Aneurysm Trial (BRAT) comparing clipping and endovascular coiling of ruptured aneurysms. There was no statistically significant difference in clinical outcomes between the two groups.

12. Luther E, McCarthy DJ, Brunet MC, et al. Treatment and diagnosis of cerebral aneurysms in the post-International Subarachnoid Aneurysm Trial (ISAT) era: trends and outcomes. *J Neurointerv Surg.* 2020;12:682–687.

    This paper uses an administrative database, the National Inpatient Sample, from 2004 to 2014 to describe trends in the treatment and clinical outcomes of ruptured and unruptured intracranial aneurysms. The authors confirm the increasing use of endovascular treatment for these lesions as well as the improved mortality and morbidity among both surgical and endovascular patients.

Landmark Article of the 21st Century

INTERNATIONAL SUBARACHNOID ANEURYSM TRIAL (ISAT) OF NEUROSURGICAL CLIPPING VERSUS ENDOVASCULAR COILING IN 2143 PATIENTS WITH RUPTURED INTRACRANIAL ANEURYSMS: A RANDOMIZED TRIAL

ISAT investigators, *Lancet.* 2002;360:1267–1274

Commentary by Jyoti Sharma

The ISAT is a multicenter, randomized trial performed in 43 centers primarily located in Europe and Canada. It compared the safety and efficacy of endovascular coiling versus neurosurgical clipping in patients with ruptured intracranial aneurysms at 2 months and 1 year. The primary measure was the proportion of patients dead or disabled as defined by the modified Rankin Scale (mRS) of 3–6. The secondary outcome measure was rebreeding. Trial enrollment was terminated early on the basis of an interim analysis, but follow-up continued. Of the 9559 eligible patients, 2143 (21.5%) were randomized. 23.7% of patients with endovascular coiling versus 30.6% with neurosurgical clipping were dependent or dead at 1 year (RR 0.774, [0.658–0.911], $p = 0.0019$)—an absolute risk reduction of 6.9%. One-year case fatality rates were similar for the two treatment groups (8.1% endovascular vs. 10.1% neurosurgery). Risk of rebreeding was low, although more common in the endovascular group at one year with no effect on mortality.

Primary recruitment in the UK and the small number of patients actually randomized (from the total assessed) limited the generalizability of ISAT to the entire population of patients with aneurysmal subarachnoid hemorrhage (selection bias). The primary outcome of functional status (dependency or death) based on the modified Rankin Scale was collected via a postal questionnaire introducing patient interpretation in selecting the appropriate category.

ISAT is a well-designed, pragmatic trial that provided a pivotal turning point in modern neurosurgery management of ruptured saccular aneurysms. Patients with low grade (WFNS [World Federation of Neurosurgical Societies] 1–2), small (<10 mm diameter), and anterior circulation ruptured aneurysms are more likely to be alive with minimal to no disability at 1 year with endovascular coiling. These findings were confirmed in additional ISAT publications in 2005 and 2009 (1- and 5-year follow-up results, respectively). ISAT II, a trial comparing the clinical outcome of surgical clipping and endovascular coiling for ruptured intracranial aneurysms not included in the original ISAT Study, was launched in 2012 with projected results available in 2024.

In the post-ISAT era, endovascular clipping has become the treatment of choice for ruptured and unruptured aneurysms especially with rapid advances in identification, operator competency, and procedural equipment. Future studies are required to determine the incidence of procedure-related complications and objective evidence-based disability from endovascular interventions.

CHAPTER 35

Delirium

Review by Ronny Munoz-Acuna and Brian O'Gara

Delirium is defined by the Diagnostic and Statistical Manual of Mental Disorders (DSM-5) as an acute fluctuating disturbance in attention, environmental awareness, cognition, and perception [1]. It remains a clinical diagnosis, commonly detected using screening tools such as the Confusion Assessment Method for the ICU (CAM-ICU) or the Intensive Care Delirium Screening Checklist (ICDSC). There are three subtypes: hyperactive (characterized by agitation, restlessness, hallucinations, or aggression), hypoactive (characterized by lethargy, inattentiveness, and motor slowness), and mixed (fluctuating between hyperactive and hypoactive subtypes). The most common phenotype encountered in clinical practice is hypoactive delirium, which is often difficult to identify [2].

INCIDENCE AND RISK FACTORS

The incidence of delirium in patients admitted to an ICU ranges from 30 to 60%, of which 80% of cases occur in patients on mechanical ventilation (MV)[2]. Delirium has been described as a multifactorial disorder with several predisposing and precipitating risk factors. Predisposing factors include advanced age, baseline cognitive impairment, increased comorbidity disease burden, frailty, alcohol, drug abuse, and high severity of presenting illness. Precipitating factors occurring during critical illness may consist of metabolic disturbances, hypotension, sepsis, inadequate pain control, MV, sleep disturbances, psychoactive medication use, and surgery. Among sedatives and analgesics, lorazepam, midazolam, meperidine, and morphine are strongly associated with a higher risk of delirium, in contrast to propofol, dexmedetomidine, and fentanyl.

COMPLICATIONS ASSOCIATED WITH DELIRIUM

Once considered a temporary nuisance, delirium has since been shown to be associated with increased MV time, ICU length of stay, excess cost, worse long-term cognitive function, and increased mortality. A prospective cohort study performed by Ely and colleagues showed that among ICU patients receiving MV, those who developed delirium spent 10 days longer in the hospital ($p < 0.001$), and had fewer median days alive and without mechanical ventilation (19 [interquartile range, 4–23] vs. 24 [19–26] days; adjusted $p = 0.03$), a higher incidence of cognitive impairment at hospital discharge (adjusted HR, 9.1; 95% CI, 2.3–35.3; $p = 0.002$), and higher 6-month mortality

DOI: 10.1201/9781003042136-35

(34% vs. 15%, $p = 0.03$) when compared to patients without delirium after adjusting for age, severity of illness, comorbid conditions, coma, and use of sedatives or analgesic medications. Cognitive decline after delirium can persist for months to years after ICU stay and is associated with patients not returning to their prior quality of life or employment. A multicenter, prospective cohort study [3] showed that patients with postoperative delirium had a larger decrease in Mini-Mental State Examination (MMSE) scores after 2 postoperative days (7.7 points vs. 2.1, $p < 0.001$), and lower MMSE scores both at 1 month (mean [SD], 24.1 vs. 27.4; $p < 0.001$) and 1 year (25.2 vs. 27.2, $p < 0.001$) after surgery than those without delirium. Furthermore, a higher proportion of patients with delirium than those without delirium had not returned to their preoperative baseline level at 6 months (40% vs. 24%, $p = 0.01$).

PREVENTION AND TREATMENT OF DELIRIUM

As numerous factors contribute to delirium, it is no surprise that multicomponent prevention measures with a multidisciplinary approach are probably the most effective strategies [4]. Inouye et al. [5] showed that the Hospital Elder Life Program, a multicomponent intervention consisting of standardized protocols for the management of cognitive impairment, sleep deprivation, immobility, visual impairment, hearing impairment, and dehydration, could decrease the incidence of delirium (42[9.9%] vs. 64[15%], $p = 0.02$) in hospitalized older patients. Similarly, the ABCDEF bundle has been associated with a reduction in the risk of delirium (adjusted odds ratio [AOR], 0.60; CI, 0.49–0.72), MV time ([AOR], 0.28; CI, 0.22–0.36), hospital death within 7 days (adjusted hazard ratio, 0.32; CI, 0.17–0.62), physical restraint use (AOR, 0.37; CI, 0.30–0.46), ICU readmission (AOR, 0.54; CI, 0.37–0.79) and discharge to a facility other than home (AOR, 0.64; CI, 0.51–0.80) [6].

Numerous pharmacological strategies for delirium prevention have been investigated, yielding inconsistent and conflicting data regarding the efficacy of any particular agent. Promising results from the DEXACET trial showed a reduction in in-hospital delirium in cardiac surgery patients when scheduled intravenous Acetaminophen was used as part of a postoperative analgesia regimen [7]. It has also been shown that dexmedetomidine achieves comparable sedation levels to midazolam in mechanical ventilated patients, and that patients sedated with dexmedetomidine as compared to midazolam had less delirium (54% vs. 76.6% [95% CI, 14%–33%]; $p < 0.001$) and spent less time on the ventilator (3.7 days [95% CI, 3.1–4.0] vs. 5.6 days [95% CI, 4.6–5.9]; $p = 0.01$) [8]. Current SCCM guidelines suggest using propofol or dexmedetomidine over benzodiazepines in mechanically ventilated patients and aim for lighter sedation levels as a preventive measure [9]. Other agents such as melatonin, corticosteroids, statins, and gabapentin have been studied, but consistent high quality evidence is lacking to fully support their role in delirium prevention.

The treatment of established delirium should be twofold: first to manage the behavioral disturbance, and secondly to find and treat the underlying medical disorder. Unfortunately, the non-pharmacological interventions mentioned above are less effective if implemented once delirium has occurred. Evidence supporting the use of pharmacologic agents for delirium treatment is inconclusive. Haloperidol remains the standard therapy in this setting. However, newer atypical antipsychotic agents such as quetiapine, risperidone, ziprasidone, and olanzapine have fewer side effects with similar efficacy, but their use has not been shown to prevent delirium in clinical trials. Given that extrapyramidal and cardiovascular complications are common side effects of both typical and atypical antipsychotics, dexmedetomidine has come to the forefront of delirium treatment in the ICU. The DahLIa study randomized patients to dexmedetomidine versus placebo, showing a hastened time to resolution of delirium in the dexmedetomidine group (median[IQR] 23.3 [13.0–54.0] vs. 40.0 [25.3–76.0] h, $p = 0.01$) and significantly fewer patients treated with antipsychotics(65.6% vs. 36.8%, 95% CI, 51.3–6.3%, $p = 0.02$) in the treatment group. Benzodiazepines are currently avoided as they may increase delirium incidence [10].

CONCLUSION

Delirium is a common and yet frequently undetected complication of critical illness and can result in significant long-term complications. Future trials should identify more sensitive instruments to diagnose delirium and to determine optimal pharmacological approaches to prevention and management. Meanwhile, preventive non-pharmacological measures involving multicomponent targeted interventions should be strongly encouraged.

ANNOTATED REFERENCES FOR DELIRIUM

1. Ely EW, Margolin R, Francis J, et al. Evaluation of delirium in critically ill patients: validation of the Confusion Assessment Method for the Intensive Care Unit (CAM-ICU). *Crit Care Med.* 2001 Jul;29(7):1370–79.

   Classic study that validated the CAM-ICU instrument against the DSM-IV criteria for delirium. Showing it is quick, valid, and reliable for diagnosing delirium in the ICU setting.

2. Krewulak KD, Stelfox HT, Leigh JP, Ely EW, Fiest KM. Incidence and prevalence of delirium subtypes in an adult ICU: a systematic review and meta-analysis. *Crit Care Med.* 2018;46(12):2029–35.

   Systematic review and meta-analysis including 48 studies (27,342 patients; 4550 with delirium) with showing overall pooled prevalence of 31%. These data show the majority of delirious ICU patients to have hypoactive delirium and delirium risk is higher in patients with greater severity of illness.

3. Saczynski JS, Marcantonio ER, Quach L, et al. Cognitive trajectories after postoperative delirium. *N Engl J Med.* 2012 Jul 5;367(1):30–9.

   Prospective study of patients 60 years of age or older undergoing coronary-artery bypass grafting or valve replacement surgery that showed that postoperative development of delirium was a risk factor for a decline in cognitive function and a prolonged period of impairment after cardiac surgery.

4. Deng L-X, Cao L, Zhang L-N, Peng X-B, Zhang L. Non-pharmacological interventions to reduce the incidence and duration of delirium in critically Ill patients: a systematic review and network meta-analysis. *J Crit Care.* 2020 Aug 31;60:241–8.

Recent systematic review and meta-analysis showing that multi-component strategies are overall the optimal intervention techniques for preventing delirium and reducing ICU length of stay in critically ill patients.

5. Inouye SK, Bogardus ST, Charpentier PA, et al. A multicomponent intervention to prevent delirium in hospitalized older patients. *N Engl J Med.* 1999 Mar 4;340(9):669–76.

Prospective randomized controlled clinical trial in a teaching institution demonstrating that an intervention consisting of standardized protocols for the management of six risk factors for delirium: cognitive impairment, sleep deprivation, immobility, visual impairment, hearing impairment, and dehydration resulted in significant reductions in the number and duration of episodes of delirium in hospitalized older patients.

6. Pun BT, Balas MC, Barnes-Daly MA, et al. Caring for critically Ill patients with the ABCDEF bundle: results of the ICU Liberation Collaborative in over 15,000 adults. *Crit Care Med.* 2019 Jan;47(1):3–14.

Prospective, multicenter, cohort study from a national quality improvement collaborative, including patients from 68 ICUs and a total of 15,226 patients, showing that a non-pharmacological approach significantly improved survival, mechanical ventilation use, coma and delirium, restraint-free care, ICU readmissions, and post-ICU discharge disposition.

7. Subramaniam B, Shankar P, Shaefi S, et al. Effect of intravenous acetaminophen vs. placebo combined with propofol or dexmedetomidine on postoperative delirium among older patients following cardiac surgery: the DEXACET randomized clinical trial. *JAMA.* 2019 Feb 19;321(7):686.

First randomized controlled trial showing a significant and meaningful reduction in the incidence of delirium with the use of scheduled IV acetaminophen in patients undergoing cardiac surgery. Additionally, delirium duration, ICU length of stay, and opioid and/or opioid equivalent use in the immediate postoperative period were lower in the intervention group.

8. Riker RR. Dexmedetomidine vs. midazolam for sedation of critically Ill patients: a randomized trial. *JAMA.* 2009 Feb 4;301(5):489.

Multicenter, prospective, double-blind, randomized trial showing that the use of dexmedetomidine vs. midazolam achieved comparable sedation levels. Patients in the dexmedetomidine group spent less time on the ventilator, experienced less delirium, and developed less tachycardia and hypertension.

9. Devlin JW, Skrobik Y, Gélinas C, et al. Clinical practice guidelines for the prevention and management of pain, agitation/sedation, delirium, immobility, and sleep disruption in adult patients in the ICU. *Crit Care Med.* 2018 Sep;46(9):e825.

Most current SCCM guidelines regarding the management of delirium in the ICU.

10. Reade MC, Eastwood GM, Bellomo R, et al. Effect of dexmedetomidine added to standard care on ventilator-free time in patients with agitated delirium: a randomized clinical trial. *JAMA.* 2016 Apr 12;315(14):1460.

This study showed a potential benefit of using dexmedetomidine, in addition to standard care, for ventilated patients with agitated delirium. There was a modest reduction in time for liberation from the ventilator and a more rapid delirium resolution. It also demonstrated sedation and opioid-sparing effects.

Landmark Article of the 21st Century

DELIRIUM AS A PREDICTOR OF MORTALITY IN MECHANICALLY VENTILATED PATIENTS IN THE INTENSIVE CARE UNIT

Ely EW et al., *JAMA*. 2004 APR 14;291(14):1753–1762

Commentary by Tara DiNitto

Ely and colleagues, proved a causal relationship between delirium and mortality.

In their study, 275 mechanically ventilated medical ICU patients were evaluated for delirium and coma by using the Confusion Assessment Method for the ICU (CAM-ICU) and Richmond Agitation-Sedation Scale (RASS). Patients neurologic status was assessed daily by study nurses and grouped into "coma" with a RASS of -4 or -5 and delirium if CAM-ICU was positive at any time while they were in the ICU.

Among the surviving 224 patients, 81.7% developed delirium (n = 1 87, 50% the hypoactive form). The primary outcome was 6-month mortality, overall hospital length of stay, and length of stay post ICU. Secondary outcomes were ventilator free days and cognitive impairment at hospital discharge. Only 18.3% of the patients never experienced delirium (n = 41); 81.7% (n = 183) experienced delirium for a median of 2 days. When looking at the alert or easily arousable patients, 54.5% exhibited delirium during their ICU stay. Evaluating the sedative/analgesic aspects between the groups, the delirium group received more benzodiazepines exclusively. There was no significant difference between the propofol, morphine, or fentanyl given to the either group. Thirty-four percent (63/183) of the patients who exhibited delirium during their ICU stay died within 6 months compared to only 15% (6/41) in the non-delirium group. After adjusting for all the covariates, including coma and medications, the delirium group had a 3-time higher risk of dying by 6 months. Each additional ICU day spent in "delirium" was associated with a 10% increased risk of death.

After multivariate analysis, patients who exhibited delirium in the ICU were nine times more likely to be discharged with cognitive impairment. Delirium was found to be an independent predictor of higher mortality and longer hospital stay even after adjusting for these and other common variants.

CHAPTER 36

Intractable Intracranial Hypertension

Review by Raphael A. Carandang

Cerebral edema and intracranial hypertension can develop in the setting of various brain pathologies including brain tumors, encephalitis, meningitis, metabolic encephalopathies, subarachnoid hemorrhage, intraparenchymal hemorrhage, malignant ischemic stroke and most often in traumatic brain injury (TBI). The Munro–Kellie doctrine, while somewhat oversimplistic, continues to frame our understanding of the relationship of the various components of the intracranial contents, volume and pressure and how pathology causes focal and diffuse changes that can result in shifts of brain tissue within the heterogenous internal surface of the cranium with its compartments separating the posterior or inferior, middle and superior cranial fossa resulting in herniation syndromes and fatal brain injury. Numerous secondary mechanisms of injury on the macrovascular and microcellular level are involved depending on the primary brain pathology including loss of cerebral autoregulation, hydrocephalus, blood–brain barrier breakdown often resulting in vasogenic edema, excitotoxicity, mitochondrial dysfunction and apoptosis resulting in cellular death and cytotoxic edema [1].

The best studied and understood of these conditions is traumatic cerebral edema, often diffuse, causing intracranial hypertension which is dangerous because it compromises cerebral perfusion [2]. The clinical assessment of these patients is difficult given the pragmatic limitations of associated polytrauma, agitation and pain requiring sedation and analgesia, shock with hemodynamic and respiratory instability, and the non-specific and acute deterioration that occurs prior to a clear clinical herniation syndrome. These difficulties highlight the need for further diagnostic tools to understand what is unfolding in the brain during these critical moments in order to initiate appropriate therapy.

The idea that swelling occurs in the head and that release of intracranial pressure may be therapeutic has been around for years dating back to ancient Egyptian times with evidence across continents of trephination being performed. Intracranial pressure (ICP) monitors have been around since the 1960s when Nils Lundberg inserted the first brain ICP monitors, measured pressures and characterized the ICP wave forms [3]. Since then the practice of ICP monitoring in severe traumatic brain injury became standard and ICP thresholds of danger were established from national traumatic coma databank data. Therapies were discovered including diuretics, osmotherapy, sedation and analgesics, hypothermia, and surgery to treat intracranial hypertension. However, despite the development of these monitoring devices coupled with advances in critical

DOI: 10.1201/9781003042136-36

211

care and newer multimodal cerebral monitoring, the mortality rate for severe TBI has not substantially changed over the past 20 years. Part of that observation can be explained by changes in mechanisms of injury in an aging demographic. Falls in the elderly have surpassed motor vehicle accidents as the most common cause of TBI. The other explanation is the lack of solid evidence-based treatments for severe TBI and intractable intracranial hypertension. Upon review of the latest consensus guidelines for management for severe TBI, the only level 1 evidence-based recommendation continues to be to NOT give steroids as it increases mortality. Nearly all the remaining treatments only have level 2 or 3 quality of evidence at best [4].

Current treatments include osmotherapy, hyperventilation, hypothermia, pentobarbital coma, augmenting cerebral perfusion pressure, and surgical decompression. All appear to be effective in lowering ICP and reversing clinical herniation. Mannitol and hypertonic saline work by shrinking the brain to create more space intracranially and prevent herniation. The former is an osmotic diuretic which causes cellular dehydration and if improperly managed can cause renal and multi-organ failure. The latter is a volume expander but can cause hyperchloremic acidosis and hypernatremia [5]. Hyperventilation exploits the sensitivity of the cerebral vasculature to CO_2 and induces vasoconstriction to reduce cerebral blood volume and ICP but has been found to cause cerebral ischemia and worsen outcomes. Hypothermia is effective in lowering ICP but causes shivering and increased metabolism and can result in increased ICP [6]. Pentobarbital coma decreases brain metabolism resulting in reduced blood flow and total blood volume thereby decreasing ICP but has severe adverse effects including refractory shock, coagulopathy, increased risk of infection, and multi-organ failure which can be fatal [7]. Augmenting mean arterial pressure (MAP) to improve cerebral perfusion pressure also makes mechanistic sense and some studies showed a trend towards decreased 2-week mortality and outcome but were complicated by a higher incidence of ARDS. Lastly, decompressive craniectomy (DC) is an option of which there are two randomized controlled trials (RTC) comparing it with medical therapy. In the DECRA study, patients were randomized to early DC in TBI patients with diffuse injury and elevated ICP versus medical management. It was a negative trial but was flawed for two major reasons: 1) despite randomization and an exclusion criteria including patients with bilateral fixed pupils, there were significantly more patients with bilateral fixed pupils in the surgical arm suggesting more herniated patients and a likelihood that outcome would be impacted significantly; and 2) the comparative ICP values in both the surgical and medical arms were well controlled (below 20 mm Hg), even in the medical arm, suggesting that this population of patients was not truly the refractory population of patients that would subjected to DC surgery in the first place. Consequently, the study was not able to answer the question of whether DC could make patients better beyond survival. The Rescue-ICP study did not have the same flaws and found that there was a mortality benefit, but it came with a higher likelihood of vegetative state and severe disability [8].

Several questions arise. Is the wrong biomarker (ICP) being targeted or is the threshold incorrect? The BEST-TRIP trial was an RCT comparing an ICP-based versus a clinical-imaging based treatment protocol and showed no difference in outcomes between both groups [9]. Is ICP an oversimplistic diagnostic marker that does not account for the complexity of the pathophysiological process in severe TBI involved in cerebral edema? A recent phase 2 trial incorporating regional oxygen monitoring with ICP and tiered standardized interventions reported a trend towards improved outcomes [10].

Various factors contribute to the current state of evidence including the heterogeneity of TBI and patients enrolled in clinical trials, underpowered studies, inadequate biomarkers to guide individualized therapy in very complex clinical situations and outcome measures that are not appropriate or sensitive enough to capture clinical benefits.

ANNOTATED REFERENCES FOR INTRACTABLE INTRACRANIAL HYPERTENSION

1. Koenig MA. Cerebral edema and elevated intracranial pressure. *Continuum*. 2018 Dec;24(6):1588–1602.

   Comprehensive review article that describes the different types and etiologies of cerebral edema and their specific treatments; the physiological concepts of elevated intracranial pressure and its measurement and management including pentobarbital coma, hypothermia and decompressive surgery and the different herniation syndromes. Describes important distinctions between vasogenic and cytotoxic edema, diffuse and focal edema, uncal, and central posterior fossa herniation syndromes.

2. Stocchetti N, Maas AI. Traumatic intracranial hypertension. *N Engl J Med*. 2014 May 29;370(22):2121–30.

   A focused review on intracranial hypertension from traumatic brain injury. Discusses pathophysiology and intracranial pressure monitoring and brief summaries of management citing evidence and offers staircase tiered management strategy.

3. Anika S, Fareed J, Bharath R, Nitesh VP, Gaurav G, Anil N. The historical evolution of intracranial pressure monitoring. *World Neurosurg*. June 2020;138: 491–7.

   A comprehensive historical review of the development of intracranial pressure monitoring.

4. Carney N, Totten AM, O'Reilly C, et al. Guidelines for the management of severe traumatic brain injury. *Neurosurgery*. 2017 Jan 1;80(1):6–15.

   Latest updated comprehensive guidelines for management of severe TBI. Notable updates include the inclusion of decompressive craniectomy and CSF drainage as treatments. Hyperosmolar therapy section focused on comparative effectiveness of different agents, additional nutritional recommendations, and reorganizing and renaming of chapters, including a separate CPP and BP threshold section and advanced cerebral monitoring and threshold section. Notable recommendations include SBP thresholds of 100–110 mm Hg, early feeding within 5 days. Of note, these guidelines came out before the results of the BOOST-2 trial were published.

5. Ropper AH. Hyperosmolar therapy for raised intracranial pressure. *N Engl J Med*. 2012;367:746–52.

   Case based review discussing the detailed physiological mechanisms of actions of mannitol and hypertonic saline, its clinical use as well as adverse effects, evidence supporting its use, as well as addressing some controversies regarding its use.

6. Clifton GL, Valadka A, Zygun D, et al. Very early hypothermia induction in patients with severe brain injury (the National Acute Brain Injury Study: Hypothermia II): a randomised trial. *Lancet Neurol.* 2011;10:131–9.

   Randomized, multicenter clinical trial of severe TBI patients assigned to hypothermia and cooled to 33°C for 48 hours and then gradually rewarmed or treated at normothermia, looking at the Glasgow outcome scale score at 6 months. This was a negative trial with no differences in outcomes, but it's notable that the hypothermia group had more episodes of ICP elevation than the normothermia group. The study was also stopped short for futility and was likely underpowered. It raised questions about the appropriate duration of hypothermia and complications of rewarming as well as differences in diffuse versus focal brain injury.

7. Roberts I, Sydenham E. Barbiturates for acute traumatic brain injury. *Cochrane Database Syst Rev.* 2012 Dec 12;12(12):CD000033

   Cochrane review of barbiturate use for acute traumatic brain injury from seven clinical trials with a total of 341 patients. They concluded that there was no outcome or mortality benefit and that a fourth of all patient receiving barbiturates develop significant hypotension that likely offsets any benefit that may have been seen.

8. Hutchinson PJ, Kolias AG, Timofeev IS, et al. Trial of decompressive craniectomy for traumatic intracranial hypertension. *N Engl J Med.* 2016 Sep 22;375(12):1119–30.

   Multicenter, international, randomized, parallel group, superiority clinical trial looking at decompressive craniectomy in traumatic brain injury, which was completed after the DECRA trial results were published showing a significant mortality benefit at 6 months but also higher rates of vegetative state and severe disability in the surgically treated patients. It differs substantially from DECRA in that it initiated surgical treatments as a last tier in truly refractory patients and included patients with intraparenchymal hematoma which compromised 20% of the patients. They also allowed for hemicraniectomy which DECRA excluded.

9. Chesnut RM, Temkin N, Carney N, et al. A trial of intracranial-pressure monitoring in traumatic brain injury. *N Engl J Med.* 2012 Dec 27;367(26):2471–81.

   The only randomized controlled trial comparing an ICP monitoring based management protocol versus a serial examination and imaging-based management protocol for severe TBI patients. Conducted in Bolivia and Ecuador because of lack of clinical equipoise and legal limitations in the US the study showed no difference in outcomes or rates of craniectomy but did result in less osmotherapy and hyperventilation and shorter duration of these treatments in the ICP monitoring group.

10. Okonkwo DO, Shutter LA, Moore C, et al. Brain tissue oxygen monitoring and management in severe traumatic brain injury (BOOST-II): a phase II randomized trial. *Crit Care Med.* 2017 Nov;45(11):1907–14.

    A two-arm, single-blind, prospective randomized controlled multicenter phase II trial assessing safety and efficacy of a management protocol optimizing $PbtO_2$ following severe TBI that showed good safety and that the addition of regional oxygen monitoring to ICP monitoring resulted in a positive trend for outcome and lower mortality.

Landmark Article of the 21st Century

DECOMPRESSIVE CRANIECTOMY IN DIFFUSE TRAUMATIC BRAIN INJURY

Cooper DJ et al., *New Engl J Med.* 2011;364(16):1493–1502.

Commentary by Andrew L.A. Garton and Jared A. Knopman

Summary: The Decompressive Craniectomy (DECRA) trial randomized 155 patients with severe traumatic brain injury (TBI) with ICPs refractory to hyperventilation, hypertonics, paralytics, and often cerebrospinal fluid diversion to either receive continued standard care management or undergo bifrontotemporal decompression after 72 hours of treatment. The randomization was stratified by treatment center as well as modality of ICP measurement (patients received either monitors or ventricular drainage catheters). There was a higher rate of complications in the surgical group (37%) than conservative (17%), skewed in part by hydrocephalus. The trial found that while decompressive craniectomy decreased ICPs effectively, it was associated with poorer functional outcomes at 6 months.

Critique: The data here only reflects patients without mass lesions, which in severe TBI (GCS: 3–8) reflects a small percentage of patients; 3478 patients were screened but with a final sample size of 155 (4.5%). Although randomization was achieved in gold-standard fashion, a higher proportion of patients in the surgical group were noted to have bilaterally unreactive pupils. There was no demonstrable evidence in radiographic edema between the two groups. This clear clinical difference could reflect worse preoperative substrate, impacting remote functional outcomes. It has also been argued that, without dividing the anterior superior sagittal sinus or the falx cerebri, the procedural efficacy was limited in DECRA. RESCUEicp, a subsequent trial on surgery in severe TBI, offered more discretion to the surgeon in peri- and intra-operative decision making. Finally, the primary outcome time point was 6 months after intervention; modern advancements in neurocognitive and physical rehabilitation may continue to offer improvements in long-term outcome in severe TBI patients, and early decompression may lead to divergent outcomes over longer intervals.

Conclusion: DECRA reflects an important attempt to offer randomized data for surgical management of refractory ICPs in severe TBI without mass lesions. In a limited subject population, decompressive craniectomies may not improve functional outcomes at short-term follow-up.

CHAPTER 37

Coagulopathy

Review by Jessica Cassavaugh

Critically ill patients, especially in the surgical intensive care units are at tremendous risk for bleeding. Bleeding is frequently either surgical, a deficit of the coagulation system or both. Coagulopathies in the intensive care unit are extremely common, and it is not unusual for multiple abnormalities to be simultaneously present. Thrombocytopenia (platelet count of $<100 \times 10^9$/L), which occurs in approximately 25% of all critically ill patients, has an increased incidence of 35–40% in surgical or trauma ICU patients [1, 2]. Likewise, laboratory measurements of coagulation time (prothrombin time [PT] and activated partial thromboplastin time [aPTT]) are also shown to be abnormal in 14–28% of critically ill patients, with a prolonged PT or aPTT occurring in over 25% of patients with traumatic injuries [2, 3]. Both thrombocytopenia and abnormal PT/aPTT have been associated with increased mortality, especially in trauma and surgical patients. According to Brohi et al., trauma patients with a coagulopathy at time of admission had an overall mortality rate of 46% compared to 11% in the non-coagulopathy group [3]. Similarly, in a study conducted by Vanderschueren et al., the mortality rate for ICU patients was 35% in patients who were thrombocytopenic at admission compared to 9% mortality for ICU patients who never developed thrombocytopenia [4].

Conventional coagulation tests (CCTs) including PT, aPTT, INR, platelet count and fibrinogen level remain widely used; however, they have significant limitations. One major limitation with CCTs is the measurement of platelet dysfunction, which is a frequent occurrence in ICU populations. While several platelet function assays exist, only a limited number are in regular use clinically. Tests based on platelet aggregation (VerifyNow) or platelet adhesion under shear stress (platelet function analyzer [PFA]) are available as rapid, point of care tests that can both be helpful in determining the presence of an antiplatelet agents (aspirin, GPIIb/IIIa antagonists, or P2Y12 inhibition) and in determining level of clot forming ability. The PFA-100 in particular, can be used to rapidly determine the absence of aspirin or GPIIb/IIIa antagonists due to its high negative predictive value. However, this the result is limited as a positive result is non-specific [5]. Considerations such as rapidity of testing, characterization of complete coagulation pathway, cumbersome nature of numerous laboratory tests, and closer association with clinical outcomes led to the development of viscoelastic measurements of whole blood (TEG, ROTEM). Since the development of these viscoelastic tests, multiple studies have shown a superior improvement in testing turnaround times, prediction of massive transfusion and mortality as well as improvement in directed transfusion [6, 7].

DOI: 10.1201/9781003042136-37

Multiple risk factors for thrombocytopenia are commonly present in critical illness including bleeding, shock, and medications. The most common cause of thrombocy-topenia in the ICU, however, is sepsis followed by trauma and disseminated intravas-cular coagulation (DIC) [1, 8]. Several studies have found an association with a higher severity of illness score (APACHE II, SOFA) and thrombocytopenia, thus suggesting that higher severity of illness is a risk for thrombocytopenia [1, 8]. DIC, one of the most common causes of ICU thrombocytopenia, is secondary to a variety of etiologies including infection, trauma, hemorrhage, and cancer. Strauss et al. demonstrated that the majority of patients (82%) with septic shock in the ICU met criteria for DIC. Other prevalent causes of thrombocytopenia include drug induced, most commonly heparin-induced thrombocytopenia (HIT), or immune mediated causes.

In addition to thrombocytopenia, platelet dysfunction which is commonly due to organ failure, hypothermia, or medications, is another significant cause of coagulopa-thy in the ICU. With the increasing use of anti-platelet medications including COX inhibitors (aspirin, NSAIDs), thienopyridines (clopidogrel, ticagrelor), glycoprotein platelet inhibitors (abciximab, eptifibatide) and others, it is not uncommon for a hemorrhagic presentation to be complicated by platelet dysfunction. This is espe-cially true for intracranial hemorrhage (ICH) whether spontaneous or secondary to trauma. The presence of an anti-platelet agent has been shown to be associated with an increase ICH volume and mortality, especially with dual antiplatelet therapy [9]. Since mortality is likely increased for patients on anti-platelet medications who have suffered ICH, the effect of platelet transfusion in this population was investigated. PATCH, a randomized study conducted in 60 hospitals throughout Europe, assessed early platelet transfusion for acute stroke patients with spontaneous cerebral hemor-rhage while on anti-platelet therapy. The PATCH investigators found increased mor-tality at 3 months and increased serious adverse events during the hospitalization for patients who received a platelet transfusion compared to standard of care [10]. While this was a small, non-blinded trial, PATCH demonstrated that platelet transfusions are at best not beneficial and at worst, are harmful for ICH in patients on anti-platelet medications.

Abnormalities of the coagulation system are another frequent cause of coagulopathy in the ICU. Such abnormalities are typically classified by a prolongation of CCTs with factor deficiencies, both acquired and innate, as well as anti-thrombotic medi-cations being the most common etiologies. A variety of medications target vari-ous components of the coagulation pathway including anti-thrombin III mediators (heparins, fondaparinux), vitamin K antagonists (warfarin), direct thrombin inhibi-tors (bivalirudin, dabigatran), and direct factor Xa inhibitors (rivaroxaban, apixaban). Deficiencies of vitamin K dependent factors remain an extremely common cause of prolonged CCTs and may be due to liver failure, vitamin K antagonists, nutritional deficiencies or in many cases, a combination of these causes. Another frequent cause of prolonged CCTs is profound coagulopathy that can occur with massive hemor-rhage and hypothermia [2]. In addition to the acquired factor deficiency that occurs with massive hemorrhage, a consumptive coagulopathy may follow, especially in trauma patients who develop DIC [3]. Having multiple, simultaneous coagulation disorders may explain, in part, the increased mortality of trauma patients who present with abnormal CCTs.

The mainstays of treatment for coagulopathies continues to be treatment of the underlying condition, replacement of deficiencies and discontinuation of any anti-thrombotic or anti-platelet medications. Guidelines for platelet transfusion vary depending on the clinical scenario; however, most guidelines support transfusion for a platelet count of $<30–50 \times 10^9$/L in high risk patients and for $<10 \times 10^9$/L in all patients [2, 8]. Plasma may be necessary when repletion of multiple coagulation factors is needed, especially during massive hemorrhage, although prothrombin complex concentrates (PCCs), isolated recombinant coagulation factors, and newer specific reversal agents may be more favorable depending on the clinical context. PCCs contain all vitamin K dependent factors (II, VII, IX, X) and should be considered for immediate reversal of a vitamin K antagonist for life-threatening bleeding, especially if a large volume transfusion would not be tolerated. In the setting of anti-Xa or anti-thrombin inhibitors, PCCs may be used, however, they have been shown to have variable outcomes and therefore may be less effective than expected [11].

Several specific reversal agents are available: idraucizumab, a monoclonal antibody that irreversibly binds dabigatran, andexenet alfa, a modified recombinant fXa protein that binds and sequesters Xa inhibitors, and ciraparantag, a small molecule that binds to and prevents heparins and Xa and thrombin inhibitors from binding to their respective targets. While these specific reversal agents are highly effective, whether or not they have an effect on outcomes has yet to be definitively shown. In addition, the cost of these agents remains a limitation as they range in the thousands of dollars per dose [11]. Recombinant factor VII is another commonly used treatment in coagulopathy, however, when used off-label it has been associated with an increase in arterial thromboembolic events [12].

ANNOTATED REFERENCES FOR COAGULOPATHY

1. Stephan F, et al. Thrombocytopenia in a surgical ICU. *Chest.* 1999;115:1363–1370.

   Prospective trial investigating incidence and outcomes associated with thrombocytopenia and surgical ICU patients. The investigators found sepsis to be the major risk factor for development of thrombocytopenia and found thrombocytopenic patients had a higher ICU mortality due to increased severity of disease.

2. Levi M, Opal SM. Coagulation abnormalities in critically ill patients. *Crit Care.* 2006;10:222.

   A comprehensive review detailing the diagnosis and etiology of major coagulopathies in critically ill patients. Describes multiple management strategies for treatment of coagulopathies with a focus on DIC.

3. Brohi K, Singh J, Heron M, Coats T. Acute traumatic coagulopathy. *J Trauma.* 2003;54.

   A retrospective study designed to determine the clinical importance of coagulopathy in severely injured trauma patients. The authors found that patients with acute coagulopathy had a significantly higher mortality rate, and the incidence of coagulopathy increased with the severity of the injury.

4. Vanderschueren S, et al. Thrombocytopenia and prognosis in intensive care. *Crit Care Med.* 2000;28:1871–1876.

   A prospective observational cohort study aimed to identify the incidence and prognosis of thrombocytopenia in the ICU. Found thrombocytopenia to be risk marker for mortality. Also found a low platelet nadir and large drop in platelet count to predict poor outcomes.

5. Paniccia R, Priora R, Liotta AA, Abbate R. Platelet function tests: a comparative review. *Vasc Health Risk Manag.* 2015;11:133–148.

   A comparative review describing current test available for assessment of platelet function with focus on modern, clinically relevant tests. Describes testing methodology and clinical applications as well.

6. Da Luz LT, Nascimento B, Shankarakutty AK, Rizoli S, Adhikari NKJ. Effect of thromboelastography (TEG®) and rotational thromboelastometry (ROTEM®) on diagnosis of coagulopathy, transfusion guidance and mortality in trauma: descriptive systematic review. *Crit Care.* 2014;18.

   Systematic review evaluating TEG and ROTEM in diagnosing early coagulopathies, guiding blood transfusion and reducing mortality. Review included 55 trials and determined TEG/ROTEM are capable of diagnosing early coagulopathies in trauma.

7. Holcomb JB, et al. Admission rapid thrombelastography can replace conventional coagulation tests in the emergency department: experience with 1974 consecutive trauma patients. *Ann Surg.* 2012;256:476–486.

   Study comparing reliability of TEG in predicting blood component transfusion when compared to CCTs in major trauma. The authors found TEG to be superior and more expedient results for transfusion component prediction.

8. Strauss R, et al. Thrombocytopenia in patients in the medical intensive care unit: bleeding prevalence, transfusion requirements, and outcome. *Crit Care Med.* 2002;30:1765–1771.

   Prospective observational studies measuring risk factors, prevalence and outcomes of thrombocytopenic patients in medical ICUs. Identified predictors of thrombocytopenia (DIC, organ failure at presentation, CPR) and determined thrombocytopenic patients are at higher risk of bleeding with increased transfusion requirements.

9. Sprügel MI, et al. Antiplatelet therapy in primary spontaneous and oral anticoagulation-associated intracerebral hemorrhage. *Stroke.* 2018;49:2621–2629.

   Study using pooled data from retrospective cohort studies and prospective single-center studies to determine the influence of concomitant antiplatelet therapy on hematoma characteristics and outcome in ICH. Results significant for anti-platelet therapy being associated with increased ICH volume and worse functional outcomes.

10. Baharoglu MI, et al. Platelet transfusion versus standard care after acute stroke due to spontaneous cerebral haemorrhage associated with antiplatelet therapy (PATCH): a randomised, open-label, phase 3 trial. *Lancet.* 2016;387:2605–2613.

    Randomized trial investigating effect of platelet transfusion on mortality in patients with ICH on anti-platelet medication. Platelet transfusion in these patients increase mortality and severe adverse events during hospitalization.

11. Ruff CT, Giugliano RP, Antman EM. Management of bleeding with non–vitamin K antagonist oral anticoagulants in the era of specific reversal agents. *Circulation*. 2016;134:248–261.

    Review article focusing on reversal of non-vitamin K antagonist oral anticoagulants including indications for use, side effects and mechanism of action.

12. Levi M, Levy JH, Andersen HF, Truloff D. Safety of recombinant activated factor VII in randomized clinical trials. *N Engl J Med*. 2010;363:1791–1800.

    The investigators studied the frequency of thromboembolic events in 35 randomized, placebo-controlled trials of rFVIIa. Using pooled data, they determined off-label use of rFVIIa is associated with increased risk of arterial thromboembolic events.

Landmark Article of the 21st Century

PLATELET TRANSFUSION VERSUS STANDARD CARE AFTER ACUTE STROKE DUE TO SPONTANEOUS CEREBRAL HAEMORRHAGE ASSOCIATED WITH ANTIPLATELET THERAPY (PATCH): A RANDOMISED, OPEN-LABEL, PHASE 3 TRIAL

Baharoglu MI et al., *Lancet*. 2016 JUN 25;387:2605–2613

Commentary by Samuel Isaac Hawkins

A key adjunct treatment for critical hemorrhage is the reversal of a medication-induced coagulopathy. For most patients with hemorrhage taking antiplatelet medications, platelet transfusions remain the principal treatment for anti-platelet effect reversal. The PATCH trial data provide the first high quality evidence from a randomized study to guide platelet transfusion practice for these patients, as prior studies had been of low quality and mostly equivocal. The key point of the study is that platelet transfusions for patients on antiplatelet agents with spontaneous intracranial hemorrhage, rather than conferring benefit, are actually harmful.

Can we extrapolate the results of the PATCH trial to patients with traumatic intracranial or extracranial hemorrhage? We should do so with caution. Spontaneous bleeding is more likely to be influenced by the presence of anatomic and structural abnormalities, such as aneurysms. These promote bleeding in such a way as to reduce the relative benefit of correcting the coagulopathy. In traumatic hemorrhage, correction of the coagulopathy may play a larger relative role and confer a larger benefit. Whether this affects the net therapeutic benefit of platelet transfusion will depend on the negative physiologic impact of transfusion, which is harder to predict with blood products than other therapeutic agents. Even purified fractionated components of whole blood contain complex macromolecules, with multiple biologically active fragments. When using blood products, we should therefore have a higher standard for the patient and disease specificity of the empiric evidence we use to support our practice.

The impact of this study is to provide clinical equipoise for the performance of randomized trials for patients on antiplatelet agents with traumatic hemorrhage.

CHAPTER 38

Postoperative Bleeding

Review by Emily E. Switzer and Kenji Inaba

Postoperative bleeding is a potentially fatal complication of elective and emergent surgery. Excessive perioperative blood loss must be identified and treated as quickly as possible to prevent morbidity and mortality. This occurrence is not uncommon with upwards of 3% of all operations complicated by excessive bleeding, which is defined as more bleeding that anticipated. In 90% of these cases, a technical defect is identified as the primary cause of bleeding. In the remaining 10% of cases, a coagulation defect is the cause (Curnow et al., 2016).

Postoperative bleeding can present in many ways. It can be insidious or obvious. Findings such as tachycardia, decreased urine output, hypotension, and narrowed pulse pressure are classic. Physical exam findings such as pallor, anxiety, obvious hematoma, increased abdominal distention, dressing saturation, sanguineous drain output, bloody nasogastric tube output, or oozing at catheter sites may also be seen. Laboratory studies including complete blood count (CBC), lactic acid, and coagulation studies should be obtained emergently. One should not be comforted by normal hemoglobin levels, as the true value can lag 4–6 hours behind the clinical presentation (Dagi, 2005). If the patient is stable, imaging studies may be helpful in identifying the source of bleeding. Hemodynamically unstable patients should be resuscitated with damage control resuscitation, a 1:1:1 ratio of packed red blood cells (pRBCs), fresh frozen plasma (FFP), and platelets. The goal is to thwart the lethal triad of hypothermia, acidosis, and coagulopathy, prevent and correct coagulopathy, avoid excessive crystalloid infusion, and allow for permissive hypotension (Holcomb et al., 2015). Early studies of whole blood resuscitation of combat casualties show promising results (Spinella et al., 2009). It is unclear how such an approach could be achieved in the civilian population. Goal directed, real time, rapid monitoring of resuscitation endpoints can be achieved with viscoelastic hemostatic assays, i.e., TEG/ROTEM. Studies have shown that use of TEG decreases the amount of overall product transfusion in both liver and cardiac operations (Fahrendorff et al., 2017).

Causes of postoperative bleeding can be broadly separated into two categories, surgical and non-surgical bleeding. Surgical bleeding is self-explanatory, while nonsurgical bleeding is caused by a disruption in the coagulation cascade which can be innate or acquired (Curnow et al., 2016).

DOI: 10.1201/9781003042136-38

Surgical bleeding is the most common cause of shock within 24 hours of surgery, thus must be at the top of the differential for the unstable postoperative patient. A methodical work-up, quickly ruling out cardiogenic, distributive, and obstructive shock is paramount. Unstable patients with surgical bleeding should be resuscitated and taken for operative or interventional exploration. Stable patients should be worked up and treated as described above (Dagi, 2005).

Once surgical bleeding has been ruled out, other potential causes of postoperative bleeding can be explored. The key to identifying possible coagulation defects is a thorough history. Common inherited causes include von Willebrand Disease (VWD) and the hemophilias. VWD is the most common congenital bleeding disorder with up to 1% of the population harboring this defect. It is caused by a qualitative or quantitative defect in von Willebrand factor (VWF), ultimately affecting platelet function. The CBC and coagulation tests are normal. VWF and Factor VIII tests are required to make the diagnosis. Treatment depends upon the type (Al-Huniti & Kahr, 2020). The hemophilias are an X-linked congenital bleeding disorder caused by a defect in Factors VIII or IX. PTT may be elevated, but specific factor assays are diagnostic. Treatment is factor based (Haider & Anwer, 2020). Acquired causes include vitamin K deficiency, medications, renal disease, liver disease, and hemorrhagic shock. A variety of medications can cause intentional or incidental platelet inhibition. Aspirin and clopidogrel are given to intentionally target platelets, while antibiotics such as penicillin and cephalosporins incidentally affect platelets (Curnow et al., 2016). Warfarin, a vitamin K dependent anticoagulant, can be reversed in a nonurgent manner with FFP and vitamin K, and emergently reversed with prothrombin complex concentrate (PCC). The novel oral anticoagulants can be reversed with the new biologics idarucizumab (dabigatran) and andexanet alfa (rivaroxaban and apixaban). These therapies are commercially available and effective, but are very expensive. If the specific reversal agents are unavailable, PCC can be used with some efficacy for all the novel anticoagulants (Levi, 2016).

The coagulation system is comprised of primary and secondary hemostasis. Platelet plug formation is the endpoint for primary hemostasis, while secondary hemostasis centers around thrombin. Thrombin is an enzyme that converts fibrinogen to fibrin and simultaneously activates platelet aggregation and the intrinsic and extrinsic pathways. Massive blood loss presents a challenge to the coagulation system. With loss of coagulation factors and thrombocytopenia comes coagulopathy (Curnow et al., 2016).

Studies on the coagulation cascade have allowed for identification and targeting of specific areas of the pathway for therapy. Tranexamic acid (TXA) is one solution that has been heavily studied. TXA is a lysine derivative, and its mechanism of action is inhibition of plasminogen. It is an anti-fibrinolytic, ultimately stabilizing the clot. It has been studied in multiple patient populations with promise, including patients with trauma, traumatic brain injury and gastrointestinal bleeding as well as perioperative cardiac surgery and ob-gyn patients (Roberts et al., 2013).

In conclusion, bleeding remains a potentially deadly complication of surgery. Early recognition of surgical versus nonsurgical bleeding is the key to successful treatment. Resuscitation efforts have changed over the past 50 years, with a shift to damage control and whole blood transfusion. Resuscitation endpoints can be monitored with TEG, which is quick and effective. Continued efforts in studying the coagulation cascade has identified adjuncts to help us control bleeding. TXA is one such promising adjunct and has been studied in many patient populations.

ANNOTATED REFERENCES FOR POSTOPERATIVE BLEEDING

Al-Huniti A, Kahr WH. Inherited platelet disorders: diagnosis and management. *Transfus Med Rev*. 2020 Sep 19;S0887-7963(20):30052–3. doi: 10.1016/j.tmrv.2020.09.006. Epub ahead of print. PMID: 33082057.

This review articles describes the different platelet disorders and works through the diagnosis including history and physical exam findings, laboratory studies, and finishes with treatment strategies.

Brenner A, Afolabi A, Ahmad SM, et al.; HALT-IT trial collaborators. Tranexamic acid for acute gastrointestinal bleeding (the HALT-IT trial): statistical analysis plan for an international, randomised, double-blind, placebo-controlled trial. *Trials*. 2019 Jul 30;20(1):467. doi: 10.1186/s13063-019-3561-7. PMID: 31362765; PMCID: PMC6668177.

This is an international, double blinded RCT of 12,000 patients with acute upper or lower GI bleed. Patients were randomized to either TXA or placebo. They found no difference in mortality, rebleeding, or arterial thrombotic events, but did find an increase in venous thrombosis. Based on these findings, the authors do not recommend TXA for GI bleeding.

CRASH-3 trial collaborators. Effects of tranexamic acid on death, disability, vascular occlusive events and other morbidities in patients with acute traumatic brain injury (CRASH-3): a randomised, placebo-controlled trial. *Lancet*. 2019 Nov 9;394(10210):1713–23. doi: 10.1016/S0140-6736(19)32233-0. Epub 2019 Oct 14. Erratum in: Lancet. 2019 Nov 9;394(10210):1712. PMID: 31623894; PMCID: PMC6853170.

The follow up study to Crash-2, Crash-3 is a multi-center international RCT that enrolled >12,000 patients. It showed that early administration of TXA to TBI patients, decreased head injury related deaths in patients with mild-moderate TBI. The risk of blood clots and seizures were similar between the two groups.

Curnow J, Pasalic L, Favaloro EJ. Why do patients bleed? *Surg J (N Y)*. 2016 Feb 24;2(1):e29–e43. doi: 10.1055/s-0036-1579657. PMID: 28824979; PMCID: PMC5553458.

This review provides an overview of reasons that patients bleed in the perioperative setting. It offers guidance on how to screen for these conditions, through appropriate patient history and examination prior to surgical intervention, as well as guidance on investigating and managing the cause of unexpected bleeding.

Dagi TF. The management of postoperative bleeding. *Surg Clin North Am*. 2005 Dec;85(6):1191–213, x. doi: 10.1016/j.suc.2005.10.013. PMID: 16326202.

This review article addresses the prompt diagnosis, differential, and management of postoperative bleeding.

Fahrendorff M, Oliveri RS, Johansson PI. The use of viscoelastic haemostatic assays in goal-directing treatment with allogeneic blood products – A systematic review and meta-analysis. *Scand J Trauma Resusc Emerg Med.* 2017 Apr 13;25(1):39. doi: 10.1186/s13049-017-0378-9. PMID: 28403868; PMCID: PMC5390346.

This meta-analysis reviews RCTs performed on patients in hemorrhagic shock, assessing the utility of the viscoelastic hemostatic assay (VHA). The VHA groups (15 RCTs) had decreased transfusion requirements and decreases blood loss compared to the control groups.

Gonzalez E, Moore EE, Moore HB. Management of trauma-induced coagulopathy with thrombelastography. *Crit Care Clin.* 2017 Jan;33(1):119–34. doi: 10.1016/j.ccc.2016.09.002. PMID: 27894492; PMCID: PMC5142763.

This RCT (TXA or placebo) enrolled 12,009 patients with mixed upper and lower GI bleeds. There was no difference in the mortality rates between groups. There was no difference in arterial complications, but the rate or VTE was higher in the TXA group.

Haider MZ, Anwer F. Acquired hemophilia. 2020 Aug 14. In: *StatPearls [Internet].* Treasure Island (FL): StatPearls Publishing; 2020 Jan. PMID: 32809329.

This review article discusses the types of hemophilias, diagnostic tests, and treatment strategies.

Holcomb JB, Tilley BC, Baraniuk S, et al.; PROPPR Study Group. Transfusion of plasma, platelets, and red blood cells in a 1:1:1 vs. a 1:1:2 ratio and mortality in patients with severe trauma: the PROPPR randomized clinical trial. *JAMA.* 2015 Feb 3;313(5):471–82. doi: 10.1001/jama.2015.12. PMID: 25647203; PMCID: PMC4374744.

680 patients from 12, level 1 trauma centers, were placed in a RCT that compared plasma, platelets, and red blood cells in a 1:1:1 ratio to a 1:1:2 ratio. Results did not show a significant difference in mortality at 24 hours or at 30 days. However, more patients in the 1:1:1 group achieved hemostasis and fewer experienced death due to exsanguination by 24 hours. Even though there was an increased use of plasma and platelets transfused in the 1:1:1 group, no other safety differences were identified between the 2 groups.

Levi M. Management of bleeding in patients treated with direct oral anticoagulants. *Crit Care.* 2016 Aug 20;20:249. doi: 10.1186/s13054-016-1413-3. PMID: 27543264; PMCID: PMC4992194.

This review article discusses the novel anticoagulants and their reversal agents.

Morrison JJ, Dubose JJ, Rasmussen TE, Midwinter MJ. Military application of tranexamic acid in trauma emergency resuscitation (MATTERs) study. *Arch Surg.* 2012 Feb;147(2):113–9. doi: 10.1001/archsurg.2011.287. Epub 2011 Oct 17. PMID: 22006852.

The MATTERs study was a military follow up study after Crash-2. The study is retrospective, 896 patients were identified and 292 received TXA within 1 hour. There was a statistically significant risk reduction in mortality, when TXA was given. All patients who received TXA also received blood products and an operation. There was an increase in blood clots in the TXA group.

Roberts I, et al. The CRASH-2 trial: a randomised controlled trial and economic evaluation of the effects of tranexamic acid on death, vascular occlusive events and transfusion requirement in bleeding trauma patients. *Health Technol Assess.* 2013;17(10):1. doi:10.3310/hta17100.

Spinella PC, Perkins JG, Grathwohl KW, Beekley AC, Holcomb JB. Warm fresh whole blood is independently associated with improved survival for patients with combat-related traumatic injuries. *J Trauma.* 2009 Apr;66(4 Suppl):S69–76. doi: 10.1097/TA.0b013e31819d85fb. PMID: 19359973; PMCID: PMC3126655.

This study retrospectively analyzed 354 patients. The two groups consisted of patients who received warm whole blood plus pRBCs and FFP and those that received pRBCs, FFP, and platelets, no whole blood. The whole blood group had a statistically significant 24 hour and 30-day survival.

WOMAN Trial Collaborators. Effect of early tranexamic acid administration on mortality, hysterectomy, and other morbidities in women with post-partum haemorrhage (WOMAN): an international, randomised, double-blind, placebo-controlled trial. *Lancet.* 2017 May 27;389(10084):2105–16. doi: 10.1016/S0140-6736(17)30638-4. Epub 2017 Apr 26. Erratum in: Lancet. 2017 May 27;389(10084):2104. PMID: 28456509; PMCID: PMC5446563.

This RCT of 20,060 women who had postpartum hemorrhage, enrolled patients to receive TXA or placebo. Death due to bleeding was the only statistically significant endpoint, with a slight reduction in the TXA group. Overall mortality, risk of hysterectomy, or complications (like VTE) were not different between the groups.

Landmark Article of the 21st Century

CRASH II TRIAL

Roberts I et al., *Lancet.* 2010 JUL 3;376(9734):23–32

Commentary by Ian Roberts

Worldwide, bleeding associated with trauma kills around 2 million people each year, with over 90% of the deaths in low and middle income countries. Tranexamic acid (TXA) is an antifibrinolytic drug that has been licensed for use for many years to treat heavy menstrual periods and for dental extraction in people with bleeding disorders. It was used sporadically to reduce blood transfusion in surgical patients. The seed that became the CRASH-2 trial was planted in 2006, when I read the results of a systematic review of randomized trials of antifibrinolytic drugs in elective surgery. Antifibrinolytics (aprotinin or TXA) reduced the need for blood transfusion by one third, reduced donor exposure by one unit, and halved the need for further surgery to control bleeding. There was also a statistically non-significant reduction in the risk of death in the antifibrinolytic treated group.

Since being cut open by a surgeon and being slashed by a machete are not completely different from a hemostatic viewpoint, we thought that TXA had the potential to reduce mortality in bleeding trauma patients. We searched the literature to see if such a trial had already been done but there was nothing at all. I had been searching for a potential intervention to reduce bleeding deaths for a long time and this looked like a winner. At that time there was a lot of interest in hemostatic drugs because Novo Nordisk was pushing recombinant activated factor seven. We had just finished the CRASH trial of corticosteroids in traumatic brain injury (10,000 patients) and had built up a large global network of collaborating centers. We realized that we could build on this network to conduct a large trial of tranexamic acid in acute traumatic bleeding.

We obtained funding support from the UK National Institute for Health Research (NIHR). The trial required a huge effort from hundreds of doctors and nurses around the world, but it was worth it. A total of 20,211 patients were recruited from 274 hospitals in 40 countries. The results showed that TXA reduces mortality with no apparent increase in side effects. If given promptly, the TXA reduces the risk of bleeding to death by about a third. On the basis of these results, it has been estimated that giving TXA to bleeding trauma patients could save up to 200,000 lives per year worldwide. Cost-effectiveness analysis showed that TXA administration is highly cost effective in high, middle, or low income countries. On the basis of the trial results, tranexamic acid was included on the WHO List of Essential Medicines and incorporated into trauma treatment guidelines in many countries. Tranexamic acid is a cheap, generic drug but has huge potential to save lives. We are fortunate to live in a country where you can obtain public funds for patient centered research despite there being little commercial interest from the pharmaceutical industry.

CHAPTER 39

Transfusion Trigger

Review by Manish S. Patel and Jeffrey L. Carson

Anemia is the most common hematological abnormality in the perioperative setting, and the majority of critically ill patients develop anemia during the course of their intensive care unit (ICU) stay. The causes of anemia in hospitalized patients are varied and include active bleeding, post-surgical blood loss, excessive phlebotomy, nutritional deficiencies, the effect of pharmacological therapeutics, or as a result of the underlying illness itself, leading to bone marrow suppression or hemolysis. The risk of death from anemia was well characterized in a retrospective cohort study of 1958 patients undergoing surgery who declined blood transfusions for religious reasons. Thirty-day mortality increased with declining preoperative hemoglobin and rose rapidly in those with hemoglobin below 6 g/dL. With a decreasing preoperative hemoglobin level, the risk of death was higher in those with cardiovascular disease compared to those without cardiovascular disease. These data suggest that patients with cardiovascular disease may be less tolerant of anemia than those without cardiovascular disease (Carson 1996).

What is less clear, however, is whether red blood cell (RBC) transfusion mitigates the risk that anemia poses. In 1942, Adams and Lundy first proposed to give a blood transfusion when the preoperative hemoglobin is below 10 g/dL or if the hematocrit is below 30%. Although this recommendation was based on little evidence, the "10/30" rule was widely used until challenged by the 1988 National Institutes of Health Consensus Conference on Perioperative Red Blood Cell Transfusions. Since that time there are over 30 randomized controlled trials (RCT) to address this question. These trials have randomized participants to either a "restrictive" transfusion strategy (transfusions are given only when the hemoglobin concentration falls below 7–8 g/dL) or a "liberal" transfusion strategy (transfusion given to maintain hemoglobin of 9–10 g/dL).

The first and classic large trial to address transfusion thresholds was the Transfusion Requirement in Critical Care (TRICC) trial. This trial randomized 838 normovolemic ICU patients to either a restrictive group (transfused for hemoglobin <7 g/dL) or a liberal transfusion group (transfused for hemoglobin <10 g/dL). There was a non-statistically significant trend towards lower 30-day mortality in the restrictive group (18.7% vs. 23.3%), as well as significantly lower rates of myocardial infarction (MI) and pulmonary edema, when compared with the liberal group (Hébert 1999). A more recent trial evaluated 998 ICU patients with septic shock and found no difference in mortality or other clinical events in those in transfused below 7 g/dL (restrictive)

DOI: 10.1201/9781003042136-39

compared to transfusion below 9 g/dL (liberal) (Holst 2014). Together, these trials suggest that a hemoglobin concentration of 7 g/dL may be used as a transfusion threshold for most critically ill patients.

Another noteworthy trial was the Functional Outcomes in Cardiovascular Patients Undergoing Surgical Hip Fracture Repair (FOCUS) trial (Carson 2011). This trial included 2016 elderly patients (mean age 81) with a history of, or risk factors for, cardiovascular disease who were undergoing hip fracture repair. Those randomly allocated to receive transfusion if hemoglobin was less than 8 g/dL or for symptoms of anemia (restrictive) had no significant difference in functional outcomes, mortality, or morbidity than those receiving transfusion if hemoglobin was less than 10 g/dL (liberal). These data support the use of 8 g/dL transfusion threshold in those undergoing orthopedic surgery and those with underlying stable cardiovascular disease (Carson 2011).

Acute upper gastrointestinal bleeding is a common cause of anemia in critical care and hospitalized patients. A notable trial evaluated transfusion thresholds in 921 patients with severe upper gastrointestinal bleeding but without massive exsanguination and compared transfusion less than 7 g/dL (restrictive) versus 9 g/dL (liberal). This is the only well powered trial to demonstrate lower mortality in the restrictive group; 45-day mortality (5% vs. 9%) and rate of re-bleeding (10% vs. 16%). This trial establishes that a restrictive transfusion strategy of 7 g/dL is safe and perhaps superior to liberal transfusion strategy in patients with upper gastrointestinal bleeding including those with underlying cirrhosis (Villanueva 2013).

Patients undergoing cardiac surgery are among the most transfused patients overall and in critical care units. The largest trial performed evaluating transfusion thresholds is the Transfusion Requirements in Cardiac Surgery (TRICS) III trial that randomly allocated 5243 patients to either a transfusion at <7.5 g/dL versus <9.5 g/dL in the operating room or ICU and <8.5 g/dL in non-ICU wards (liberal). There was no difference in the 28-day mortality (3% in the restrictive group vs. 3.6% in the liberal group), stroke, MI, or renal failure between the two groups (Mazer 2017). Follow-up at 6 months also showed no difference in outcomes (Mazer 2018). These results are consistent with The Transfusion Indication Threshold Reduction (TITRe2) trial (Murphy 2015). Taken together, these trials suggest that a restrictive transfusion threshold of hemoglobin level of 7.5 g/dL is safe in those undergoing cardiac surgery.

Patients with traumatic brain injury do not appear to benefit from a liberal transfusion strategy. A RCT using a 2×2 factorial design evaluating erythropoietin administration and transfusion strategies showed no difference in 6-month mortality between liberal (<10 mg/dL) and restrictive (<7 mg/dL) approaches. Furthermore, the incidence of adverse events was higher in the liberal transfusion group (Robertson 2014).

Despite extensive research that has defined optimal transfusion thresholds, there remain areas of uncertainty. An important and common issue is whether patients with underlying cardiovascular disease should be transfused at higher hemoglobin thresholds. Definitive trials have not been performed although there is some evidence that support liberal transfusion strategy (Carson 2013). A definitive answer awaits completion of ongoing studies such as the Myocardial Ischemia and Transfusion trial (MINT: www.minttrial.org).

In conclusion, there are now more than 47 RCTs that enrolled over 20,000 patients evaluating RBC transfusion thresholds. Recent systematic reviews have concluded that a restrictive transfusion strategy utilizing a hemoglobin concentration of 7–8 g/dL did not impact the 30-day mortality or morbidity when compared with a more liberal transfusion strategy among a wide-ranging patient population (Carson 2018, 2021). There is insufficient evidence to recommend a transfusion threshold in patients with acute coronary syndrome, acute stroke, and other disorders. Finally, it is always good practice to take into account each patient's unique clinical circumstance, in addition to the hemoglobin level, when making the decision to transfuse.

ANNOTATED REFERENCES FOR TRANSFUSION TRIGGER

Carson JL, Duff A, Poses RM, et al. Effect of anaemia and cardiovascular disease on surgical mortality and morbidity. *Lancet.* 1996;348(9034):1055–1060.

A retrospective cohort study in 1958 patients undergoing surgery who refused blood transfusions that shows the natural history and perioperative consequences of anemia. The 30-day mortality was 33.3% in those with a preoperative hemoglobin <6 g/dL, as opposed to 1.3% in patients with a preoperative hemoglobin of 12 g/dL or higher. In those patients with underlying cardiovascular disease, the risk of death increased precipitously with preoperative hemoglobin levels <10 g/dL compared to those without cardiovascular disease.

Carson JL, Terrin ML, Noveck H, et al. Liberal or restrictive transfusion in high-risk patients after hip surgery. *N Engl J Med.* 2011;365(26):2453–2462.

The FOCUS trial is one of the largest RCTs evaluating transfusion triggers. It enrolled 2016 patients with a history of, or underlying risk factors for, cardiovascular disease undergoing surgical hip fracture repair and randomized them into a restrictive (hemoglobin <8 g/dL or symptomatic of anemia) transfusion strategy versus a liberal transfusion strategy (hemoglobin <10 g/dL). There was no difference in the primary outcome of death or the ability to walk across the room between the restrictive and liberal groups (OR 1.01, 95% CI 0.84–1.22), in-hospital death or acute coronary syndrome (4.3% vs. 5.2%), or 60-day mortality (6.6% vs. 7.6%).

Carson JL, Brooks MM, Abbott JD, et al. Liberal versus restrictive transfusion thresholds for patients with symptomatic coronary artery disease. *Am Heart J.* 2013;165:964–971.

The MINT pilot trial enrolled 110 patients admitted for acute coronary syndrome and randomized to either a restrictive threshold group (hemoglobin <8 g/dL or symptoms of anemia) or liberal group (hemoglobin <10 g/dL). The 30-day mortality rate was lower in the liberal transfusion group when compared to the restrictive group (1.8% vs. 13%, p = 0.032). The results of this pilot trial should be interpreted cautiously since small trials need to be confirmed with larger studies.

Carson JL, Stanworth SJ, Alexander JH, et al. Clinical trials evaluating red blood cell transfusion thresholds: an updated systematic review and with additional focus on patients with cardiovascular disease. *Am Heart J.* 2018; 200:96–101.

This most recent systematic review is an updated one to the 2016 Cochrane review and includes a total of 37 trials and 19,049 patients, focusing on new data in patients with cardiovascular disease. The 30-day mortality in cardiac surgery was no different between restrictive and liberal transfusion strategies (RR 0.99, 95% CI 0.74–1.33). Overall, in 26 trials with 15,681 patients, there was no difference in 30-day mortality between the two strategies (RR 1.00, 95% CI 0.86–1.16).

Carson JL, Stanworth SJ, Roubinian N, et al. Transfusion Thresholds for guiding red blood cell transfusion. *Cochrane Database Syst Rev.* 2021;10:CD002042.

This Cochrane database systematic review and meta-analysis summarized trials evaluating restrictive versus liberal RBC transfusion thresholds including 47 RCTs and 20,599 patients. Restrictive transfusion strategies reduced RBC transfusions by 41% (RR 0.59, 95% CI 0.53-0.66) and did not change the 30-day mortality (RR 1.0, 95% CI 0.86–1.16) when compared with liberal transfusion strategies. Updated reviews have found nearly identical results.

Hébert PC, Wells G, Blajchman MA, et al. A multicenter, randomized, controlled clinical trial of transfusion requirements in critical care. Transfusion requirements in critical care investigators, Canadian Critical Care Trials Group [see comments]. *N Engl J Med.* 1999;340(6):409–417.

The TRICC trial was the first RCT evaluating transfusion thresholds utilizing a restrictive vs. liberal transfusion strategy. The trial enrolled 838 euvolemic ICU patients and found a non-significant lower 30-day mortality between the restrictive (hemoglobin <7 g/dL) and the liberal (hemoglobin <10 g/dL) transfusion groups (18.7% vs. 23.3%, p = 0.11). However, the restrictive group did have fewer cases of MI (0.7% vs. 2.9%, p = 0.02) and pulmonary edema (5.3% vs. 10.7%, p <0.01).

Holst LB, Haase N, Wetterslev J, et al. Lower versus higher hemoglobin threshold for transfusion in septic shock. *N Engl J Med.* 2014;371:1381–1391.

The TRISS trial is a RCT comparing a restrictive (hemoglobin <7 g/dL) transfusion strategy vs. a liberal (hemoglobin <9 g/dL) in 998 ICU patients with septic shock. The 90-day mortality did not differ between the restrictive (43%) and liberal (45%) transfusion groups (RR 0.94, 95% CI 0.78–1.09; p = 0.44).

Murphy GJ, Pike K, Rogers CA, et al. Liberal or restrictive transfusion after cardiac surgery. *N Engl J Med.* 2015;372:997–1008.

2003 cardiac surgery patients in the TITRe2 trial were randomized to a restrictive group (hemoglobin <7.5 g/dL) or a liberal group (hemoglobin <9 g/dL). The 30-day mortality did not differ between the restrictive (2.6%) and the liberal (1.9%) group, the 90-day mortality was statistically favored the liberal transfusion group (2.6% vs. 4.2%; OR 1.64, 95% CI 1.00–2.67; p = 0,045).

Mazer CD, Whitlock RP, Fergusson DA, et al. Red-cell transfusion threshold for cardiac surgery. *N Engl J Med.* 2017;377:2133–2144.

Mazer CD, Whitlock RP, Fergusson DA, et al. Six-month outcomes after restrictive or liberal transfusion for cardiac surgery. *N Engl J Med.* 2018;379:1224–1233.

The TRICS III trial randomly allocated 5243 patients undergoing cardiac surgery to restrictive transfusion threshold of hemoglobin <7.5 g/dL and liberal threshold of hemoglobin

<9.5 in OR/ICU patients and <8.5 g/dL in non-ICU patients. This trial found no differences in 28-day mortality rates between the two groups (3% in restrictive vs. 3.6% in liberal; OR 0.85, 95% CI 0.62–1.16). Six-month follow-up confirmed the short-term results.

Robertson CS, Hannay HJ, Yamal, J-M, et al. Effect of erythropoietin and transfusion threshold on neurologic recovery after traumatic brain injury: a randomized controlled trial. *JAMA.* 2014;312: 36–47.

The investigators used a 2 × 2 factorial design to determine if one of two transfusion strategies and administration of erythropoietin or placebo would result in improved neurologic outcome in patients with traumatic brain injury. Compared to placebo, erythropoietin had no effect on favorable outcomes. Thromboembolic events were higher in the erythropoietin group. Outcomes were similar in the two transfusion strategy groups. Adverse outcomes were higher the liberal transfusion group.

Villanueva C, Colomo A, Bosch A, et al. Transfusion strategies for acute upper gastrointestinal bleeding. *N Engl J Med.* 2013;368(1):11–21.

This RCT enrolled 832 patients with acute upper gastrointestinal bleeding and randomized them to a restrictive strategy (hemoglobin <7 g/dL) or a liberal strategy (hemoglobin <9 g/dL). The likelihood of survival at 45 days was higher in the restrictive group when compared with the liberal group (95% vs. 91%; HR 0.55, 95% CI 0.33–0.92; p = 0.02). This trial was notable for being the first transfusion trial showing a mortality benefit using a restrictive transfusion strategy.

Landmark Article of the 21st Century

A MULTICENTER, RANDOMIZED, CONTROLLED CLINICAL TRIAL OF TRANSFUSION REQUIREMENTS IN CRITICAL CARE

Hébert PC et al., *N Engl J Med.* 1999 FEB 11;340(6):409–417

Commentary by Paul C. Hébert

It has been 22 years since the publication of the TRICC trial [1]. Since then, 47 randomized trials of transfusion triggers have been published, all generally demonstrating that a restrictive transfusion strategy decreases red cell transfusions by 40% without any negative consequences on clinically important outcomes [2]. If anything, outcomes were better in some subgroups in the restrictive arm.

The journey started in 1991, where as a research fellow, I wondered about exploring whether a much more liberal strategy (threshold held greater than 12.0 g/dL) versus a much more restrictive one (transfusion threshold less than 7.0 g/dL) would improve oxygen delivery sufficiently to save lives of supply dependent patients with septic shock. I wrote up the study as part of a clinical trials course for my Master degree. I continued to refine the protocol over the next 2 years. Then, I presented the study at the Canadian Critical Care Trials Groups (CCCTG) in the Spring of 1993. During my presentation to Canada's leading intensivists, every part of the trial was scrutinized and questioned.

First, the premise. My colleagues were far less interested in the concept of driving up oxygen delivery to save lives but far more interested in simply understanding how and when to transfuse red cells. They then pointed out that red cell transfusions may have important effects on immune and inflammatory responses, causing worsened organ injury and possibly increased rate of infection. Through our discussions, it became clear that both arms of the trial had its proponents, with half believe enhance oxygen transport and support for the sick heart would save lives whilst others believing that red cells had important adverse biological effects in critically ill patients. Unfortunately, it also became clear that each side was entrenched in their respective views and practices. The discussion became very animated with one side stating the other was engaged in malpractice. Then, one wise member of our group stood up to say that the divergent views in a largely data free zone were in fact exactly why we needed to do the trial. And thereafter, we had a few more hours of constructive debate. All of the trial design element were discussed and improved.

After assembling a team of critical care physicians—a world class biostatistician, Dr. George Wells, and a transfusion medicine expert, Morris Blajchman—we received a Medical Research Council grant on our first submission. And then, we implemented the project, attempting to recruit 2300 patients over the next 5 years. After 4 years, fewer patients and physicians were agreeing to participate in the study. Canadians were hearing about contaminated blood scandals on a daily basis because of an ongoing Royal Commission (equivalent to Senate hearings or investigations in the US). Despite our best efforts, we were unable to increase enrollment rates. We finally decided to close out the study after 838 patients, an insufficient number to properly ensure that both arms of the trial were equivalent.

A few months later, after all of data was in and cleaned, the trial statistician and I proceeded to go through the primary analysis together. To our surprise, the restrictive group seemed to do a bit better. I could not believe my eyes. I asked to check the coding. Could we have mislabeled the group? He said no. He had already checked. And then, I wanted to know a lot more. Were there subgroups more affected than other? Were results consistent? What about secondary outcomes? What about high risk groups, like patients with heart disease? The enthusiasm of that day is still with me. To be looking at data that no one else had seen! And especially, with results that were so unexpected. We thought we were going to find nothing in an underpowered study. Instead, we were looking at data from a study that challenged existing norms. We followed this work with several other studies to explore why red cell transfusion may have adversely affected outcomes including studies leucoreduction (JAMA papers) led by Dean Fergusson and a major Age of Blood study (ABLE) led by myself, Jacques Lacroix, Dean Fergusson and Alan Tinmouth (NEJM). With my pediatric colleague, Jacques Lacroix, Finally, Jacques Lacroix myself and others led a major pediatric critical care trials also demonstrating that a restrictive transfusion strategy decreased red cell transfusions while not increasing the rates of organ failure in children.

It then took over another decade and many other studies with similar findings before red cell transfusion practice changed. It is personally very gratifying to have been part of such an important team effort, especially as a young scientist. I am humbled by the long term impacts of our work. The drastic decrease in red cell use accompanied by few clinically important consequences is gratifying. I am most proud of the fact that we opened up a field of research where the true clinical impacts of transfusions are still being explored. It has spread well beyond critical care and red cells. I only hope our next generation considers a career in clinical research.

REFERENCES

1. Hébert PC, Wells G, Blajchman MA, et al., the Canadian Critical Care Trials Group. Transfusion requirements in critical care: a multicentre randomized controlled clinical trial. *N Engl J Med.* 1999;340:409–417.
2. Carson JL, Stanworth SJ, Roubinian N, et al. Transfusion Thresholds for guiding red blood cell transfusion. *Cochrane Database Syst Rev.* 2021;10:CD002042.

CHAPTER 40

Massive Transfusion

Reviewed by Dina M. Filiberto and Martin A. Croce

Management of severely injured trauma patients has evolved over the years with regard to operative techniques and resuscitation. Resuscitative strategies have shifted among whole blood, crystalloid, and variable blood components, with the goal of avoiding the lethal triad of hypothermia, acidosis, and coagulopathy.

Massive transfusion (MT) is generally defined as greater than or equal to 10 units of blood over 24 hours, although alternative volumes have been described. This threshold identifies a population of potentially salvageable, severely injured patients. Massively transfused patients represent a small fraction of trauma patients; however, they utilize a great deal of resources and have a high mortality. At a large level one trauma center, of patients that were transfused one unit of blood, only 3% of those patients received greater than 10 units of packed red blood cells. Yet they received 71% of all transfused packed red blood cells, and had a mortality of 39%. This subgroup of patients is the focus of a large body of research to improve clinical outcomes (Como et al., 2004).

The utilization of intravenous fluids as initial resuscitation combined with the supranormal resuscitation paradigm led to higher cardiac index and delivery of oxygen in patients. Despite these improved values, aggressive fluid resuscitation may actually worsen patients' acidosis and coagulopathy, increasing their risk of abdominal compartment syndrome, acute respiratory distress syndrome, multiple system organ failure, and mortality (Balogh et al., 2003). Later research investigating a hypotensive resuscitation strategy demonstrated how the pendulum had swung the other way. Patients with a low mean arterial pressure goal (50 mm Hg) who received fewer products and intravenous fluids, were less likely to develop postoperative coagulopathy, and had a lower mortality compared to patients with a high mean arterial pressure (65 mm Hg) (Morrison et al., 2011).

While the utility of limited crystalloid resuscitation became apparent, military studies demonstrated the survival benefit of packed red blood cell and plasma transfusion in a 1:1 to 1:1.5 ratio (Borgman et al., 2007). For patients that require continued transfusion, the development of massive transfusion protocols allow the surgeon to notify the blood bank of their need for delivery of coolers with packed red blood cells and thawed plasma and delivery of platelets at room temperature. Subsequently, a more tailored approach to severely injured patients has emerged. The two-pronged approach is comprised of damage control surgical techniques, which aim to limit contamination and

DOI: 10.1201/9781003042136-40

hemorrhage at the index operation. The second prong is damage control resuscitation which consists of permissive hypotension and balanced volume repletion with packed red blood cells, thawed plasma, and platelets (Holcomb et al., 2007). A retrospective before and after study of the implementation of damage control resuscitation in patients undergoing damage control laparotomy demonstrated less fluid and blood product administration, less coagulopathy and improved 30-day survival (Cotton et al., 2011).

The traditional definition of MT is merely a static volume that does not account for different rates of transfusion over time and potentially different underlying patho-physiology. Using a broad volume-based definition results in survivor bias. Patients who do not meet the specified threshold prior to death will be excluded from the population, removing a subset of critically ill patients who are potentially salvage-able. Rethinking the way MT is defined in which survivor bias, volume, and rate of transfusion are addressed, can provide more granular data when investigating resus-citation in hemorrhagic shock. Savage et al. redefined MT as a critical administration threshold (CAT) of 3 units of blood transfused per hour. This definition allowed for a better matching of volume of hemorrhage with rate of resuscitative transfusions. In the population studied, 46% of patients met the CAT threshold and 22% met the traditional MT threshold. When CAT criteria was met with increasing frequency, mortality predictably increased as well. CAT identified 75% of all deaths, while MT only identified 33% of all deaths. CAT is a prospective variable that is twice as predic-tive of mortality when compared to the traditional definition of MT. The concept of CAT was subsequently applied prospectively with subtle changes in the methodology to better study a patient population with hemorrhagic shock. CAT remained predic-tive of mortality with an increasing frequency of CAT episodes resulting in increased morbidity and mortality. Importantly, 29% of patients were captured by CAT that did not reach the traditional MT threshold. This cohort was significantly injured, with one third of patients CAT+ more than once, and 10% that died in their hospitalization. The traditional definition of MT misses this population (Savage et al., 2015).

Building on these studies, Meyer et al. sought to further refine the definition of massive transfusion to better predict mortality and represent the severity of illness. Traditional MT, CAT, and resuscitation intensity (RI, the total products given in the first 30 minutes [1 U PRBC, 1 U plasma, 1L crystalloid, 500 mL colloid]), were com-pared. CAT and RI captured 23% of patients that died who did not meet the traditional MT criteria. RI and CAT were similar in predicting early mortality, however, when RI is used as a continuous variable, it is also able to quantify risk of death, with each unit increase associated with a 20% increase in mortality (Meyer et al., 2018).

Current guidelines for damage control resuscitation in patients with severe traumatic hemorrhage recommend development and utilization of massive transfusion proto-cols and damage control resuscitation that target a high ratio of plasma and platelets to packed red blood cells. Evidence suggests these protocols can prevent traumatic coagulopathy and hemorrhagic death (Cannon et al., 2017). Continued evolution in resuscitation challenges clinicians to better characterize severely injured patients, allowing for earlier intervention and therapies.

ANNOTATED REFERENCES FOR MASSIVE TRANSFUSION

Balogh Z, Mckinley BA, Cocanour CS, et al. Supranormal trauma resuscitation causes more case of abdominal compartment syndrome. *Arch Surg.* 2003 Jun;138(6):637–642.

This analysis compared supranormal resuscitation with normal resuscitation in 156 patients. Supranormal resuscitation was associated with increased crystalloid administration, decreased intestinal perfusion, and increased intra-abdominal hypertension, abdominal compartment syndrome, multiple organ failure, and death.

Borgman MA, Spinella PC, Perkins JG, et al. The ratio of blood products transfused affects mortality in patients receiving massive transfusions at a combat support hospital. *J Trauma.* 2007 Oct;63(4):805–813.

The authors compared three groups of patients with different plasma to RBC ratios who received massive transfusion. High plasma:RBC ratio (1:1.4) is independently associated with survival.

Cannon JW, Khan MA, Raja AS, et al. Damage control resuscitation in patients with severe traumatic hemorrhage: a practice management guideline from the Eastern Association for the Surgery of Trauma. *J Trauma Acute Care Surg.* 2017 Mar;82(3):605–617.

Guideline published by the Eastern Association for the Surgery of Trauma using available evidence to recommend the use of massive transfusion and damage control resuscitation protocols with a high plasma and platelet to packed red blood cell ratio.

Como JJ, Dutton RP, Scalea TM, Edelman BB, Hess JR. Blood transfusion rates in the care of acute trauma. *Transfusion.* 2004 Jun;44(6):809–813.

The authors evaluated patterns of packed red blood cell use at a large level one trauma center over the course of 1 year. Three percent of patients received more than 10 units of packed red blood cells and received 71% of all packed red blood cells given. Most of these patients received plasma and platelets to treat coagulopathy.

Cotton BA, Reddy N, Hatch QM, et al. Damage control resuscitation is associated with a reduction in resuscitation volumes and improvement in survival in 390 damage control laparotomy patients. *Ann Surg.* 2011;254:598-605.

An analysis of 390 patients who underwent damage control laparotomy. Patients were divided into pre-damage control resuscitation and damage control resuscitation groups. Patients that underwent damage control resuscitation received less products and fluids, were less coagulopathic, and were associated with a 2.5-fold increased odds in 30-day survival.

Holcomb JB, Jenkins D, Rhee P, et al. Damage control resuscitation: directly addressing the early coagulopathy of trauma. *J Trauma.* 2007;62:307–310.

A discussion on traumatic coagulopathy and the introduction of balanced blood component resuscitation.

Meyer DE, Cotton BA, Fox EE, et al. A comparison of resuscitation intensity and critical administration threshold in predicting early mortality among bleeding patients: a multicenter validation in 680 major transfusion patients. *J Trauma Acute Care Surg.* 2018;85:691–696.

A study with 680 patients from 12 trauma centers compared resuscitation intensity and critical administration threshold. Both are similar predictors of mortality in patients massively transfused and capture more patients than the traditional massive transfusion definition.

Morrison CA, Carrick MM, Norman MA, et al. Hypotensive resuscitation strategy reduces transfusion requirements and severe postoperative coagulopathy in trauma patients with hemorrhagic shock: preliminary results of a randomized controlled trial. *J Trauma.* 2011;70:652–663.

A randomized controlled trial with 90 patients that compared a hypotensive resuscitation strategy to a standard resuscitation strategy. Patients with a lower mean arterial pressure received less blood products and fluids, and had decreased postoperative coagulopathy and mortality.

Savage SA, Sumislawski JJ, Zarzaur BL, Dutton WP, Croce MA, Fabian TC. The new metric to define large-volume hemorrhage: results of a prospective study of the critical administration threshold. *J Trauma Acute Care Surg.* 2015;78:224–230.

The authors evaluated 316 patients who received at least 1 unit of PRBC. They compared the traditional definition of massive transfusion to an alternate definition of critical administration threshold (CAT). CAT+ patients were associated with a two-fold increased risk of death. CAT utilizes rate and volume of transfusion, which allows for early identification of injured patients at greatest risk of death.

Landmark Article of the 21st Century

REDEFINING MASSIVE TRANSFUSION WHEN EVERY SECOND COUNTS

Savage SA et al., *J Trauma Acute Care Surg.* 2013;74:396–402

Commentary by Stephanie A. Savage

The concept of massive transfusion, defined as 10 or more units of packed red blood cells given in a 24-hour period, was the topic of ongoing discussion when I joined the faculty at the Presley Trauma Center in Memphis, Tennessee. Everyone felt this was a flawed metric to identify massively bleeding patients. The focus on a static volume, given at some point in a 24-hour period, meant patients could be considered "massively transfused" if they received blood products quickly or slowly and persistently over an entire day. Those bleeding too rapidly to reach the arbitrary 10-unit cut-off were never identified. The foundational metric for our retrospective trauma research was fundamentally flawed.

My partners and I spent hours spit-balling models that would account for both rate and volume of hemorrhage. Elegant studies by M. Abrahamowicz et al. modeled cumulative effects of time-dependent exposures to a drug (blood in this case) and were our inspiration. Ultimately, these models were too complex for bedside application, as Dr. Fabian so wisely pointed out. Instead, we focused on aberrant surgical behavior as a key. At the time, we routinely ordered two units at a time for transfusion in most routine indications. The decision to give a third unit in a short time period represented a warning that something more profound was occurring (bleeding) and retrospectively represented a non-routine transfusion. Using time-dependent hazard models, we were able to demonstrate that the critical administration threshold (CAT) was superior to the old massive transfusion definition and accounted for survival bias as well! The CAT was out of the bag for future hemorrhage-related research.

CHAPTER 41

Burns

Review by Brian Brisebois and Joyce McIntyre

Burn injuries remain one of the most common cause of trauma worldwide, disproportionately affecting low- or middle-income countries. In the United States, burn injuries result in the hospitalization of about 40,000 patients every year, with three quarters receiving treatment in a specialized burn center. In the United States, burn prevalence is distributed bimodally based on age, with the greatest incidence in young children and adults 20–59 years old (Greenhalgh). Treatments for burns have been described since ancient times including depictions in early cave paintings, as well as descriptions in early Chinese and Greek texts. The Egyptian Ebers papyrus, written around 1500 BC, describes a topical mixture of dung, wax, horn, and porridge soaked in resin as a burn treatment. It wasn't until the middle of the 20th century that advances in burn care resulted in remarkable improvements in mortality (Liu).

Burn wounds produce a wide array of systemic effects including massive inflammation and a hypermetabolic state that can persist for years (Lundy). In a large case series of 242 children with severe burns, all patients experienced significant hypermetabolism, muscle loss, bone mineral content loss, serum protein abnormalities, cardiac abnormalities, and insulin resistance (Jeschke). The destruction of natural barriers, inflammation, and subsequent leaking of protein into the extravascular space results in rapid fluid shifts capable of causing severe edema and hypovolemic shock (Liu). In the United States, 67% of burns are small (<10% total surface body area, or TBSA) (Greenhalgh).

Immediate management of the severely burned patient prioritizes the ABCs (airway, breathing, circulation) typical of modern trauma care. Early intubation should always be considered in patients with >40% TBSA (>30% TBSA if burns are deep), as swelling can rapidly obstruct the airway. Other indicators that should trigger consideration of early intubation are burns to the head, face, mouth, smoke-inhalation injury, altered level of consciousness, change in voice, or the possibility of delay in transfer to a burn center (Greenhalgh). Between 5% and 35% of all patients with burns will also have some degree of inhalation injury, although over-intubation among burn patients is common (Lundy). A 2016 study demonstrated one third of hospitalized burn patients were extubated within 1 day (Greenhalgh). There are significantly higher rates of complications for intubated burn patients, so risk-benefit should be carefully considered (Lundy).

DOI: 10.1201/9781003042136-41

Smoke inhalation injury should be considered in any patient with possible extended exposure to smoke. Bronchoscopic or laryngoscopic evidence of soot or injury below the vocal cords is diagnostic (Greenhalgh). Although highly specific, a negative inspection does not rule out the presence of smoke inhalation injury (Lundy). Individuals exposed to flash explosions (i.e., cigarette igniting supplemental oxygen) do not usually suffer smoke inhalation injury (Lundy, Greenhalgh). CO poisoning can be confirmed by elevated levels of carboxyhemoglobin (ABG and pulse oximeter won't be helpful). Suspected CO poisoning should be treated with 100% oxygen while carboxyhemoglobin levels are obtained (Greenhalgh).

Early and adequate fluid resuscitation is critical to prevent hypovolemic shock (Liu), although over-resuscitation, or "fluid creep," has been associated with increased morbidity (Lundy). The "Rule of Nines" can be used to estimate TBSA burned; each arm 9%, head 9%, anterior trunk 18%, posterior trunk 18%, each leg 18%. Although quick and easy, it is not very accurate. The Lund-Browder chart adjusts for age and is commonly used in burn centers (Greenhalgh). The Parkland formula (4 mL/kg/% TBSA; half over first 8 hours; remaining half over 16 hours) is the most widely used formula to determine initial resuscitation rates, although some centers use the modified Brooke formula (2 mL/kg/% TBSA; half over first 8 hours; remaining half over 16 hours) (Lundy, Greenhalgh). Recent ABA consensus statements suggest these two equations establish appropriate limits for initial resuscitation (Lundy). Children need greater fluid/kg/% TBSA burned than adults. Delayed resuscitation, smoke inhalation, and alcohol intoxication all greatly increase fluid requirements. These equations are useful starting points, but infusion rates should be carefully adjusted based on urine output (UO). A target UO of 1 mL/kg/h for children <30 kg and 0.5 mL/kg/h for adults is ideal. When at or just below target UO, fluids should be gradually decreased until steady state is achieved (Greenhalgh).

The ideal endpoint for fluid resuscitation remains somewhat controversial, although most burn centers (95%) use UO as the gold standard. Use of hemodynamic monitoring endpoints have grown in popularity, although recent meta-analysis of RTCs comparing it to UO found no survival advantage (Paratz). Hyperosmolar fluids such as 5% albumin or fresh frozen plasma are increasingly used at burn centers for fluid maintenance in severely burned patients (>30% TBSA) (Greenhalgh, Lundy). Several studies have demonstrated the association of albumin with reduced fluid requirements (Greenhalgh). Colloid or FFP should not be administered for the first 12–24 hours post burn, as the protein could be lost to the interstitium and exacerbate edema (Lundy).

Patients with <20% TBSA enter a profound and long-lasting hypermetabolic state that leads to muscle wasting, organ failure, and death if not treated. Adjusting room temperature close to 18°C, pain control, sedation, and preventing sepsis are current strategies for preventing or mitigating the hypermetabolic response (Greenhalgh). The efficacy of propranolol to mitigate catabolic muscle wasting was demonstrated in a small cohort of children (Herndon) and remains a promising therapy modality.

Administration of oxandrolone and other anabolic agents like insulin, IGF-1, and GH have also demonstrated efficacy (Greenhalgh). Multimodal pain relief should be initiated within the first 24–48 hours. Use of opiates as the primary method of treating burn pain, as recommended by the Society of Critical Care Medicine (SCCM), is currently controversial considering recent evidence regarding tolerance, addiction, and opioid-induced hyperanalgesia. Useful non-opioid agents include ketamine, acetaminophen, clonidine, dexmedetomidine, benzodiazepines, and quetiapine. NSAIDs increase bleeding and rates of AKI in burn patients and should be avoided (Lundy).

Enteral nutrition is ideal and should be started within the first 24 hours for any patient with >30% TBSA burns. The ideal enteric formulation is calorie-dense with a high carbohydrate to fat ratio (Lundy). Caloric requirements can be calculated using any of the various resting energy expenditure equations (Harris-Benedict, Toronto, Milner) multiplied by a factor of 1.5 (Greenhalgh). It should be noted that these equations tend to be less effective at predicting caloric needs after 1 month (Lundy). Protein should be provided to offset muscle catabolism. Children should get 2.5–3.0 g/kg/day and adults 1.5–2.0g/kg/day, adjusted based on the outcome of nitrogen-balance studies. Supplementation of glutamine, vitamin C, selenium, and zinc are common, as these are often depleted after burn injury (Lundy).

Rapid removal of eschar and either grafting or application of dermal covering are a primary strategy to reduce metabolic stress (Greenhalgh). Ambroise Pare described early burn wound excision as early as the 16th century (Liu). A 2006 RTC meta-analysis demonstrated a significant reduction in mortality and time in hospital associated with early burn excision (Ong). Circumferential chest, abdominal, and extremity burns can result in compartment syndrome with subsequent ischemia and tissue damage. Compartment syndrome typically develops 12–18 hours post burn and are associated with initial over-resuscitation in addition to circumferential burns (Greenhalgh). This feared complication can be managed by escharotomy in the operating room or at bedside in the unit. Using cautery for hemostasis, a simple incision is made through the burned skin which relieves the restrictive pressure of the burned skin.

The traditional Baux score formula, which tends to overpredict mortality and doesn't account for inhalation injury, has received an update. The formula retains ease of use, but accounts for inhalation injury and was recalibrated using patient data from the national burn registry to more accurately predict outcome (Osler). Hospitalization duration can be estimated at 1 day for every 1% TBSA, with longer stays required for larger burns (Greenhalgh).

Acute lung injury (ALI) or acute respiratory distress syndrome (ARDS) is a common complication in burn patients, occurring in 2–17% of all burns (Oda). Use of conventional low tidal volumes has been associated with inadequate oxygenation in as many as a third of burn patients in a recent single center RTC, with a higher failure rate among those with smoke inhalation injury (Lundy). High-frequency percussive ventilation (HFPV) has been demonstrated to be beneficial specifically for inhalation injury. It helps clear debris and mucous, as well as reduce rates of pneumonia. Some burn centers report success with high-frequency oscillatory ventilation (HFOV) for severe ARDS (Lundy). The use of extracorporeal membrane oxygenation (ECMO) in the setting of burn injuries is questionable. A recent meta-analysis suggests ECMO provides no survival benefit for patients with burn and inhalation injuries who experience respiratory failure (Asmussen). ALI after burn surgery has been positively correlated with intraoperative hypothermia, independent of extent of excision, transfusions, or surgery length and may be suggestive of the degree of invasiveness (Oda).

Infection and sepsis are involved in 75–85% of all burn injury deaths (Liu). Defining sepsis in burn patients is problematic due to the always present concurrent hypermetabolic response. Systemic inflammatory response syndrome (SIRS), the typical hallmark of sepsis, is present in most burn patients and therefore not helpful. The 2007 American Burn Association Consensus Conference defined sepsis in burns as three or more changes in temperature, heart rate, respiration rate, platelet abnormalities, hyperglycemia, or inability to continue enteral feedings which should trigger a search for infection (Greenhalgh). Typical causes of bacteremia include *Staphylococcus aureus*, *Klebsiella pneumoniae*, *Escherichia coli*, *Enterococci*, *Acinetobacter*, and perhaps the most well know burn-associated pathogen, *Pseudomonas aeruginosa*. Resistant organisms are becoming more common (Lundy). It should be noted that burn patients are often excluded from major sepsis trials (Greenhalgh), greatly limiting our understanding of sepsis in burn injuries.

Acute kidney injury (AKI) is commonly associated with both burns and sepsis (Chung). Preventing hypoperfusion and avoiding nephrotoxins are key strategies to avoid AKI. Treatment options are limited (Lundy). A recent major multi-center RCT examining the efficacy of high-volume hemofiltration (HVHF) on reduction of AKI mortality demonstrated no improvement in survival, although it should be noted the study was terminated early due to slow enrollment (Chung). The study did demonstrate a significant decrease in vasopressor dependency index at 48 hours and a decrease in multiple organ dysfunction syndrome at 14 days for patients in the intervention arm. There was also no difference in adverse events between study arms (Chung).

Arguably the biggest development in ICU burn care in the 21st century is negative pressure wound therapy (NPWT), which has resulted in significantly improved rates of graft take and decreased hospitalization time (Llanos), even when compared to conventional modern dressings (Petkar). NPWT is particularly helpful when wound bed or grafting conditions are poor (Petkar). NPWT can be easily and affordably implemented in any hospital that has central vacuum system access bedside (Llanos). The efficacy of amniotic membrane transplantation has been demonstrated in cases of mild to moderate acute ocular burns, where it was shown to rapidly restore corneal and conjunctival surfaces (Meller). While there have been advancements in biological dressings over the past 50 years, cost and accessibility remain prohibitive.

The long-term effects of burn injuries and treatments are debilitating and distressing. The BSHS-B is an abbreviated outcome scale designed to quantify degree of disability in burn patients allowing for comprehensive assessment. The questions include important elements regarding sexuality and hand function that were excluded from previous scales (Kildal). Finally, a common concern is whether burn injuries predispose an individual to malignant cancer, as is sometimes observed in Marjolin ulcers. A large study involving 16,900 burn patients concluded that burn wounds are not associated with an increased risk of developing cancer for at least 25 years after the injury (Mellemkjaer).

ANNOTATED REFERENCES FOR BURNS

Asmussen S, Maybauer DM, Fraser JF, et al. Extracorporeal membrane oxygenation in burn and smoke inhalation injury. *Burns.* 2013;39(3):429–435.

The authors performed a meta-analysis of six clinical studies to determine the effectiveness of ECMO at improving survival for patients who experience acute respiratory failure with burn and inhalation injury. The results suggest there is no improvement in survival for these patients (Survival rate 0.542, 95% CI 0.404–0.641). The authors note that there were only a few clinical trials, and they all had limited number of patients, so the role of ECMO in the treatment of burns remains somewhat unclear.

Chung KK, Coates EC, Smith DJ Jr, et al. Randomized controlled Evaluation of high-volume hemofiltration in adult burn patients with Septic shoCk and acUte kidnEy injury (RESCUE) Investigators. High-volume hemofiltration in adult burn patients with septic shock and acute kidney injury: a multicenter randomized controlled trial. *Crit Care.* 2017;21(1):289.

This multi-center, prospective randomized trial examined the impact of HVHF/CVVH on hemodynamic profile, organ function and overall survival in burn patients (n = 37) who developed septic shock with AKI. Vasopressor dependency index decreased significantly (p = 0.007) at 48 hours and multiple organ dysfunction syndrome score decreased at 14 days (p = 0.02) for subjects in the HVHF group. There was no difference in survival or adverse events between the two groups. It should be noted that the trial was terminated early due to slow enrollment.

Greenhalgh DG, Saffle JR, Holmes JH 4th, et al. American Burn Association consensus conference to define sepsis and infection in burns. *J Burn Care Res.* 2007;28(6):776–790.

Authors 2007 conference to define sepsis and infection criteria in burn patients. The SIRS criteria is too non-specific to be useful in burns. Triggers for sepsis concern are at least three of the following; Temp >39° or <36.5°C, progressive tachycardia, progressive tachypnea, thrombocytopenia after day 3, hyperglycemia, or decreased enteral feeding. Authors recommend not initiating multiple organ dysfunction syndrome (MODS) assessment until after completion of initial resuscitation and scores should grade organ failure over range of values.

Greenhalgh DG. Management of burns. *N Engl J Med.* 2019;380(24):2349–2359.

Author presents an excellent overview of burn care, including immediate and long-term management strategies. Special considerations for burn patients are outlined, such as fluid resuscitation protocols (Rule of Nines, Lund-Browder chart, and the Parkland formula), the hypermetabolic state, sepsis, wound healing, and wound care.

Herndon DN, Hart DW, Wolf SE, Chinkes DL, Wolfe RR. Reversal of catabolism by beta-block-ade after severe burns. *N Engl J Med.* 2001;345(17):1223–1229.

This randomized trial of 25 children with severe (>40% TBSA) burns showed that β-blockade blunted the typical hypermetabolic response and muscle wasting typical of burn injuries. Administration of propranolol resulted in decreased heart rate (p <0.001) and decreased resting energy expenditure (p = 0.1). It also improved net muscle protein balance from baseline (p = 0.002) in 12 of the 13 patients in the study group.

Jeschke MG, Chinkes DL, Finnerty CC, et al. Pathophysiologic response to severe burn injury. *Ann Surg.* 2008;248(3):387–401.

This large case series of 242 severely burned (>30% TBSA) pediatric patients describes the pathophysiologic changes that occurred within their patient population from triage to discharge. All demonstrated hypermetabolism with significant muscle loss (muscle protein net balance of −0.05% ± 0.007 nmol/100 mL leg/min), loss of lean body mass (−4.1% ± 1.9%; p <0.05), decreased bone mineral content (3% ± 1%), decreased bone mineral density (2 ± 1%), serum protein abnormalities (p <0.05), cardiac function abnormalities (p <0.05), and significant changes to all 17 of the serum cytokines measured in the study. The authors noted that severe burns affect the expression of acute phase proteins, result in changes to serum triglycerides levels, and have dramatic effects on several important hormonal axis (GH-IGF-I, FTI-T4, cortisone-cortisol, insulin-glucose, PTH-osteocalcin, and sex hormones).

Kildal M, Andersson G, Fugl-Meyer AR, Lannerstam K, Gerdin B. Development of a brief ver-sion of the Burn Specific Health Scale (BSHS-B). *J Trauma.* 2001;51(4):740–746.

Authors used questionnaire data from 248 burn patients to verify validity of the brief version of the burn specific health scale (BSHS-B) as compared to the older BSHS-A. The BSHS-B is a simplified outcome scale based on 40 questions and covers seven domains of burn related disability; simple functional abilities, work, body image, interpersonal relationships, affect, heat sensitivity, and treatment regimens.

Liu HF, Zhang F, Lineaweaver WC. History and advancement of burn treatments. *Ann Plast Surg.* 2017;78(2 Suppl 1):S2–S8.

Authors review the evolution of burn care over the course of human history. Excellent descriptions of early burn care including treatments recommended by ancient Egyptians, Chinese, and Greeks.

Llanos S, Danilla S, Barraza C, et al. Effectiveness of negative pressure closure in the integra-tion of split thickness skin grafts: a randomized, double-masked, controlled trial. *Ann Surg.* 2006;244(5):700–705.

This double blind, randomized trial of 60 burn patients who received split thickness skin grafts demonstrated the effectiveness of negative pressure closure (NPC) dress-ings in decreasing the area of graft loss, decrease in need for secondary procedures, and decreasing hospital stay. The median area of graft loss in the NPC group was 0.0 cm² versus 4.5 cm² in the control group (p = 0.001). The NPC group also had fewer days from grafting to discharge (8 days in NPC group vs. 12 days in controls) and was less likely to require a second coverage procedure (16% in NPC group vs. 40% in controls).

Lundy JB, Chung KK, Pamplin JC, Ainsworth CR, Jeng JC, Friedman BC. Update on Severe Burn Management for the Intensivist. *J Intensive Care Med.* 2016;31(8):499–510.

This outstanding 2016 review article focuses on advancements in critical care for burn patients. It includes details on resuscitation, inhalation injury, ventilation, sedation and analgesia, infectious disease, nutrition support, organ dysfunction, wound failure and end of life considerations.

Mellemkjaer L, Hölmich LR, Gridley G, Rabkin C, Olsen JH. Risks for skin and other cancers up to 25 years after burn injuries. *Epidemiology.* 2006;17(6):668–673.

Authors examined records of 16,903 burn patients to determine long term cancer risks associated with burn injuries. Results suggest there is no increased risk for skin or any other type of cancer in burn injuries for at least 25 years following injury.

Meller D, Pires RT, Mack RJ, et al. Amniotic membrane transplantation for acute chemical or thermal burns. *Ophthalmology.* 2000;107(5):980–990.

This early 21st century prospective case series (n = 13) demonstrated the effectiveness of amniotic membrane transplantation (AMT) in promoting re-epithelialization and preventing scar formation in acute ocular burns. AMT quickly restored corneal and conjunctival surfaces (23.7 ± 9.8 days) in cases of mild to moderate burns.

Oda J, Kasai K, Noborio M, Ueyama M, Yukioka T. Hypothermia during burn surgery and postoperative acute lung injury in extensively burned patients. *J Trauma.* 2009;66(6):1525–1530.

The authors of this case series (n = 16) demonstrated that the degree of intraoperative hypothermia during burn surgery is associated with the development of acute lung injury post-operatively as well as increased polymorphonuclear neutrophil cell counts 24 hours after surgery. The study also demonstrated that there was no significant association between the development of lung injury and blood loss during surgery, transfusions received, extent of injury or duration of surgery.

Ong YS, Samuel M, Song C. Meta-analysis of early excision of burns. *Burns.* 2006;32(2):145–150.

The authors conducted a meta-analysis of six RTCs and demonstrated a significant reduction in mortality associated with early excision and grafting, but only in patients without inhalation injury (RR 0.36, 95% CI 0.20–0.65). Early excision was also associated with shorter hospital stay and greater blood transfusion requirement.

Osler T, Glance LG, Hosmer DW. Simplified estimates of the probability of death after burn injuries: extending and updating the Baux score. *J Trauma.* 2010;68(3):690–697.

Authors present a much-needed update to the Baux score, the traditional method used to calculate percent mortality after a burn injury. While quick and simple, the Baux score tends to overpredict mortality and doesn't reflect the advances in burn care or the effects of inhalation injury. Data from 39,888 burn patients was used to recalibrate the score to more accurately reflect mortality statistics as well as account for inhalation injury. The original equation is only slightly modified to account for inhalation injury, maintaining its ease of use, but the rough score can then be used to calculate an accurate percent mortality using the revised Baux score equation.

Paratz JD, Stockton K, Paratz ED, et al. Burn resuscitation–hourly urine output versus alternative endpoints: a systematic review. *Shock.* 2014;42(4):295–306.

The authors performed a systematic review of 20 studies to determine the ideal endpoint for fluid resuscitation during early burn management. They examined studies that compared traditional measures of hourly urine output with hemodynamic monitoring and other alternative endpoints. Use of hemodynamic monitoring was associated with

*increased survival (RR 0.77; CI 0.42–0.85; p <0.004), but inclusion of only the random-
ized trials demonstrated no appreciable differences in mortality between endpoints (RR
0.72; CI 0.43–1.19; p = 0.19) suggesting that more large scale studies are needed.*

Petkar KS, Dhanraj P, Kingsly PM, et al. A prospective randomized controlled trial comparing negative pressure dressing and conventional dressing methods on split-thickness skin
grafts in burned patients. *Burns.* 2011;37(6):925–929.

*This randomized trial of 40 split thickness skin grafts compared mean percentage of graft
take in patients treated with negative pressure dressings versus conventional dressings. They
found negative pressure closure was associated with higher rates of graft take, with a mean
96.7% versus 87.5% in those treated with conventional dressings (p <0.001). They also note
a significant decrease in the mean days required for graft take from 11 days for those in the
control group to 8 days for those treated with negative pressure dressings (p <0.001).*

Landmark Article of the 21st Century

EFFECTIVENESS OF NEGATIVE PRESSURE CLOSURE IN THE INTEGRATION OF SPLIT THICKNESS SKIN GRAFTS: A RANDOMIZED, DOUBLE-MASKED, CONTROLLED TRIAL

Llanos S, Danilla S, Barraza C et al., *Ann Surg.* 2006;244(5):700–705

Commentary by Steven Blau

Split thickness skin grafts remain an important part of the surgeon's armamentarium,
but graft loss consequent to infection, shear, and seromas and other fluid collections preventing graft inosculation continues to occur. In this paper, Llanos and his
colleagues in Chile present a well-designed, double-blind study of skin grafting in
60 patients using negative pressure therapy maintained for 5 days post procedure
which demonstrates the success of this therapy. This is neither the first (Moisidis) nor
the most recent (Joo) report on this therapy but it is the largest and nearly all have
reached similar conclusions with regard to graft quality and quantity (that is, survival
of the entire graft). The technique represents a trade-off, though, between the time
to produce a bulky tie-over bolster and the cost of the commercial product to provide
the controlled negative pressure. These authors have circumvented some of the costs
by connecting the device to a hospital wall suction—a workaround which might not
pass muster with US hospital administration. The grafts in this study were small,
averaging about 32 cm^2 and they were meshed 1:1.5 or pie-crusted and graft size may
impact the 100% graft success reported here. In the last 2 months, though, we've
used this technique on four patients with graft sizes of about 400–600 cm^2 with great
success (skin grafts meshed 1:1.5 or 1.2 on granulating "open" abdomen wounds).
Negative pressure therapy is not standardized in these papers with regard to timing
(3 or 5 or 6 days) to first graft exposure or final treatment or the amount of suction
(-75 to -100 units mmHg) when the commercial product is used or the type of foam
used. Although most of these studies were on meshed grafts, there might be a role for
this therapy on unmeshed grafts to better fixate the graft, especially in areas where
bulky dressings may be contraindicated.

REFERENCES

Joo HS, Lee SJ, Lee S-Y, Sung KY. The efficacy of negative pressure wound therapy for split-thickness skin grafts for wounds on the trunk or the neck: a randomized controlled trial. *Wounds*. 2020;32(12):334–338.

Moisidis E, Heath T, Boorer C, Ho K, Deva AK. A prospective, blinded, randomized, controlled clinical trial of topical negative pressure use in skin grafting. *Plast Reconstructr Surg*. 2004 Sep 15;114(4):917–922.

REFERENCES

CHAPTER 42

ICU Issues with Thoracic Trauma

Review by Morgan Crigger and Natasha Keric

Traumatic thoracic injuries often do not require operative intervention; however, these injuries portend a high mortality risk, especially if not identified and treated early [1]. Critical care management of these injuries has evolved to improve outcomes.

One of the most common traumatic thoracic injuries is a pneumothorax (PTX), with a subset of patients sustaining an occult pneumothorax (OPTX). Positive pressure ventilation (PPV) presents a unique treatment challenge to an OPTX in that there is a risk of progression to a tension PTX, which if untreated, has a mortality approaching 90% [2]. Multiple studies have shown that these patients can be managed safely without the need for a tube thoracostomy (TT), and if they do progress to failure, the likelihood of developing a tension PTX is very low [2, 3]. Factors associated with failure include hemothorax, increase in size of the OTPX, respiratory distress, ventilator associated pneumonia and ventilator days >7 days. While PPV is an overall risk factor for failure, the use of peak inspiratory pressure >30 cm H_2O and tidal volumes >6 mL/kg were not associated with the need for a TT [2, 3].

Traditionally, any size hemothorax (HTX) is managed with a TT, however, placement of a chest tube is not without complications. Current studies suggest that a HTX with <300 mL of blood, or 1.5 cm on the CT chest, can be managed with conservative treatment. Twenty-three percent of patients treated with conservative measures progress to failure and require more invasive treatments [5]. Factors contributing to failure include worsening respiratory failure, ongoing mechanical ventilation, progression of the HTX size >300 cc and development of a PTX and retained HTX [5]. Retained HTX has been shown to lead to longer ICU stays, increased hospital length of stay, increased ventilator days, increased risk of pneumonia and worse functional outcomes at discharge [4]. Operative intervention for retained HTX with either video assisted thoracoscopic surgery or thoracotomy has been shown to have more successful chest drainage when compared with a second chest tube placement or thrombolytic therapies [4].

Single, multiple, or flail segment rib fractures are associated with multiple thoracic injuries including PTX, HTX, and pulmonary contusions. Pulmonary contusions are complex injures that are associated with ventilation/perfusion (V/Q) mismatch, increased pulmonary shunting, reduced CO_2 clearance and decreased oxygenation creating a picture similar to acute respiratory distress syndrome (ARDS) [6]. The morbidity and mortality associated with rib fractures, especially flail segments and pulmonary contusions, warrant aggressive treatment. Current recommendations state

DOI: 10.1201/9781003042136-42

that if a patient is 65 years or older with comorbid conditions and two or more rib fractures; or at a lower age with increased frailty and pulmonary dysfunction; or with a flail chest, should be admitted to the ICU for monitoring [7]. Initial multimodal pain control is crucial, and includes oral and or acetaminophen and NSAIDs, muscle relaxants, rib blocks with local anesthesia, and an epidural if needed [7]. If epidural analgesia is contraindicated, paravertebral blocks are another option. Mechanical ventilation should be used to support respiratory failure. Current recommendations for management of pulmonary contusions and flail chest are to use positive end-expiratory pressure (PEEP) [8]. Use of airway pressure release ventilation (ARPV) within 1 day of intubation for treatment of pulmonary contusion has been shown to increase lung recruitment and blood flow to dependent alveolar units improving oxygenation and V/Q mismatch which has been shown to decrease rates of ventilator associated pneumonia [9]. Early operative intervention of both flail and non-flail segments with rib fixation has been shown to decrease ventilator days, narcotic use, and pulmonary complications [10].

Blunt traumatic aortic injury carries a significant mortality in the pre and post hospital setting approaching 50–70% [11]. Treatment has evolved with the implementation of thoracic endovascular stent grafts becoming much more common place over open repair. In the landmark paper by Dr. Riyad Karmy-Jones, patients with aortic rupture underwent endovascular stent graft (EVSG). This treatment was selected as these patients had sustained multi system traumas or carried comorbid conditions such that an open repair would not be possible. Treatment with EVSG resulted in positive outcomes with 72% of patients eventually discharging home [12]. There were four cases of an endoleak with the main cause being lateral expansion of the endograft into the rupture resulting in shortening of the graft and a decreased landing zone [12]. These endoleaks were amenable to repair with cuff extenders and multiple stent grafts, with only one patient requiring an open repair [12]. This observation led to widespread adoption of endovascular repair of traumatic aortic ruptures. Based on the following grading system: intimal tear (grade 1), intramural hematoma (grade 2), pseudoaneurysm (grade 3), and rupture (grade 4); current recommendations are to repair any grade 2 injury or higher [13]. However, there are newer reports that grade 2 injuries can be managed without initial operative intervention [13]. Non-operative management consists of intensive care admission with beta blockade and other antihypertensive agents aiming for a goal systolic blood pressure between 100–120 mm Hg, mean arterial pressure <80 mm Hg, and heart rate 60–80 beats/min with continued long-term surveillance with CT after discharge [14]. Close monitoring of grade 1 and 2 injury is essential as an acute aortic rupture is most likely to occur within the first 4 to 6 hours after injury [14].

Blunt trauma to the chest rarely leads to blunt cardiac injury (BCI). Screening for BCI includes a 12-lead ECG, which has a high negative predictive value of 95% [15]. There is still not a consensus on what to do with abnormal troponin values. Should they be trended, how often, and to what value? However, troponin I is valuable if it is within normal limits along with no ECG changes, essentially ruling out BCI [15]. A patient with ECG findings of a new arrhythmia, ST elevation, ischemia, or heart block should be admitted for continuous monitoring to telemetry or the ICU and an echocardiogram obtained [15]. Treatment remains supportive for BCI.

With advances in critical care and minimally invasive procedures, augmenting the postoperative and nonoperative care, many traumatic thoracic injuries continue to be managed successfully with improved outcomes for patients.

ANNOTATED REFERENCES FOR ICU ISSUES WITH THORACIC TRAUMA

1. Meredith JW, Hoth JJ. Thoracic trauma: when and how to intervene. *Surg Clin North Am.* 2007;87(1):95–118. doi:10.1016/j.suc.2006.09.014

   A review of the algorithms that applies to managing thoracic trauma patients with discussion of considerations and variables that enter into the decision-making process. Also discussed various scenarios in which these treatments apply. Covers technical considerations of multiple thoracic operative procedures.

2. Kirkpatrick AW, Rizoli S, Ouellet J, et al. Occult pneumothoraces in critical care. *J Trauma Acute Care Surg.* 2013;74(3):747–755. doi:10.1097/ta.0b013e3182827158

   Interim analysis of the Occult Pneumothoraces in Critical Care which is a unblinded, multicenter, prospective randomized control trial comparing pleural drainage to close clinical observation among trauma patients with occult pneumothorax requiring positive pressure ventilation. Discusses positive and negative outcomes of conservative management of occult pneumothorax.

3. Moore FO, Goslar PW, Coimbra R, et al. Blunt traumatic occult pneumothorax: is observation safe?—Results of a prospective, AAST multicenter study. J Trauma: *Injury Infect Crit Care.* 2011;70(5):1019–1025. doi:10.1097/ta.0b013e318213f727

   A prospective, observational, multicenter study from 16 trauma centers over 2 years to identify patients with occult pneumothorax and discussed the possibility of conservative management. They found that observations resulted in a 6% failure rate in non-intubated patients and a 14% failure rate in patients on positive pressure ventilation. None of the 448 patients observed progressed to tension pneumothorax.

4. Prakash PS, Moore SA, Rezende-Neto JB, Trpcic S, Cannon JW. Predictors of retained hemothorax in trauma: results of an Eastern Association for the Surgery of Trauma multi-institutional trial. *J Trauma Acute Care Surg.* 2020 Oct;89(4):679–685. doi: 10.1097/TA.0000000000002881. PMID: 32649619.

   A prospective, observational, multi-institutional study from 17 centers within the United States and Canada of adult trauma patients diagnosed with an hemothorax over 2 years. They found that the retained hemothorax rate was 29% which was associated with larger hemothorax on presentation. They also noted that patients with a retained hemothorax had higher rates of pneumonia and longer hospital length of stay.

5. Gilbert RW, Fontebasso AM, Park L, Tran A, Lampron J. The management of occult hemothorax in adults with thoracic trauma: a systematic review and meta-analysis. *J Trauma Acute Care Surg.* 2020;89(6):1225–1232. doi:10.1097/ta.0000000000002936

   A systematic review that evaluates the clinical outcomes of conservatively managed occult hemothorax. The primary outcome of this review is failure of conservative management. Six studies were included over 70 years of publications. They determined that a hemothorax of less than 300 cc can be safely managed without TT in certain situations.

6. Sutyak JP, Wohltmann CD, Larson J. Pulmonary contusions and critical care management in thoracic trauma. *Thorac Surg Clin.* 2007;17(1):11–23. doi:10.1016/j.thorsurg.2007.02.001

An in-depth discussion of the pathophysiology of pulmonary contusions, current ventilator strategies and methods to combat morbidities associated with pulmonary contusions including ventilator associated pneumonia.

7. Brasel KJ, Moore EE, Albrecht RA, et al. Western Trauma Association critical decisions in trauma: management of rib fractures. *J Trauma Acute Care Surg.* 2017;82(1):200–203. doi:10.1097/ta.0000000000001301

Multiple management algorithms from the Western Trauma Association addressing the management of adult patients with rib fractures. This paper discusses work up, pain control options, operative and non-operative treatments, and follow-up recommendations.

8. Simon B, Ebert J, Bokhari F, et al. Management of pulmonary contusion and flail chest: an Eastern Association for the Surgery of Trauma practice management guideline. *J Trauma Acute Care Surg.* 2012;73(5):S351–S361. doi:10.1097/ta.0b013e31827019fd

The Eastern Association for the Surgery of Trauma (EAST) practice management guidelines for patients with pulmonary contusions and flail chest. There are multiple level 2 and 3 recommendations made for diagnosis and treatments of pulmonary contusions and flail chest. They also discuss the historical treatments and discuss how these have evolved over time.

9. Walkey AJ, Nair S, Papadopoulos S, Agarwal S, Reardon CC. Use of airway pressure release ventilation is associated with a reduced incidence of ventilator-associated pneumonia in patients with pulmonary contusion. *J Trauma: Injury Infect Crit Care.* 2011;70(3). doi:10.1097/ta.0b013e3181d9f612

A retrospective cohort study looking at 68 patients treated with airway pressure release ventilation (APRV) for pulmonary contusions. They found that APRV when used in treatment of pulmonary contusions is associated with a decrease in ventilator associated pneumonia. They also noted that APRV was not associated with increased hospital mortality or change in ventilator days.

10. Pieracci FM, Leasia K, Bauman Z, et al. A multicenter, prospective, controlled clinical trial of surgical stabilization of rib fractures in patients with severe, nonflail fracture patterns (Chest Wall Injury Society NONFLAIL). *J Trauma Acute Care Surg.* 2020 Feb;88(2):249–257. doi: 10.1097/TA.0000000000002559. PMID: 31804414.

A multicenter, prospective, controlled, clinical trial over 12 centers comparing surgical rib fixation within 72 hours to medical management. They found that patients who underwent surgical rib fixation early had better quality of life, decreased narcotic consumption, and decreased pleural space complications than the medical management group.

11. Cheng D, Mcnickle AG, Fraser DR, et al. Early characteristics and progression of blunt traumatic aortic injuries at a single level I trauma center. *Vasc Endovasc Surg.* 2021;55(2):105–111. 15385744209660645. doi:10.1177/1538574420966450

A retrospective review of the University Medical Center of Southern Nevada trauma registry of 32 patients with blunt aortic injury managed either operatively or non-operatively. They discussed grading systems of injury and current treatments of each grade. They note that grade 1 and 2 injury have been managed non-operatively successfully and discuss the failure rates and follow-up needed for treatment.

12. Karmy-Jones R, Hoffer E, Meissner MH, Nicholls S, Mattos M. Endovascular stent grafts and aortic rupture: a case series. *J Trauma*. 2003 Feb;55(5):805–10. doi: 10.1097/01. TA.0000094429.98136.29. PMID: 14608148.

Retrospective review over 6 years at a single institution describing 11 patients with thoracic aortic rupture treated with endovascular stent instead of open repair. This paper discussed the technical considerations for stent placement as well as the types of stents that lead to the most successful treatment. They also discuss pitfalls of treatment and ways to treat endoleaks or stent grafts that are not seated correctly.

13. Lee WA, Matsumura JS, Mitchell RS, et al. Endovascular repair of traumatic thoracic aortic injury: clinical practice guidelines of the Society for Vascular Surgery. *J Vasc Surg*. 2011;53(1):187–192. doi:10.1016/j.jvs.2010.08.027

A systematic review discussing practice guidelines for endovascular repair of thoracic aortic injury. This paper polled experts and came to a consensus on a select number of issues to guide clinical practice. They describe a grading system for injury, and discusses treatment guidelines for timing of repair, medical management of injury, current grafts available, repair related to the age of the patient, vascular access, coverage of the left subclavian artery, systemic heparinization, and placement of a spinal drain to aid in paraplegia prevention.

14. Rabin J, Dubose J, Sliker CW, O'Connor JV, Scalea TM, Griffith BP. Parameters for successful nonoperative management of traumatic aortic injury. *J Thorac Cardiovasc Surg*. 2014;147(1):143–150. doi:10.1016/j.jtcvs.2013.08.053

Retrospective review of 97 patients from the University of Maryland over 4.5 years. They discuss current medical management techniques for grades 1 and 2 aortic injury as well as current surgical techniques for grades 3 and 4 injury.

15. Clancy K, Velopulos C, Bilaniuk JW, et al.; Eastern Association for the Surgery of Trauma. Screening for blunt cardiac injury: an Eastern Association for the Surgery of Trauma practice management guideline. *J Trauma Acute Care Surg*. 2012 Nov;73(5 Suppl 4):S301–S306. doi: 10.1097/TA.0b013e318270193a. PMID: 23114485.

The Eastern Association for the Surgery of Trauma (EAST) practice management guideline updates the original from 1998 recommendations on blunt cardiac injury. This guideline has multiple level 1, 2, and 3 recommendations for screening and workup of blunt cardiac injury.

Landmark Article of the 21st Century

ENDOVASCULAR STENT GRAFTS AND AORTIC RUPTURE: A CASE SERIES

Karmy-Jones R, Hoffer E, Meissner MH et al., *J Trauma*. 2003;55(5):805–810

Commentary by Riyad C. Karmy-Jones

The paper was written at a time when thoracic specific devices were not widely available and were designed for aneurysmal disease. It was also a time of struggle both within and without the vascular community as too who would "control" these emerging technologies.

This series constituted patients who were critically ill and could not be repaired by open techniques. This high risk group was in contradistinction to many European and Canadian studies which limited TEVAR to stable patients with small injuries.

The paper reviewed the specific anatomic concerns relative to TEVAR, and compared "off the shelf" constructed stents to commercially available abdominal grafts. With reference to the left subclavian and stroke risk, we suggested that in young patients, the subclavian could be covered. Now we know this is true although older patients may be at increased risk, although as much from wire manipulation in the arch as impacting vertebral perfusion. Newer approaches, including fenestration and kissing stents permit preservation of the left subclavian with greater ease. We mentioned sizing "10–20%". We now know that oversizing can lead to increased endocollapse. We also recognize that in patients with a pliable aorta, if in shock, aortic diameters can increase by as much as 30% which requires some judgement as to appropriate sizing. We stressed the need to try and avoid lack of apposition along the inner wall and discussed "ballooning" the endograft. Currently, we rarely do this as we are concerned about creating a dissection. Later studies confirm that the point of curvature has the maximal stress in the aorta, and if any endograft "juts up away from the inner wall" there is increased likelihood of collapse. We noted that all of us were awaiting more thoracic specific devices, including those with smaller diameters, and perhaps shorter lengths. Now we have longer delivery systems, smaller sheath sizes permitting percutaneous access, and more flexible endografts to fit the aortic curvature (with much lower incidence of lack of wall apposition). Nonetheless, we are still waiting for shorter endografts to become more available. However, the current devices are so much more stable and predictable in deployment that the use of adenosine is rarely required. The paper also presaged the hybrid room and the occasional uses of TEVAR as a bridge to definite management (especially in younger patients).

Much has been clarified. Medical management is accepted in specific patients, and is associated with improved outcome if intervention is required. TEVAR has become the favored approach, offering a less morbid option than open repair, which tends to be relegated to ascending and arch of the aorta (although that will soon change). It appears that TEVAR is as durable as open repair, and the majority of any complications are managed percutaneously. Procedures are performed in hybrid suites, with percutaneous approaches, and can be combined with other procedures. In patients deemed to have increased risk of stroke, percutaneous approaches are available to preserve vertebral perfusion.

CHAPTER 43

ICU Issues with Abdominal and Pelvic Trauma

Review by Allison J. Tompeck and Ara J. Feinstein

Care of the polytrauma patient begins in the trauma bay and often quickly transitions to the intensive care unit. In patients with ongoing physiologic derangements or unresolved shock, communication between the intensive care and trauma or surgical team is imperative. A thorough handoff, including mechanism of injury, initial resuscitation, imaging findings, and injuries should be performed. In the setting of ongoing resuscitation requirements, particular attention must be paid to clues that the abdomen may be the source of decompensation.

Evaluation of a patient requiring ongoing resuscitation begins with a thorough tertiary exam. One must consider the mechanism of injury and force trajectory. A direct blow to the epigastrium is most often inflicted by a steering wheel in motor vehicle crashes, or a handlebar in bicycle crash [1]. This mechanism threatens injury to the pancreas, duodenum, liver, and extra-hepatic biliary tree. Patients presenting with a positive abdominal seatbelt sign are at increased risk for hollow viscus and mesenteric injures. Laboratory data should be trended to assess coagulopathy, end organ perfusion (lactate, base deficit), and rhabdomyolysis. As these inquiries begin to differentiate inadequate resuscitation versus unaddressed etiologies, repeat imaging may be indicated. This includes focused assessment with ultrasound and CT with additional contrast phases. Particular attention should be given to increases in intrabdominal fluid, especially if solid organ injury was noted on previous imaging. Increased size of pelvic or retroperitoneal hematoma should be noted. In the adequately resuscitated, normothermic patient without evidence of hemorrhage, ongoing impaired perfusion mandates the intensivist urgently search for unrecognized injuries.

Intra-abdominal injuries following blunt trauma may be unrecognized during the initial assessment due to altered mental status, endotracheal intubation, distracting injuries, false negative imaging, and/or examination.[2] Blunt small bowel injury has an estimated incidence of 5–15%, with an associated increase in mortality if diagnosis is delayed greater than 8–24 hours [3, 4]. In addition, mural hematomas or mesenteric devascularization injuries progress to bowel necrosis and perforation over time, thus delaying clinical presentation [5]. The diagnostic value of a CT scan for hollow viscus injury at initial presentation has an estimated sensitivity of 50–94% [4]. The most common indirect CT scan finding of blunt bowel or mesenteric injury is free fluid in the absence of solid organ

DOI: 10.1201/9781003042136-43

injury, followed by bowel wall thickening, hematoma, and mesenteric stranding. In addition, modern non-operative management of blunt solid organ injury in hemodynamically stable patients limits intra-operative diagnosis of concomitant hollow viscus injuries which can occur in up to 13% of patients [5, 6]. McNutt et al. demonstrated that unrecognized blunt bowel and mesenteric injuries are statistically associated with oliguria, persistent systemic inflammatory response >24 hours, ileus, new abdominal tenderness, tachycardia, and bandemia [3]. Therefore, worsening abdominal examination, new or persistent sepsis or worsening CT scan findings warrants concern for missed hollow viscus injury and consideration of operative exploration [2, 3].

Duodeno-pancreatic and extrahepatic biliary tree injuries are relatively uncommon, and deceptively subtle during initial evaluation. Early definitive diagnosis is limited by anatomic location and frequent association with hepatic and major abdominal vascular injuries [1]. Serum amylase and lipase only offer 50% sensitivity for pancreatic injury, but normal serum levels have a 95% negative predictive value [7]. Pancreatic injuries manifest over time and therefore combined serial measurements of serum amylase and lipase should be considered if there is clinical suspicion [1, 7]. CT scan with IV contrast is the radiographic test of choice. However, if initially negative and clinical suspicion remains high, a repeat CT 8–24 hours following injury is more likely to reveal duodeno-pancreatic pathology [1, 7]. Magnetic resonance cholangiopancreatography (MRCP) is a second-line noninvasive diagnostic modality for suspected injury of pancreatic parenchyma, the pancreatic duct, and biliary tree [1]. Finally, a high index of clinical suspicion paired with hemodynamic instability demands surgical exploration to expose the duodeno-pancreatic complex [1, 7].

Not infrequently, patients with combined abdomino-pelvic trauma have ongoing resuscitation needs without evidence of ongoing bleeding or serious organ injury. Traumatic shock (TS), also known as vasoplegic syndrome (VS), describes a state of persistent hypotension, normal or increased cardiac output, and decreased systemic vascular resistance [8, 9]. A key component of this clinical diagnosis is the absence of alternative etiologies such as sepsis, uncontrolled hemorrhage, missed injuries, abdominal compartment syndrome, or hypovolemia. Risk factors shown to increase the incidence of TS include blood transfusion, pelvic or long bone fractures, burns over a significant body surface area, traumatic injuries with an elevated injury severity score (ISS), and conditions with significant systemic inflammation such as pancreatitis. The exact pathogenesis is unclear. It is likely due to the presence of overlapping mechanistic pathways affecting vascular reactivity, which clinically culminate in persistent failure of vascular homeostasis [8, 9]. The persistent hypotension of TS uniquely results in oliguria yet normal capillary refill and oxygen arterial saturation [8].

Management begins with volume replacement, however this alone fails to restore hemodynamics and achieve end-points of resuscitation. Failure to recognize this phenomenon as a loss of tone historically led to the over-resuscitation of trauma patients. Large volumes of crystalloid contributed to coagulopathy, abdominal compartment syndrome, and acute respiratory distress syndrome (ARDS). Adjuncts, such as ultrasound and stroke volume variation can assist the clinician in ensuring that adequate volume resuscitation has been undertaken before starting vasopressors. Patients with TS may require pressors, specifically norepinephrine, at significantly higher doses and for a prolonged duration relative to other etiologies of shock. Surprisingly, the increased total dose of vasoconstricting medications does not result in the same degree of peripheral ischemia as seen in other types of shock. Vasopressin, which induces vascular smooth muscle contraction, is indicated as a second agent and may reduce the overall dose of catecholamines [8]. Finally, methylene blue, a guanylate cyclase inhibitor or Giapreza (Angiotensin II), should be considered for catecholamine resistant TS, however the literature is sparse and availability is limited [8].

ANNOTATED REFERENCES FOR ICU ISSUES WITH ABDOMINAL AND PELVIC TRAUMA

1. Coccolini F, Kobayashi L, Kluger Y, et al. Duodeno-pancreatic and extrahepatic biliary tree trauma: WSES-AAST guidelines. *World J Emerg Surg*. 2019;14:56.

   http://doi.org/10.1186/s13017-019-0278-6.

   This consensus paper outlines the optimal evaluation and management of duodeno-pancreatic and extra-hepatic biliary tree trauma for both pediatric and adult populations. The recommendations are further emphasized by the sequelae of late presentation and associated increased morbidity and mortality.

2. Tisherman SA, Stein DM. ICU management of trauma patients. *Crit Care Med*. 2018;46:1991–1997.

   The authors provide a concise definitive review of the initial assessment and intensive care management of critically ill trauma patients. First ventilator management, massive transfusion, and coagulopathy are addressed. Next, the authors highlight specific injuries and challenges inherent to each organ system. Finally, this paper exposes care as a continuum and the challenges of overlapping management.

3. McNutt MK, Chinapuvvula NR, Beckmann NM, et al. Early surgical intervention for blunt bowel injury: The Bowel Injury Prediction Score (BIPS). *J Trauma Acute Care Surg*. 2015;78:105–111.

   The author describes a new simple score to identify blunt bowel injuries that require early surgical intervention. Retrospective analysis of 110 patients at a single center identified 3 predictors: admission CT scan grade of mesenteric injury, white blood cell count, and abdominal tenderness. A score greater than or equal to 2 strongly predicted blunt hollow viscus injury for which early surgical intervention is indicated.

4. Fakhry SM, Allawi A, Ferguson PL, et al. Blunt small bowel perforation (SBP): An Eastern Association for the Surgery of Trauma multicenter update 15 years later. *J Trauma Acute Care Surg*. 2019;86:642–650.

   After reviewing 127,919 trauma admission and 94,743 activations, these authors show initial CT scans continue to miss SBP. They recommend that any intraperitoneal abnormalities on initial CT scan should indicate high suspicion and recommend repeat CT or therapeutic intervention at 8 hours if uncertainty remains.

5. Harmston C, War JBM, Patel A. Clinical outcomes and effect of delayed intervention in patients with hollow viscus injury due to blunt abdominal trauma: A systematic review. *Eur J Trauma Emerg Surg.* 2018;44:369–376.

These authors review patients with blunt hollow viscus injury who underwent early versus later surgical intervention. Overall mortality was 17%, and there was no difference in mortality between groups. The authors conclude that there is insufficient data to suggest a higher mortality when surgery is delayed 24 hours.

6. Swaid F, Peleg K, Alfici R, Matter I, Osha O, Ashkenazi I, Givon A, Israel Trauma Group, Kessel B. Concomitant hollow viscus injuries in patients with blunt hepatic and splenic injuries: An analysis of a National Trauma Registry database. *Injury.* 2014;45:1409–1412.

A retrospective cohort study of 57,130 patients with blunt torso injury. Authors show that blunt splenic and or blunt hepatic injury, particularly if combined, predicts the presence of hollow viscus injury (HVI). Isolated blunt splenic injury clearly correlates with an increased incidence of HVI, however isolated hepatic injury may not.

7. Jurkovich GJ. AAST invited lecture: Pancreatic trauma. *J Trauma Acute Care Surg.* 2019;88(1):19–24.

This author reviews pancreatic physiology, four diagnostic components of pancreatic trauma and controversies of management. During his discussion of management, he highlights variations in peripancreatic anatomy and surgical options for injuries grade III or greater.

8. Liu H, Yu L, Yang L, Green MS. Vasoplegic syndrome: An update on perioperative considerations. *J Clin Anesth.* 2017;40:63–71.

The authors review the risk factors, mechanistic pathways, clinical presentation, and management strategies of vasoplegic syndrome (VS). In addition, they suggest ways to differentiate VS from other diagnoses such as reperfusion syndrome.

9. Lambden S, Creagh-Brown BC, Hunt J, Summers C, Forni LG. Definitions and pathophysiology of vasoplegic shock. *Crit Care.* 2018;22:174.

http://doi.org/10.1186/s13054-018-2102-1

This reviews the features of VS, explores the pathophysiology and associated causes of vasoplegia. The author concludes that without a clear definition, investigation is limited.

Landmark Article of the 21st Century

BLUNT SPLENIC INJURY IN ADULTS: MULTI-INSTITUTIONAL STUDY OF THE EASTERN ASSOCIATION FOR THE SURGERY OF TRAUMA

Peitzman AB, *J Trauma Acute Care Surg.* 2000;49:177–189

Commentary by Andrew B. Peitzman

The paradigm shift toward nonoperative management of blunt abdominal solid organ injury evolved rapidly in the late 1980s and 1990s. The EAST multi-institutional trial of blunt splenic injury in adults was conceived because of concerns with the studies on nonoperative management of solid organ injuries to that point: 1) Studies had included injury to the spleen and liver. We thought the natural history of injury to the spleen was different than the liver; spleens were more likely to bleed during observation. 2) Studies had included both adults and children. We thought that pediatric spleens behaved differently and skewed the observations. 3) Some studies included both penetrating and blunt injury. 4) Grade 4 and especially grade 5 injuries comprise only 15% of blunt splenic injuries in adults. Thus, single institutional studies had insufficient high grade injuries to make accurate observations. Dr. Brian Heil, a resident in plastic surgery at the time, generated the computer data entry forms and maintained the database.

Adults ($n = 1488$) with blunt splenic injury from 27 level I and II trauma centers were studied retrospectively. In this multi-institutional study, 38.5% of adults with blunt splenic injury went directly to laparotomy; 61.5% were admitted with planned observation. Angiography/embolization was rarely utilized in this study. Ultimately, 55% of patients were successfully managed nonoperatively. The failure rate of observation was 10.8%; increasing with grade of injury and quantity of hemoperitoneum. Sixty-one percent of failures occurred in the first 24 hours. Successful nonoperative management was associated with higher blood pressure and hematocrit on admission, less severe injury based on ISS, Glasgow Coma Scale, grade of splenic injury, and quantity of hemoperitoneum.

In addition, several important observations were made from this multi-institutional trial with larger numbers that could not have been made from a single institutional study. This was most noteworthy in the patients who failed nonoperative management (studied in detail in J Am Coll Surg 2005;201:179–187). These observations were: 1) Several unstable patients were managed nonoperatively with high rates of failure; 2) although used infrequently at that time, the false negative rate for FAST was 40%; 3) of the 12 deaths in the patients who failed nonoperative management, 60% were preventable, based on the previous two observations; 4) grade 5 splenic injury failed nonoperative management in 75% (3 of 4). More importantly, 74 of 78 grade 5 splenic injuries underwent splenectomy on admission.

CHAPTER 44

Extremity Trauma

Review by Sanjeev Kaul, Saraswati Dayal, and Javier Martin Perez

EPIDEMIOLOGY OF VASCULAR INJURY

Vascular injury in patients suffering from trauma to the extremity can lead to death from exsanguination, shock, tissue injury, and metabolic derangements. Vascular assessment of injured extremities is thus a critical component of the evaluation and management of trauma patients with blunt or penetrating trauma. Hard signs of vascular injury include active hemorrhage, an expanding hematoma, bruit over the wound, an absence of distal pulse, and ischemia in the extremity. In an observational study of penetrating extremity trauma at an urban trauma center, all patients that were taken immediately to surgery as a result of hard signs ultimately had a major arterial injury requiring repair, implying a 100% positive predictive value for when penetrating trauma shows hard signs of arterial injury. For patients who do not present with hard signs of vascular injury, an injured extremity index (IEI), which is analogous to the ankle-brachial index (ABI) and arterial pressure index (API) but applies to any extremity, should be performed. The IEI can be computed as follows: *IEI = highest systolic pressure in extremity that is injured/systolic pressure in proximal vessel of an uninjured extremity*, where an abnormal IEI measures less than 0.9. In studies exploring the predictive value for ABI and API in identifying vascular injury requiring surgical intervention, the sensitivity, specificity, and positive predictive value of an ABI lower than 0.90 were 100%, and an API less than 0.90 had a sensitivity of 87% and a specificity of 97% for arterial disruption. Patients who undergo revascularization of an injured extremity are at risk for ischemia reperfusion injury as reperfusion paradoxically can cause further damage, ultimately threatening the viability of organs, and can cause significant metabolic derangement such as hyperkalemia and acidosis. There are several therapeutic strategies being explored to limit ischemia reperfusion injury including ischemic preconditioning. However, when these strategies have been applied to clinical practice, outcomes have been ambiguous. Timely reperfusion of the ischemic area at risk is the most widely accepted strategy to prevent ischemia reperfusion injuries and related complications such as multiorgan dysfunction syndrome (MODS).

MANAGEMENT OF EXTREMITY TRAUMA

The optimal management of extremity trauma continues to remain a challenge and of great interest to present-day trauma surgeons. The critically ill trauma patient should be considered for transfer to a level 1 or level 2 trauma center. Limb loss, infection,

DOI: 10.1201/9781003042136-44

and nonunion are feared complications of the extremity as well as systemic complications of shock, renal failure, sepsis, respiratory failure and death. The critical care management of the acutely ill trauma patient with extremity trauma needs to take into account the risk versus benefit ratio of limb salvage against the possible threat to life from limb salvage operations.

A framework of critical care aspects of the management of extremity trauma are discussed here. The variables affecting prognosis can be broadly divided into patient related and injury related. The patient variables are underlying physiology, age, gender, comorbidities, and underlying medications. The injury variables are severity, energy of injury, morphology of fracture, bone loss, soft tissue injury, blood supply, location, and other significant associated injuries like brain injury.

Early diagnosis of fractures, soft tissue injury, vascular injury, and nerve injury is essential followed by a damage control approach of management of extremity trauma in a critically ill patient.

Since a history is often unreliable, a careful inspection and palpation followed by appropriate radiological studies of the extremity may be necessary to diagnose open and closed fractures, soft tissue trauma, vascular injuries, and nerve injuries.

Various classifications have been used for fractures. The Gustilo classification which is most used in open fractures takes into account the degrees of soft tissue injury, contamination, and vascular injury. The AO classification details the degree of skin, muscle, and neurovascular injury. All individuals with injuries to more than one system or the injury severity score (ISS) greater than 16 should be considered polytrauma cases.

Early administration of antibiotics, tetanus toxoid, surgical cleaning, and meticulous debridement are essential in exposed fractures. The systemic conditions of patients with multiple trauma and the local conditions of the limb affected need to be taken into account. This is especially relevant in traumatic brain injury, hemorrhagic shock and or hypoxemia with a P/F ratio less than 200. Early skeletal stabilization is necessary. Definitive fixation should be considered when possible, and temporizing fixation methods should be used when necessary. Early closure should be the aim, and flaps can be used for this purpose if needed for large defects.

Immediate definitive fixation of the fracture may be performed if the local and the systemic conditions are permissive in the form of minimal soft tissue trauma, major contamination, and clinical instability. Recently literature has shown that definitive fixation and debridement can be done within a 24-hour period without any increase in infection.

In cases where definitive fixation is not possible, external fixation with debridement may be the most appropriate form of damage control surgery. During this period, avoidance of hypotension, hypothermia, acidosis, and coagulopathy is a must with active resuscitation. There is a need for great communication between the anesthesiologists, trauma surgeons, orthopedic surgeons, and other surgeons working on the patient either concurrently or sequentially in the operating room to avoid prolonged surgery as well as sharing of relevant clinical, physiological, and lab data.

The timing of repeat surgery with debridement is dependent on the degree of contamination and the physiological recovery of the patient. The internalization of hardware has a window of opportunity between the first and the second week after which the risk of infection is higher.

Small skin defects can be closed early, and larger soft tissue defects may need temporizing dressings such as negative pressure therapy followed by skin grafts or muscle flaps.

Severe soft tissue and bony injuries may require a review of the advantages and disadvantages at attempting limb salvage. This may be stratified into risk of life from attempted limb salvage versus expected degree of function after multiple operative procedures. There are no universally accepted guidelines. One of the traditional scoring systems used to predict the likelihood of amputations is a MESS (Mangled Extremity Severity Score) score greater than 7 even though recent literature question its predictability of amputation.

The critical care management of the severely ill trauma patient with extremity trauma needs to take into account the risk to life from attempted limb salvage versus the likelihood of a viable functional limb.

EXTREMITY COMPARTMENT SYNDROME

Acute compartment syndrome of the extremity may result from crush injury, penetrating trauma with concomitant arteriovenous injuries, electrical injury, and thermal injury. These injuries may exist concomitantly with associated fractures, skin loss, and degrees of muscle injury. Associated secondary conditions such as soft tissue infection, rhabdomyolysis, and osteomyelitis may result. The true incidence of acute compartment syndrome (ACS) in the extremity is unknown and may only be confirmed upon fasciotomy. The associated delays in diagnosis of ACS may result in increased cost, prolonged hospital stays, and decreased limb function and quality of life. Given that early diagnosis of ACS is essential, a high clinical index of suspicion is warranted based on clinical history. Despite the physical examination being the primary method of diagnosis, there is limited evidence only in awake patients regarding diagnostic performance. Given the limitations of the physical examination, there is evidence for the utility of repeated or continuous intra-compartmental pressure (ICP) monitoring where a threshold value (diastolic blood pressure minus ICP) of >30 mm Hg is used to guide definitive intervention. Laboratory values such as lactate, troponin, and urine myoglobin have a role in the diagnosis of ACS. Biomarkers may be utilized for late presentation or missed cases of ACS but not to screen for ACS and determine the need for fasciotomy. No evidence supports a specific technique of fasciotomy, but a complete decompression of all involved compartments is considered optimal. Post-operative wound care favors negative pressure wound dressing for reduced time to final closure and skin grating. Rhabdomyolysis is associated with ACS and leads to acute kidney injury due to volume depletion, impairment of glomerular filtration, intra-renal vasoconstriction, direct/ischemic tubular injury, and tubular occlusion. Creatinine kinase levels of as low as 5000 U/L may lead to kidney injury; however, CK levels of greater than 20,000 U/L are more likely to lead to AKI. Primary treatment remains aggressive volume resuscitation. Alkalization with sodium bicarbonate has been utilized in the treatment of rhabdomyolysis with limited evidence supporting improved clinical outcomes. In a study of trauma patients, there was no benefit on the incidence of renal failure, need for dialysis, or death. Furthermore, there are limited data supporting mannitol and loop diuretics in the treatment of rhabdomyolysis.

ANNOTATED REFERENCES FOR EXTREMITY TRAUMA

Hauser CJ, Adams CA Jr, Eachempati SR. Surgical infection society guideline: prophylactic antibiotic use in open fractures: an evidence-based guideline. *Surg Infect (Larchmt).* 2006;(74):379–405.

This study systematically reviews the effects of prophylactic antibiotic administration on the incidence of infection in complicating open fractures. As the paper states, prolonged courses of broad-spectrum antibiotics were often cited as the standard of care for prevention of infective complications at the time of its publication. Results support the conclusion that a short course of first-generation cephalosporins, begun as soon as possible after injury, significantly lowers the risk of infection when used in combination with prompt, orthopedic fracture wound management.

Higgins TF, Klatt JB, Beals TC. Lower Extremity Assessment Project (LEAP): the best available evidence on limb-threatening lower extremity trauma. *Orthop Clin North Am.* 2010;41(2):233–239.

This paper is a review of the Lower Extremity Assessment Project (LEAP), a prospective observational study exploring a score-based methodology in deciding whether to amputate or salvage a limb, and the various subsequent papers that leveraged the LEAP study population which explore, among other topics, long-term persistent disability, psychological distress, complications, the effects of smoking on fracture healing and complications, and the outcomes of rotational flaps vs. free tissue transfers in patients requiring flap coverage. This review highlights how the original LEAP study and subsequent papers collectively give surgeons an enhanced insight into factors that drive outcomes, and present statistics that can be used to help counsel patients at time of initial hospitalization.

Jorge-Mora A, Rodriguez-Martin J, Pretell-Mazzini J. Timing issue in open fractures debridement: a review article. *Eur J Orthop Surg Traumatol.* 2013;23(2):125–129.

This review article highlights several studies that discuss the impact of the timing of debridement of open fractures on the incidence of infection. The article concludes that the 14 cited studies do not establish a link between delayed surgery and infection rates, but that debridement and irrigation on the whole are important factors in reducing the prevalence of infection following an open fracture.

Townsend RN, Lheureau T, Protech J, Riemer B, Simon D. Timing fracture repair in patients with severe brain injury (Glasgow Coma Scale score <9). *J Trauma*. 1998 Jun;44(6):977–982; discussion 982–983.

This study evaluated all patients admitted to a level 1 trauma center over a 10 year window, who sustained a femur fracture and severe closed head injury—having a GCS score of 8 or less upon admission or during the first 8 hours after admission, and discusses the timing of operative repair of fractures and subsequent risk of secondary brain injury. The study concludes that timing of the operation was a strong predictor of operative hypotension, with 60% of the patients operated on within 2 hours experiencing hypotension. Only 1 of 12 patients (8.3%) operated on after 24 hours experienced episodes of hypotension. Eighty-nine percent of patients with severe head injury and femur fractures who had no abdominal or pelvic injuries were hypotensive if operated on in less than 2 hours.

Landmark Article of the 21st Century

RESUSCITATIVE ENDOVASCULAR BALLOON OCCLUSION OF THE AORTA (REBOA) AS AN ADJUNCT FOR HEMORRHAGIC SHOCK

Stannard A, Eliason JE, Rasmussen TE, *J Trauma*. 2011;71(6):1869–1872

Commentary by Todd E. Rasmussen

The 2011 manuscript "Resuscitative Endovascular Balloon Occlusion of the Aorta (REBOA) as an Adjunct for Hemorrhagic Shock" was submitted at the prompting of then Editor-in-Chief of the *Journal of Trauma*, Dr. Basil A. Pruitt, who recognized the changing landscape of hemorrhage control and resuscitation and the growing role of endovascular techniques in this space. At the time, two epidemiologic studies had been performed by the US military, identifying the lethality of non-compressible torso hemorrhage and a third, the Eastridge "Death on the Battlefield" project, was underway. The military had initiated a research program to assess resuscitative endovascular balloon occlusion of the aorta as an alternative to direct aortic clamping via laparotomy or thoracotomy. By 2011 initial porcine models had shown the endovascular approach held promise and a new device was in the early prototype stage. The inability of traditional open surgical approaches to reduce mortality from this injury scenario also created an urgency for a new approach, one that could be rendered more effectively as a stabilizing maneuver and earlier in the course of hemorrhagic shock.

Although the publication christened the term REBOA and defined the aortic occlusion zones, the maneuver itself was hardly new. In 1954, then Major Carl Hughes published a case series from the Korean War in which a rudimentary endovascular balloon device was inflated inside of the aorta as an intraoperative rescue maneuver and several case series, still using antiquated technologies, appeared in publication in the 1980s and 1990s. It wasn't until after the revolution of endovascular technologies had occurred between 1990 and 2010, that REBOA could be legitimately reappraised for its potential to shift the management of bleeding and shock. Remember, at this time the seemingly immovable mortality from ruptured abdominal aortic aneurysms was for the first time in five decades being positively affected by the use of endovascular approaches, including REBOA. There was a sense, an enthusiasm, and a plausible clinical model showing that REBOA would work in severely injured and shocked patients.

Understanding the potential for this paper to be a landmark reference, and because it was aimed at opening the aperture of endovascular skills to other disciplines (i.e., to the general and trauma surgery communities), it was written deliberately as a procedure note. The paper outlines five steps in the performance of REBOA as well as the materials available at that time needed for each step. Out of caution, the manuscript also listed considerations and potential hazards of each of the steps in this procedure. Notably, although more agile REBOA technologies are now available, the zones, the steps, and the potential hazards outlined in this original manuscript are still relevant for those establishing standard procedures for the performance of this resuscitative maneuver.

By some counts the manuscript has been cited nearly 1000 times and its appeal is a testament to the vision of Dr. Pruitt as he encouraged the paper for the *Journal of Trauma* during his final months as Editor-in-Chief. As an indication to interest in the paper, and as one can read in the publication fine print, the paper was submitted to the journal on October 31, 2011, it was accepted the next day on November 1st and it was published the following month, December 2011. While the role of endovascular balloon occlusion of the aorta in the management of bleeding and shock is not yet fully determined, this publication occurred at a unique juncture in time and will always be recognized as the REBOA paper. It's my hope that the manuscript continues to have enduring value and that it will serve as a guide for those considering this and other endovascular approaches in the management of the severely injured or ill patient.

CHAPTER 45

Traumatic Brain Injury

Review by John K. Bini

Traumatic brain injury (TBI) is a major cause of death and disability in both children and adults in the most productive years of their lives [3]. In the United States an estimated 1.7 million traumatic brain injuries occur every year and account for 275,000 hospitalizations and over 50,000 deaths [3]. It is estimated that these injuries are responsible for leaving over 500,000 individuals with permanent neurological sequelae resulting in an economic burden exceeding US$64 billion annually [3].

Although the primary structural damage to the brain results in morbidity and mortality, the vast majority cases of disability may be attributed to secondary injury. Thus, the primary goal for treating patients with traumatic brain injuries is to prevent secondary injury by avoiding hypotension, hypoxia, and elevated intracranial pressure. Intracranial hypertension occurs in up to 70% of patients and is responsible for a substantial proportion of TBI-related deaths [6, 9].

Because of the significant impact of secondary injury, the Brain Trauma Foundation (BTF) has published management guidelines. These recommendations synthesize the available evidence and translate it into recommendations for treatment, monitoring and thresholds. They recommend management of severe TBI patients using information from intracranial pressure (ICP) monitoring to reduce two-week post injury mortality. In addition, they recommend that ICP monitoring should be used in all salvageable patients with severe TBI and ICP monitoring in patients with severe TBI with a normal CT scan if two or more of the following features are noted on admission: age over 40, unilateral or bilateral motor posturing, or systolic blood pressure at less than 90 [2].

Despite these evidence-based guidelines, it is apparent that the application of these guidelines is inconsistent, and significant clinical equipoise with regard to appropriate management of severe traumatic brain injuries still exists. In the 7 years between the 3rd and 4th editions of BTF Guidelines, 94 new studies were added to the library of evidence. Although there have been numerous new publications, many of them repeat the same methodological flaws found in previous research [2]. Talving et al. assessed compliance with the BTF Guidelines for the Management of Severe TBI and the effect on outcomes. A total of 216 patients met the BTF guideline criteria for ICP monitoring yet compliance with BTF guidelines was 46.8%. The authors concluded that patients managed according to the BTF ICP guidelines experienced significantly improved survival [10].

DOI: 10.1201/9781003042136-45

Alali et al. [1] evaluated the relationship between ICP monitoring and mortality in centers participating in the American College of Surgeons Trauma Quality Improvement Program (TQIP). The association between ICP monitoring and mortality was determined after adjusting for important confounders. The authors stratified hospitals into quartiles based on ICP monitoring utilization. Hospitals with higher rates of ICP monitoring use were associated with lower mortality: The adjusted odds ratio (OR) of death was 0.52 (95% CI, 0.35–0.78) in the quartile of hospitals with highest use, compared to the lowest [3]. These findings are consistent with an early large retrospective Canadian registry study conducted by Lane, which also found that ICP monitoring was associated with significantly improved survival [6].

Farahvar et al. used a large, prospectively collected database containing information on patients admitted to one of 20 level 1 and 2 level II trauma centers. The authors examined the effect on 2-week mortality of ICP reduction therapies administered to patients with severe TBI treated either with or without an ICP monitor. They found that patients of all ages treated with an ICP monitor in place had lower mortality at 2 weeks ($p = 0.02$) than those treated without an ICP monitor [3]. Using the same database, Gerber examined the trends in adherence to the guidelines and the effect of time period on case-fatality. During the time period studied, adherence to the guidelines increased and use of ICP monitoring increased and case fatality decreased [4].

Shafi et al. used the National Trauma Data Bank and looked at patients with blunt TBI. They identified 708 patients who underwent ICP monitoring and 938 who did not. Multivariate logistic regression was used to determine the relationship between ICP monitoring and survival while controlling for overall injury severity, Only 43% of patients meeting BTF criteria had ICP monitoring. They concluded that ICP monitoring was associated with a reduction in survival [9].

Other studies have produced mixed results and recommendations either showing a negative impact of monitoring or no difference in outcome. These findings are consistently inconsistent across the entire spectrum of management options for TBI [5, 7]. Interestingly, prior to 2012, the use of ICP monitoring to direct treatment and its influence on important outcomes had never been tested in a randomized clinical trial.

In 2012 Chesnut and colleagues published the results of a large randomized clinical trial in their landmark paper comparing outcomes with and without ICP monitoring. This is a randomized controlled multicenter clinical trial which enrolled 324 patients who had severe TBI. The primary outcome measure was a composite score of survival time, impaired consciousness, and functional status at 3 months and 6 months and neuropsychological status at 6 months [11].

The investigators found no significant between-group difference in the composite primary outcome (score, 56 in the pressure-monitoring group vs. 53 in the imaging–clinical examination group; $p = 0.49$), or 6-month mortality (39% in the pressure-monitoring group and 41% in the imaging–clinical examination group; $p = 0.60$).

This is the first large randomized clinical trial comparing ICP monitoring versus standard care to guide management. This study was performed in less developed countries where ICP monitoring was not standard and limitations in prehospital care, ICU care and rehabilitation services impact their primary outcome variables [11].

In conclusion, TBI presents a significant public health problem. Despite current published guidelines, variability in adherence to those guidelines and clinical equipoise still exist. The landmark paper presented may contribute to the ongoing clinical equipoise. Regarding TBI there is a paucity of class 1 data to support current practices and the majority of high-quality investigations in this arena refute what was routine clinical management for many decades. This is true for steroid use, hyperventilation, fluid restriction (rather than euvolemia) and more recently, decompressive bifrontal craniectomy, induced hypothermia, CSF drainage, and barbiturate burst suppression. Hyperosmolar therapy which is a mainstay is unsubstantiated in any large prospective trial.

The landmark study by Chesnut and colleagues does, however, conclusively demonstrate that quality randomized clinical trials can be performed and should be conducted with the goal of reducing the burden of this public health epidemic.

ANNOTATED REFERENCES FOR TRAUMATIC BRAIN INJURY

1. Alali AS, Fowler RA, Mainprize TG, et al. Intracranial pressure monitoring in severe traumatic brain injury: Results from the American College of Surgeons Trauma Quality Improvement Program. *J Neurotrauma*. 2013;30(20):1737–1746. doi:10.1089/neu.2012.2802

    The authors evaluated the relationship between ICP monitoring and mortality in centers participating in the American College of Surgeons Trauma Quality Improvement Program (TQIP). Data on 10,628 adults with severe TBI were derived from 155 TQIP centers from 2009–2011. The association between ICP monitoring and mortality was determined after adjusting for important confounders. Overall mortality (n = 3769) was 35%. Only 1874 (17.6%) patients underwent ICP monitoring, with a mortality of 32%. The adjusted odds ratio (OR) for mortality was 0.44 [95% confidence interval (CI), 0.31–0.63], when comparing patients with ICP monitoring to those without. The authors stratified hospitals into quartiles based on ICP monitoring utilization. Hospitals with higher rates of ICP monitoring use were associated with lower mortality: The adjusted OR of death was 0.52 (95% CI, 0.35–0.78) in the quartile of hospitals with highest use, compared to the lowest. The authors concluded that ICP monitoring utilization was associated with lower mortality and variability in ICP monitoring rates contributed only modestly to variability in institutional mortality rates.

2. Carney N, Totten AM, O'Reilly C, et al. Guidelines for the Management of Severe Traumatic Brain Injury, Fourth Edition. *Neurosurgery*. 2017;80(1):6–15. doi: 10.1227/NEU.0000000000001432. PMID: 27654000.

    This is the most recent Brain Trauma Foundation effort to synthesize the available evidence and to translate it into recommendations. The authors only make recommendations when there is evidence to support them and they do not necessarily constitute complete protocols for clinical use. They intended that their recommendations be used by others to develop specific treatment protocols. These current evidence-based recommendations are grouped into three areas: treatments, monitoring and thresholds. Treatments include: decompressive craniectomy, prophylactic hypothermia, hyperosmolar therapy, cerebral spinal fluid drainage, ventilation therapies, anesthetics analgesics and sedatives, steroids, nutrition, infection prophylaxis, deep vein thrombosis prophylaxis, and seizure prophylaxis. The area on monitoring includes monitoring of intracranial pressure, cerebral perfusion pressure, and advanced cerebral monitoring. The section on thresholds talks about blood pressures, intracranial pressure, swivel perfusion pressure, and advanced cerebral monitoring.

With regard to intracranial pressure monitoring, they recommended management of severe traumatic brain injury patients using information from ICP monitoring to reduce 2-week post injury mortality. They also recommend that intracranial pressure monitoring should be used in all salvageable patients with severe traumatic brain injury and also recommend that ICP monitoring is indicated in patients with severe TBI with a normal CT scan if two or more of the following features are noted on admission: age over 40, unilateral or bilateral motor posturing, or systolic blood pressure at less than 90.

Details of these guidelines can be found at: https://www.braintrauma.org/coma/guidelines

3. Farahvar A, Gerber LM, Chiu Y, Carney N, Härtl R, Ghajar J. Increased mortality in patients with severe traumatic brain injury treated without intracranial pressure monitoring. *J Neurosurg.* 2012;117(4):729–734. Retrieved Nov 26, 2020, from https://thejns.org/view/journals/j-neurosurg/117/4/article-p729.xml

This study uses a large, prospectively collected database containing information on patients admitted to one of 20 level I and two level II trauma centers, part of a New York State quality improvement program administered by the Brain Trauma Foundation between 2000 and 2009. The authors examined the effect on 2-week mortality of ICP reduction therapies administered to patients with severe TBI treated either with or without an ICP monitor. The study population included 2134 patients with severe TBI (Glasgow Coma Scale [GCS] Score <9), 1446 patients were treated with ICP-lowering therapies; 1202 had an ICP monitor placed. They found that age, initial GCS score, hypotension, and CT scan findings were associated with 2-week mortality. They also found that patients of all ages treated with an ICP monitor in place had lower mortality at 2 weeks (p = 0.02) than those treated without an ICP monitor, after adjusting for parameters that independently affect mortality. They concluded that in patients with severe TBI treated for intracranial hypertension, the use of an ICP monitor is associated with significantly lower mortality.

4. Gerber LM, Chiu Y, Carney N, Härtl R, Ghajar J. Marked reduction in mortality in patients with severe traumatic brain injury. *J Neurosurg.* 2013;119(6):1583–1590. Retrieved Nov 27, 2020, from https://thejns.org/view/journals/j-neurosurg/119/6/article-p1583.xml

The authors conducted a retrospective database review and analyzed 2-week mortality due to severe traumatic brain injury (TBI) from 2001 through 2009 in New York State and examined the trends in adherence to the guidelines. Univariate and multivariate logistic regression analyses were performed to evaluate the effect of time period on case fatality. From 2001 to 2009, the case-fatality rate decreased from 22% to 13% (p <0.0001) and remained significant after adjusting for factors that independently predict mortality. During the time period studied, adherence to the guidelines increased and use of ICP monitoring increased from 56% to 75% (p <0.0001). Adherence to cerebral perfusion pressure treatment thresholds increased from 15% to 48% (p <0.0001). The proportion *of patients having an ICP elevation greater than 25 mmHg dropped from 42% to 29% (p = 0.0001). Based on the author's findings they suggested a causal relationship between adherence to the evidence based guidelines and improved outcomes as represented by decreased 2-week mortality.*

5. Kostić A, Stefanović I, Novak V, Veselinović D, Ivanov G, Veselinović A. Prognostic significance of intracranial pressure monitoring and intracranial hypertension in severe brain trauma patients. *Med Pregl.* 2011;64(9–10):461–465. PMID: 22097111.

This is a small Serbian prospective randomized clinical trial that looked at the prognostic value of intracranial pressure monitoring and intracranial pressure-oriented therapy in severe traumatic brain injured patients. Thirty-two patients were randomized to undergo intracranial pressure monitoring while 29 patients were managed without ICP monitoring. In the intracranial pressure monitoring group, mortality was 47% while in the other group mortality was 66%. Because of the small sample size these large differences did not meet statistical significance. They did find however, that in the group of patients who died, there was an average intracranial pressure of 27 mm Hg compared to an intracranial pressure of 18 in the survival group and these findings were statistically significant. Based on their results these authors recommended instituting intracranial pressure-oriented therapy at 18 mm Hg after 2 hours of monitoring.

6. Lane PL, Skoretz TG, Doig G, Girotti MJ. Intracranial pressure monitoring and outcomes after traumatic brain injury. *Can J Surg.* 2000;43(6):442–448.

This is an early large retrospective Canadian registry study that looked at differences between traumatic brain injured patients treated using ICP monitors and those treated without ICP monitors over a 6-year period. The population included cases with an Injury Severity Score (ISS) greater than 12 from the 14 trauma centers in Ontario. Cases with a Maximum Abbreviated Injury Scale score in the head region (MAIS head) greater than 3 were selected for further analysis. Logistic regression analyses were conducted to investigate the relationship between ICP and death. Of the 5507 identified, 541 had an ICP monitor inserted. Their average ISS was 33.4 and 71.7% survived. Multivariate analyses controlling for MAIS head, ISS and injury mechanism indicated that ICP monitoring was associated with significantly improved survival (p <0.015). This finding strongly supports the need for a prospective randomized trial of management protocols, including ICP monitoring, in patients with severe TBI.

7. Mauritz W, Steltzer H, Bauer P, Dolanski-Aghamanoukjan L, Metnitz P. Monitoring of intracranial pressure in patients with severe traumatic brain injury: An Austrian prospective multicenter study. *Intensive Care Med.* 2008;34(7):1208–1215. doi: 10.1007/s00134-008-1079-7. Epub 2008 Mar 26. PMID: 18365169.

This is an Austrian multicenter prospective cohort study. The authors looked at 88,274 patients admitted to 32 medical/surgical and mixed Austrian ICU's between 1998 and 2004. The authors were looking at reasons why patients either received or did not receive intracranial pressure monitoring and identified factors influencing hospital mortality after TBI. The study found 1856 patients (2.1% of all ICU admissions) with severe TBI (GCS <9). Of these, 1031 (56%) received intercranial pressure monitoring. They found that younger patients, female patients, and patients with isolated traumatic brain injuries were more likely to receive intracranial pressure monitoring. Interestingly, they found that patients in medium sized centers were more likely to receive intracranial pressure monitoring and those patients in large centers. The authors concluded that ICP monitoring may possibly have beneficial effects on outcomes and they also concluded that patients *with severe traumatic brain injuries should be admitted to experience centers with high patient volumes since based on their data this seem to improve outcomes.*

8. Cremer OL, van Dijk GW, van Wensen E, et al. Effect of intracranial pressure monitoring and targeted intensive care on functional outcome after severe head injury. *Crit Care Med.* 2005;33:2207–2213.

This is a retrospective cohort study perform at two level I trauma centers in the Netherlands on 333 brain injured patients. Allocation was determined by which center the patients were admitted. In one center, mean arterial pressure was maintained at approximately 90 mm Hg in therapeutic interventions, based on clinical observations in CT findings. At the other center, management was aimed at maintaining ICP less than 20 any CPP greater than 70. Their primary outcome measure was an extended Glascow Outcome Score after 12 months. Only 67% of the patients in the ICP center had an intracranial pressure monitor placed. No difference was found between groups for functional outcome or in hospital mortality.

9. Shafi S, Diaz-Arrastia R, Madden C, Gentilello L. Intracranial pressure monitoring in brain-injured patients is associated with worsening of survival. *J Trauma.* 2008;64(2):335–340. doi: 10.1097/TA.0b013e31815dd017. PMID: 18301195.

This study used the National Trauma Data Bank (1994-2001) and looked at patients with blunt TBI, head-abbreviated injury score (AIS) 3 to 6, age 20 to 50 years, GCS </=8, abnormal brain computed tomographic scan, and intensive care unit admission for 3 days or more. Early deaths (<48 hours) and delayed admissions (>24 hours after injury) were excluded. They identified 708 patients who underwent ICP monitoring and 938 who did not. Multivariate logistic regression was used to determine the relationship between ICP monitoring and survival while controlling for overall injury severity, TBI severity, craniotomy, associated injuries, comorbidities, and complications. Only 43% of patient meeting BTF criteria had ICP monitoring. After adjusting for admission GCS, age, blood pressure, head AIS, and injury severity score (ISS), ICP monitoring was associated with a reduction in survival (OR = 0.55; 95% CI, 0.39–0.76; p <0.001). The study did not address management in response to elevated intra cranial pressure or the brain specific treatments received by patients in each group.

10. Talving P, Karamanos E, Teixeira P, et al. Intracranial pressure monitoring in severe head injury: Compliance with Brain Trauma Foundation guidelines and effect on outcomes: A prospective study. *J Neurosurg.* 2013;119(5): 1248–1254. Retrieved Nov 26, 2020, from https://thejns.org/view/journals/j-neurosurg/119/5/article-p1248.xml

This study assessed compliance with the Brain Trauma Foundation's Guidelines for the Management of Severe Traumatic Brain Injury and the effect on outcomes. This is a prospective, observational study including patients with severe blunt TBI (Glasgow Coma Scale score ≤8, head Abbreviated Injury Scale score ≥3) between January 2010 and December 2011. The study population was stratified into two study groups: ICP monitoring and no ICP monitoring. Primary outcomes included compliance with BTF guidelines, overall in-hospital mortality, and mortality due to brain herniation. Multiple regression analysis was used to determine the effect of ICP monitoring on outcomes. A total of 216 patients met the BTF guideline criteria for ICP monitoring. Compliance with BTF guidelines was 46.8%.

Hypotension, coagulopathy, and older age were negatively associated with the placement of ICP monitoring devices. In-hospital mortality was significantly higher in patients who did not undergo ICP monitoring (53.9% vs. 32.7%, adjusted p = 0.019). Mortality due

to brain herniation was significantly higher for the group not undergoing ICP monitoring (21.7% vs. 12.9%, adjusted p = 0.046). The authors concluded that patients managed according to the BTF ICP guidelines experienced significantly improved survival.

11. Chesnut R. A trial of intracranial-pressure monitoring in traumatic brain injury. *New Engl J Med.* 2012;367:2471–2481.

Landmark Article of the 21st Century

A TRIAL OF INTRACRANIAL-PRESSURE MONITORING IN TRAUMATIC BRAIN INJURY

Chesnut R, *New Engl J Med.* 2012;367:2471–2481

Commentary by Randall M. Chesnut

In 1995, Jam Ghajar et al. published a US trauma center survey, revealing that ICP monitoring was relatively infrequent in traumatic brain injury (TBI). Shortly thereafter, Ghajar, Don Marion, and I hypothesized that we could change TBI practice if we demonstrated the scientific necessity of ICP monitoring. This led to the first edition of the *Guidelines For The Management Of Severe TBI In Adults*, wherein we discovered the very weak nature of the evidence supporting ICP monitoring. We ended the ICP-monitoring guidelines section with a call for an RCT, noting that such was unlikely, as nobody would support a non-monitored control group.

During our ongoing observational TBI studies in LMICs, our Latin American co-PIs suggested that they could do such an RCT, as non-monitored care was standard practice in resource-limited countries. Scientific equipoise was unchanged, but the visceral response was opposite. These physicians provided excellent, attentive clinical care but without the "toys" we enjoy. The BEST TRIP trial was born.

When the results showed no benefit for the ICP-monitor-guided management cohort, we became ICP-pariahs, having difficulty demonstrating that we hadn't tested monitoring but, rather, the universal one-size/one-threshold-fits-all TBI management technique applied to monitored patients. As the furor settled (and we could remove our Kevlar), the implication that we don't manage ICP (or TBI) optimally became obvious and we finally recognized the necessity of multimodality-monitoring-based targeted therapy (precision medicine) as our future. TBI ≠ ICP; ICP is but one window in the ommatidia that comprise TBI.

CHAPTER 46

Pressure Wounds

Review by Paulette Seymour-Route

Over 100 years have passed since the presence of bedsores, now defined as pressure injury, were noted by nursing and medicine. The need for cleanliness, special surfaces, position changes, and a dedicated ward was identified in the mid-1800s as a way to prevent pressure injuries. Nightingale is credited for identifying the need for a system of care, unit organization, and the need to keep statistics [1]. We continue to address this seemingly intractable patient problem in 2020.

International guidelines define a pressure injury as localized damage to the skin and/ or underlying tissue as a result of pressure or pressure in combination with shear. In addition to the skin, pressure injury can be found on a mucous membrane. Mucus membrane pressure injuries are usually related to a medical device [2].

An estimated 2.5 million patients develop a hospital-acquired pressure injury (HAPI) during their hospitalization thereby increasing morbidity and contributing to 60,000 deaths [3]. Recent modeling estimates the national hospital incremental cost of treating HAPIs to be approximately $26.8 billion [4]. Pressure injuries are known to be high in critical care populations due to patient complexity and severity of illness. The overall prevalence of pressure injury occurring in adult ICU patients has recently been reported as 26.6% with an ICU acquired prevalence of 16.2% [5].

Patient acuity itself can be a barrier to implementing pressure injury prevention strategies in the critical care population. Though the skin is the largest organ in the body, it is not routinely a high care priority. Lifesaving interventions necessary to treat the patient's condition take precedence [6]. Patient factors such as age, past medical history, nutrition and sensory and mobility issues increase the risk. The critical care admitting diagnosis can include organ failure, sepsis, trauma and other diagnoses with hemodynamic instability compounding the risk. Critical care interventions routinely include the use of medical devices such as endotracheal tubes and other respiratory devices, cervical collars and other immobilization devices, tubes, and catheters. The estimated pooled incidence of adult and pediatric medical device related pressure injury is reported as 12% [7]. Prevention measures to mitigate risk associated with medical devices are a key continuing need.

Competing priorities to avoid complications (e.g., balancing the need to keep the head of bed (HOB) no greater than 30 degrees to prevent HAPI, while also trying to prevent

DOI: 10.1201/9781003042136-46

ventilator-associated pneumonia) is a challenge. Vasopressor drugs and organ support measures can limit mobility in the already unstable patient. The ability to turn and the adherence to a turning schedule for ICU patients are both critical and at times hard to achieve. The development of a wearable patient sensor that measures patient turning by assessing relative position within a three-dimensional space and that alerts the nurse to change the patient position has demonstrated potential for reducing HAPIs [8].

Deep tissue injury (DTI) is a significant and underappreciated risk for critical care patients. Injury can occur in hours to days depending on the complexity of the patient diagnosis and hemodynamic stability. Since DTIs develop from the inside out, by the time they manifest themselves, the tissue damage and cellular death has begun. Biomedical engineers and scientists are key collaborators to address early diagnostic imaging techniques and injury prevention product development. Thermal imaging, performed on admission at the bedside, has been demonstrated to be useful in identifying critical care patients at high risk for DTI development in vulnerable anatomical areas such as heels, coccyx, and sacrum. This imaging can allow for early preventative interventions and a decrease in DTIs [9]. Computer modeling can guide product design for prophylactic dressings that can mitigate risk for critical care patients [10]. Combining technological advances such as these demonstrate promise. The need for care team collaboration to employ and test evidence-based prevention strategies in the critical care population is imperative.

Looking forward, generating a sustained interest by clinicians in critical care pressure injury prevention remains a challenge. Continued research is needed to advance the science related to a systematic approach to pressure injury prevention including the use of technology, and the inclusion of evidence-based pressure injury prevention modalities in appropriate clinical practice bundles. Periodic review of critical care HAPIs by the critical care team can inform the science and improve patient outcomes.

ANNOTATED REFERENCES FOR PRESSURE WOUNDS

1. Levine, JM. 100 years of bedsores: How much have we learned? *Adv Skin Wound Care.* 2018;31(3):139–140.

   https://doi.org/10.1097/01.ASW.0000530066.59878.2b

   The commentary describes the history, risks, and treatment of bed sores and the reality that we still have a long way to go to address the issues that remain around prevention, resource allocation and interdisciplinary collaboration.

2. European Pressure Ulcer Advisory Panel; National Pressure Injury Advisory Panel: Pan Pacific Pressure Injury Alliance. *Prevention and Treatment of Pressure Ulcers/Injuries: Clinical Practice Guideline.* 3rd ed. The International Guideline; 2019.

   This international and interprofessional guideline provides up-to-date information related to pressure injury classification, injury pathways, and staging. The guideline also provides an evidenced-based review of current prevention and treatment interventions appropriate for use in various populations.

3. Padula W, Pronovost P, Makic, M, et al. Value of hospital resources for effective pressure injury prevention: A cost-effectiveness analysis. *BMJ Qual Saf* 2019;28(2):132–141.

https://dol.org/10.1136/bmjqs-2017-007505

The authors performed a cost-utility analysis using Markov modeling to evaluate 34,787 patient records. The analysis suggests that pressure injury prevention for all inpatients is cost effective and hospitals should invest in compliance with international prevention guidelines.

4. Padula W, Delarmente B. The national cost of hospital-acquired pressure injuries in the United States. *Int Wound J*. 634–640.

https://dol.org/10.1111/iwj.13071

The authors used a Markov model to simulate the accumulation of costs (in 2016 dollars) attributed to treating patients with hospital acquired pressure injuries and estimated the incremental cost of treating a HAPI at about $10,708 per patient and suggests that the national cost attributable to HAPIs could be approximately $26.8 billion dollars. Costs are disproportionately attributable to Stage 3 and Stage 4 full-thickness wounds.

5. Labeau S, Alfonso E, Benbenishty J, et al. Prevalence, associated factors and outcomes of pressure injuries in adult intensive care unit patients: The DecubICUs study. *Intensive Care Med*. 2020;47(2):160–169.

https://doi.org/10.1007/s00134-020-0634-9

The authors of the international DecubICUs study examined data from 13,254 patients in 1117 ICUs from 90 countries. There were 6747 pressure injuries of which 3997 or 59.2% were hospital acquired and overall prevalence was 26.6%. Sacrum and heels were most common sites.

6. Coyer F, Cook L, Doubrovsky A, Campbell J, Vann A, McNamara G. Understanding contextual barriers and enablers to pressure injury prevention practice in an Australian intensive care unit: An exploratory study. *Aust Crit Care*. 2019;32(2):122–130.

https://doi.org/10.1016/j.aucc.2018.02.008

The authors describe the results of the first phase of a multiphase project (SUSTAIN study), whereby a descriptive cross-sectional cohort survey of attitudes, barriers, and enablers of pressure injury prevention was completed by 204 nurses. Subjects identified high patient acuity as a significant barrier to pressure injury prevention.

7. Jackson D, Sarki A, Betteridge R, Brooke J. Medical device-related pressure ulcers: A systematic review and meta-analysis. *Int J Nurs Stud*. 2019;92:109–120.

https://doi.org/10.1016/j.ijnurstu.2019.02.006

The authors reviewed observational studies reporting medical device-related pressure injuries. Meta-analysis of the final 29 studies was used to calculate the estimated pooled incidence and prevalence. The medical device related results demonstrated as estimated pooled incidence of 12% (95% CI 8–18) and 10% prevalence (95% CI 6–16). The results were reported with caution due to the heterogeneity observed between the studies. Common devices included respiratory devices, cervical collars, tubing devices, splints, and intravenous catheters.

8. Pickham D, Berte N, Pihulic M, Valdez A, Mayer B, Desai M. Effect of a wearable patient sensor on care delivery for preventing pressure injuries in acutely ill adults: A pragmatic randomized clinical trial (LS-HAPI study). *Int J Nurs Stud*. 2018;80:12–19.

https://doi.org/10.1016/j.ijnurstu.2017.12.012

The authors evaluated the clinical effectiveness of a wearable patient sensor to improve compliance with turning in a randomized sample of 1312 patients in two adult intensive care units. Results support the use of the sensor to improve turning compliance and reduced incidence of HAPIs.

9. Koerner S, Adams D, Harper S, Black J, Langemo D. Use of thermal imaging to identify deep-tissue pressure injury on admission reduces clinical and financial burden of hospital-acquired pressure injuries. *Adv Skin Wound Care*. 2019;32(7):312–320.

   https://doi.org/10.1097/01.ASW.0000559613.83195.f9

   This study included 114 consecutive adult ICU patients who received a thermal imaging and clinical assessment of areas known to be high risk for deep tissue injury (heels, sacrum, and coccyx) upon admission. The thermal assessment was performed using an FDA approved long-wave infrared thermography scanning device. Of the 308 anatomical areas of interest scanned in 114 patients, 12 thermal anomalies were identified in 9 unique patients that were consistent with nonvisual signs of DTIPIs on admission. Once identified, the patients were started on therapeutic interventions known to mitigate DTI. The majority of the anomalies (9 of 12) were found on a heel. Two of the 12 anomalies manifested as a DTI. Based on historical incidence, five would have been predicted to occur. Prevention efforts initiated based on the thermal assessment reduced the DTI rate.

10. Gefen A, Alves P, Creehan S, Call E, Santamaria N. Computer modeling of prophylactic dressings: An indispensable guide for healthcare professionals, *Adv Skin Wound Care*. 2019;32(7S):S4–S13.

    https://doi.org/10.1097/01.ASW.0000558695.68304.41

    The authors reviewed the published literature to date employing computer finite element modeling for efficacy research of prophylactic dressings related to pressure injury development. Computer models inform the process of engineering prophylactic dressings and may be useful to provide guidance for clinical use.

Landmark Article of the 21st Century

EFFECT OF A WEARABLE PATIENT SENSOR ON CARE DELIVERY FOR PREVENTING PRESSURE INJURIES IN ACUTELY ILL ADULTS: A PRAGMATIC RANDOMIZED CLINICAL TRIAL (LS-HAPI STUDY)

Pickham D et al., *Int J Nurs Stud.* 2018;80:12–19

Commentary by Barbara Mayer

As an amateur historian, I found it fascinating that the first known report of a pressure injury was recorded by an Egyptian physician in the 17th century BC. More than 3000 years later, the 16th century French surgeon, Ambroise Paré suggested using "… a little pillow of down to keep his buttock in the air, without his being supported on it" for treating sacral ulcers [1]. Three hundred years later, Édouard Brown-Séquard, a physiologist and neurologist known for his work on spinal cord physiology, recognized prolonged compression could result in ulceration of the skin [2]. Fast forward to today, nearly 4000 years after the first report, and we continue to struggle with preventing these injuries and the pain and indignity experienced by our patients. There is evidence, however, that suggests multiple variables affect nurse compliance with turning protocols: low prioritization, lack of an accepted definition of what constitutes an "effective" turn, ineffective methods to monitor a patient's position, and lack of reminders when a turn is due. My own research and personal experience have found that nurses do view pressure injury prevention as a high priority, but methods relying on manual reminders and self-report have little success in facilitating and improving compliance.

Understanding why we do what we do, and how we do it has permeated my 42 years of nursing practice, particularly with prevention of pressure injuries. Why, despite a lack of empirical evidence to support it, do we continue the practice of turning our patients every two hours? We have leveraged technological advances to solve other clinical issues and improve care and outcomes. Could we do the same to answer the questions about turning effectiveness in preventing pressure injuries and subsequently increase compliance? We conducted a randomized clinical trial using a proprietary wearable patient sensor (Leaf Healthcare, Inc.) that measures body position, records duration and frequency of turns, and provides real time visual confirmation and feedback on turning compliance in critically ill patients. This study demonstrated that this electronic solution could, indeed, increase compliance and reduce the incidence of pressure injuries. We continue to use the monitoring system and have sustained the level of compliance demonstrated by the study. Further, this wearable sensor has been implemented in other facilities as well. Together, practice expertise and technology will continue to save countless patients from experiencing the debilitating consequences of pressure injuries.

REFERENCES

1. Levine JM. Historical notes on pressure ulcers: The cure of Ambroise Pare, *Decubitus*. 1992;5(2):23–26.
2. Levine JM. Historical perspective: The neurotrophic theory of skin ulceration, *J Amer Ger Soc*. 1992;40(12):1281–1283.

CHAPTER 47

ICU Monitoring

Review by Daniel Walsh

A common reason for admission to the intensive care unit (ICU) is for the patient to be in a more closely monitored setting. Despite a growth in monitoring technologies over the last 50 years, there is little evidence that these technologies improve major outcomes. For some technologies there are only observational studies to assess their effect on outcomes. It makes intuitive sense that having the type of physiologic data that many monitors provide would help provide effective care tailored specifically to each patient. This is likely why these technologies are adopted so widely even before evidence of their effectiveness.

More than one third of ICU patients are monitored with an arterial catheter [1]. So far there is a lack of randomized trials assessing impacts of arterial catheters, and there have only been observational studies assessing associations of this monitoring technology and outcomes. The largest study showed no association between arterial catheters and mortality in the total cohort, though the cohort of patients with arterial catheters that required vasopressors had an increase in mortality [1]. This observation is quite possibly related to sicker patients who required higher doses of pressors and were more often monitored with arterial catheters. Without randomized trials causal information is unobtainable.

Two monitors that almost every ICU patient receives are telemetry and pulse oximetry. There is some evidence to suggest that telemetry can decrease mortality for in-hospital cardiac arrest, especially asystole or ventricular fibrillation arrests. A recent retrospective observational study comparing monitoring of patients with telemetry versus no telemetry demonstrated higher survival for patients with in-hospital cardiac arrests when telemetry was used. Such studies show a correlation that may not be causal. Again, prospective and randomized data are lacking [2]. The use of pulse oximetry has been widely adopted in the perioperative and ICU settings. The largest randomized trial studying the utility of pulse oximetry entered more than 20,000 patients. Although a 19-fold increase in the incidence of diagnosed hypoxemia with pulse oximetry was observed, it still failed to show a difference in respiratory, cardiovascular, or neurologic outcomes. It is estimated that more than a 20-fold increase in enrollment would have been required to show a change in outcomes for this trial [3]. It is important to note that both of these technologies are non-invasive with very little risk of serious complications. However, one of the possible adverse effects of routine monitoring

DOI: 10.1201/9781003042136-47

with these devices can be alarm fatigue. It has been estimated that 77–99% of clinical alarms are false. In one 5-year period, 500 patient deaths related to alarm fatigue were documented. Strategies to reduce alarm fatigue include avoidance of over-monitoring, judicious selection of alarm limits and use of multimodal alarms may reduce the incidence of false alarms. Whether or not these interventions reduce that risk of alarm fatigue and adverse patient outcome is unknown [4]. The safe use of alarms is a 2021 National Patient Safety Goal promulgated by the Joint Commission.

One of the more invasive monitors that is used in the ICU is the pulmonary artery catheter (PAC). The initial description of the PAC in 1970 was followed by quick adoption of the technology [5]. In patients with acute myocardial infarction, use of the PAC increased from 7% in 1975 to almost 20% in 1984 [6]. By the 1990s, almost 40% of ICU patients were instrumented with a PAC [7]. This widespread adoption occurred without clear evidence that the use of the PAC improved clinical outcomes and without clear agreement on how to interpret findings or how to use these findings to provide nuanced patient care. The PAC-Man trial was far from the first investigation suggesting lack of benefit of the PAC, but it was the largest and best-powered trial showing lack of benefit of PAC use in a general ICU patient population [8]. As such, it effectively completed the inquiry into the effectiveness of the PAC in the general ICU population and prompted intensivists to continue decreasing the use of the PAC without looking back. As a result of the PAC-Man trial and those before it, the PAC has become one of the most well-studied monitors. The use of the PAC in general ICU patients had declined to about 6% by 2008 [9].

The use of the PAC was so widespread and thought to be so essential to patient care that for some time it was difficult to perform rigorous trials assessing the impacts of the PAC on clinical outcomes. An attempt at a randomized trial failed to enroll an adequate number of patients as more eligible patients were excluded than enrolled as care teams felt that it was ethically mandated to use the PAC [10]. This is an example of how our beliefs can influence the scientific study of medical interventions. The use of the PAC had been steady during the early 1990s, but began declining after a landmark observational trial in 1996 suggesting increased risk of death in ICU patients receiving PAC [7, 11]. This observational trial cast enough doubt on the benefits of the PAC to finally allow equipoise for randomized trials. Prior to the PAC-Man trial, there were two randomized trials in general ICU patients. The first was designed as a pilot study with the goal of recruiting 200 patients to allow power calculations for future studies. This study showed no difference in mortality [12]. The second trial, though larger than the first, failed to meet its power goals though it also showed no difference in mortality [13]. These trials cast enough doubt on the PAC that trends in use had continued to further decline [11]. The PAC-Man trial, with almost 50% more enrollment than the previous trial, was better powered to answer this question and was seen as a more conclusive answer.

The PAC-Man trial had a pragmatic design examining the effectiveness of the PAC as it did not have any protocolization for the management of patients within the PAC intervention group [8]. This was done as there had been no consensus on optimal management protocols and so would give an assessment of what the real-world use may be of the PAC. While this can be seen as a limitation compared to a trial examining the efficacy of the PAC with a rigid management protocol, many see it as more generalizable given the lack of consensus on management, especially as this was a multicenter study assessing care across 65 ICUs. In addition to the primary outcome of mortality, the secondary outcomes of ICU length of stay, hospital length of stay, and organ-days of support in ICU also showed no difference between the PAC treatment group and the control group [8]. Similar to the pragmatic management in the treatment group, the inclusion criteria were very pragmatic as simply being identified by the treating team as someone who was thought to benefit from a PAC [8]. The mortality rate in both groups was particularly high at 66–68% [8]. This could have been a population that had a severity of illness that was too great to be able to be impacted by PAC management. However, in the two prior studies of PAC, in general, ICU patients had lower mortality rates around 50% and also showed no difference between groups [12, 13]. There was a 10% incidence of direct complications related to PAC placement in the treatment group [8]. The majority were minor such as hematoma at insertion site or arterial puncture during placement. But 3% of patients in the PAC treatment group had arrhythmias requiring treatment within 1 hour of placement and a small number of patients had pneumo or hemothoraces. This highlights that the use of the PAC is not without risk and must be done with careful consideration. It is notable that the suggestion of increased risk of death from the PAC in the observational trial was not shown in any of the randomized trials. The use of the PAC should be done judiciously as the PAC-Man trial demonstrated no benefit to mortality or length of stay by using the PAC, and there are risks related to PAC insertion,. This judicious use by clinicians is reflected in the decreasing use of the PAC over time.

With the decreasing use of the PAC, interest has grown in less invasive methods to monitor cardiac output. There are several methods available with some form of Doppler or bioreactance being the most frequently used. A variety of studies have focused on validation of the accuracy of the measurements of these techniques compared to invasive measures from a PAC but their effect on outcomes has been less thoroughly evaluated. The doppler-based techniques seem to have similar accuracy as measures from the PAC. The bioreactance technique has slightly decreased accuracy relative to the PAC though has a high accuracy in assessing trends in cardiac output [14]. More randomized trials are needed to evaluate the potential impact on outcomes that these monitors may have.

ANNOTATED REFERENCES FOR ICU MONITORING

1. Gershengorn HB, Wunsch H, Scales DC, Zarychanski R, Rubenfeld G, Garland A. Association between arterial catheter use and hospital mortality in intensive care units. *JAMA Intern Med.* 2014;174(11):1746–1754.

Retrospective propensity-matched cohort analysis of over 13,000 patients with an arterial catheter in the ICU across more than 100 hospitals. There was no association between arterial catheter use and hospital mortality. In a subgroup that was receiving vasopressors the use of an arterial catheter was associated with an increased odd of death (OR, 1.08; 95% CI 1.02–1.14).

2. Cleverley K, Mousavi N, Stronger L, et al. The impact of telemetry on survival of in-hospital cardiac arrests in non-critical care patients. *Resuscitation.* 2013;84(7):878–882.

Retrospective review of 668 cardiac arrests across six hospitals within the same health system. Patients on telemetry versus no telemetry had higher survival rates both immediately following arrest (66% vs. 34%, OR = 3.67, p = 0.02) and to hospital discharge (30% vs. 6%, OR = 7.17, p = 0.01). This effect was especially present for those with asystole or ventricular fibrillation.

3. Jubran A. Pulse oximetry. *Crit Care.* 2015;19:272.

This is a general review on the technology of pulse oximetry. It reviews the principles and mechanisms behind the technology. It reviews the data showing the accuracy of the SpO_2 relative to the SaO_2. It reviews trials that have investigated a benefit to outcomes from the use of pulse oximetry and the lack of shown benefit.

4. Ruskin KJ and Hueske-Kraus D. Alarm fatigue: Impact on patient safety. *Curr Opin Anaesthesiol.* 2015;28:685–690

Review paper on prevalence and dangers of false medical alarms and alarm fatigue. Healthcare professionals may be exposed to as many as 1000 false alarms per shift. The US Food and Drug Administration has reported over 500 deaths related to false alarms over a period of 5 years.

5. Swan HJ, Ganz W, Forrester J, Marcus H, Diamond G, Chonette D. Catheterization of the heart in man with use of a flow-directed balloon-tipped catheter. *N Engl J Med.* 1970;283(9):447–451.

Initial description of the PAC. Discusses design and construction of the catheter. Discusses technique for placement and gives placement data for 100 passes in 70 patients. Describes waveforms obtained by catheter.

6. Gore JM, Goldberg RJ, Spodick DH, Alpert JS, Dalen JE. A community-wide assessment of the use of pulmonary artery catheters in patients with acute myocardial infarction. *Chest.* 1987;92(4):721–727.

Population based observational study across multiple hospitals in a single metro area. 3000 patients with acute myocardial infarction were assessed from 3-year time points across a 12-year period. Incidence of PAC use was assessed and was shown to be increasing over the 12-year period. Use of the PAC was associated with increased mortality and increased length of stay, though as this was observational it is difficult to say if this is simply because the patients that received a PAC were more ill.

7. Connors AF, Speroff T, Dawson NV, et al. The effectiveness of right heart catheterization in the initial care of critically ill patients. SUPPORT Investigators. *JAMA.* 1996;276(11):889–897.

Prospective cohort study looking at outcomes associated with PAC use in general ICU patients. Over 5700 patients across five hospitals over a 5-year period were observed. The use of a PAC was associated with an increased 30-day mortality (odds ratio 1.24; 1.03–1.49). Use of the PAC was also associated with increased mean hospital stay cost and increased ICU length of stay. Authors conclude these results justify a randomized controlled trial for use of the PAC.

8. Harvey S, Harrison DA, Singer M, et al. Assessment of the clinical effectiveness of pulmonary artery catheters in management of patients in intensive care (PAC-Man): a randomised controlled trial. *Lancet.* 2005;366(9484):472–477.

   Randomized controlled trial with over 1000 patients across 65 ICUs in the UK. See text above for further details regarding trial.

9. Gershengorn HB, Wunsch H. Understanding changes in established practice: pulmonary artery catheter use in critically ill patients. *Crit Care Med.* 2013;41(12):2667–2676.

   Retrospective cohort study assessing use of PAC from 2001–2008 across ICUs that participated with Project IMPACT database. Total PAC use decreased from 10.8% of patients to 6.2% during this time period.

10. Guyatt G. A randomized control trial of right-heart catheterization in critically ill patients. Ontario Intensive Care Study Group. *J Intensive Care Med.* 1991;6(2):91–95.

    This was an attempt at a randomized controlled trial for PAC use. Only able to enroll 33 patients. There were 52 otherwise eligible patients that were excluded from enrollment as the attending physician felt that use of the PAC was ethically mandated. Not enough equipoise to complete trial.

11. Wiener RS, Welch HG. Trends in the use of the pulmonary artery catheter in the United States, 1993–2004. *JAMA.* 2007;298(4):423–429.

    Retrospective observational trial assessing use of the PAC between 1993–2004 across ICUs in nine different states. Rates of PAC utilization were steady between 1993–1995 and then beginning in 1996 (after Connors, et al. trial) the use began to decrease. Overall, use of the PAC decreased about 65% from 1996–2004.

12. Rhodes A, Cusack RJ, Newman PJ, Grounds RM, Bennett ED. A randomised, controlled trial of the pulmonary artery catheter in critically ill patients. *Intensive Care Med.* 2002;28(3):256–264.

    Pilot single-center, randomized control trial with goal to enroll 200 patients to allow further power calculations. Enrolled 201 patients to management with either a PAC or without a PAC. Found no difference between groups in 28 day mortality. The PAC treatment group received more fluids and had increased renal failure.

13. Richard C, Warszawski J, Anguel N, et al. Early use of the pulmonary artery catheter and outcomes in patients with shock and acute respiratory distress syndrome: a randomized controlled trial. *JAMA.* 2003;290(20):2713–2720.

    Multicenter, randomized trial across 36 ICUs in France. Enrolled 676 patients to receive treatment either with PAC or without PAC. No difference between groups in 28 day mortality, organ failure, hospital length of stay, mechanical ventilation use, or use of vasoactive agents.

14. Thiele RH, Bartels K, Gan TJ. Cardiac output monitoring: a contemporary assessment and review. *Crit Care Med.* 2015;43(1):177–185.

    This paper reviews various technologies available to make non-invasive assessments of cardiac output. It gives a review of the concept behind the Fick equation and how cardiac output can be measured invasively with a PAC. It reviews the principles and clinical considerations behind several alternative non-invasive methods.

Landmark Article of the 21st Century

ASSESSMENT OF THE CLINICAL EFFECTIVENESS OF PULMONARY ARTERY CATHETERS IN MANAGEMENT OF PATIENTS IN INTENSIVE CARE (PAC-MAN): A RANDOMISED CONTROLLED TRIAL

Harvey S, Harrison D, Singer M et al., *Lancet.* 2005;366:472–477

Commentary by Mervyn Singer

At the turn of the century the utility of the pulmonary artery catheter (PAC) in critical care was being seriously questioned. Introduced into clinical practice in the 1970s without formal evaluation of clinical or cost-effectiveness, it certainly enabled a more detailed understanding of cardiovascular physiology. However, it was an invasive procedure with a recognized complication rate. Furthermore, user expertise was often suboptimal leading to data misinterpretation and misapplication of therapy. Non-randomized studies also suggested worse outcomes were associated with PAC use, even after risk adjustment. Government funding was thus provided to perform an academic-led randomized controlled trial in 65 ICUs within the United Kingdom.

Patients deemed to require PAC insertion on clinical grounds were randomized to receive care with or without the PAC. There was no consensus among participating sites as to whether the control group should receive non-invasive cardiac output monitoring. This was resolved by creating two strata, either no option (Stratum A) or retaining the option (Stratum B) to use alternative monitors. Two-thirds opted for Stratum B. The trial was powered to detect a 10% absolute reduction in mortality.

In total, 1040 patients were enrolled, two thirds of whom were medical. No differences were seen in hospital mortality (66% control, 68% PAC), length of ICU or hospital stay, or days of organ support. Subset analysis indicated no clear signal for benefit/harm in any of the underlying clinical conditions (sepsis, heart failure, respiratory failure) nor for Strata A and B. We thus concluded there was no advantage to using PAC in the critically ill. Other multicenter studies confirmed this finding and the impact was a huge reduction in PAC use worldwide.

CHAPTER 48

Alcohol Withdrawal

Review by Akhil Patel and Kunal Karamchandani

In recent decades, alcohol has become one of the most commonly abused substances in the world. In the United States, about 17 million people annually are diagnosed with alcohol use disorder which is associated with more than 80,000 alcohol related deaths. The financial costs are estimated to be greater than $249 billion annually [1].

Alcohol is a psychotropic depressant of the central nervous system (CNS) and acts via stimulation of gamma-aminobutyric acid (GABA), the main inhibitory neurotransmitter of the CNS, and the inhibition of glutamate, the main central excitatory neurotransmitter. It increases the activity of GABA, by increasing chloride channel openings at the GABA receptors. Such alterations in neurotransmission are responsible for many of the symptoms associated with alcohol withdrawal. Acute alcohol ingestion causes increased GABA-ergic transmission and blockade of glutamate at the NMDA receptors leading to somnolence. Increases in the concentration of GABA within the CNS over time will result in down-regulation of the $GABA_A$ receptors and upregulation of the NMDA receptors [2]. When a chronic alcohol user abruptly ceases intake, there is an imbalance between the excitatory and inhibitory pathways in the brain, leading to alcohol withdrawal syndrome (AWS). An acute reduction in alcohol use leads to decreased neurotransmission in the $GABA_A$ pathways and increased neurotransmission in NMDA pathways. Similarly, there is upregulation of noradrenergic and dopaminergic pathways which causes the autonomic hyperactivity and hallucinations associated with alcohol withdrawal. Symptoms of AWS typically occur 3–10 days from last use, but may start as soon as a few hours after the last drink. Development of alcohol withdrawal symptoms has been correlated with increased hospital stay, risk of mechanical ventilation, costs, risk of readmission with withdrawal, and mortality [1].

While a majority of individuals experience only minor, uncomplicated withdrawal symptoms, such as increased anxiety, headache, nausea, vomiting, insomnia, and mild tremors, which self-resolve, a small subgroup of these individuals experience a more complicated syndrome that includes hallucinations, seizures, delirium, and/or more severe autonomic hyperactivity. Patients with such severe symptoms usually require intensive care unit (ICU) admission. The Revised Clinical Institute Withdrawal

DOI: 10.1201/9781003042136-48

Assessment for Alcohol scale (CIWA-Ar) is one of the most commonly used tools to address withdrawal severity as well as treatment effects amongst these patients. It is a 10-item scale that tracks the degree of nausea and vomiting, headache, tremor, diaphoresis, anxiety, agitation, disorientation, and auditory, visual, and tactile disturbances [3]. The CIWA-Ar scale requires patient interaction to accurately assess patient symptomology and allow active medication titration. The scale is used for its therapeutic use as it can be continued throughout the withdrawal process. Other scales such as the Riker Sedation-Agitation scale and Richmond Agitation-Sedation scale can be used for patients that require mechanical ventilation or are unable to communicate [1].

Since the advent of CIWA-Ar, treatment protocols have favored multiple assessments and administrations based on scores. As compared to a scheduled treatment regimen, a symptom-triggered therapy individualizes treatment, decreases treatment duration as well as the amount of benzodiazepine used, and is as efficacious as a standard fixed-schedule therapy for alcohol withdrawal [4]. Unlike preventive medicine, which is typically first line treatment in many disease processes, symptom-based treatment seems to be more effective for the management of AWS. Benzodiazepines (BZD) have been the mainstay of treatment for AWS and they act on the GABA receptor, simulating the action of alcohol by increasing the frequency of chloride channel opening. Benzodiazepines decrease symptom severity, the risk of delirium, and the length and frequency of seizures associated with AWS. However, the use of BZDs is associated with increased risk of excessive sedation, motor and memory deficits and respiratory depression, and the risk of abuse and dependence. The potential adverse effects of benzodiazepines have created a space for alternatives.

Barbiturates, especially phenobarbital have been studied as a viable alternative to benzodiazepines, and have shown promising results [5, 6]. In patients affected by severe AWS and who are approaching the need for mechanical ventilation, the combination of benzodiazepines and barbiturates can decrease the need of mechanical ventilation and may decrease ICU length of stay [7]. In critically ill patients requiring high doses of BZDs to control AWS symptoms or developing DT, barbiturates are an option either by themselves or as adjuncts to BZDs. Although a GABA receptor potentiator, phenobarbital can prolong calcium channel opening without the need for pre-synaptic GABA. Another benefit is the long half-life of 80–120 hours in comparison to 14–20 hours for long-acting benzodiazepines. A recent study comparing the use of phenobarbital and lorazepam in the emergency department, and at 48 hours, found that phenobarbital was as effective as lorazepam for AWS [5]. Similarly, Tidwell et al. [6] compared the use of phenobarbital and benzodiazepine treatment and found a decrease in hospital and ICU length of stay with the use of phenobarbital. They also found a decrease in mechanical ventilation and the use of other antipsychotics or sedatives for agitation. Despite these encouraging results, the use of barbiturates in the treatment of AWS has been limited, given their narrow therapeutic window, the risk of excessive sedation, and the interference with the clearance, of many drugs.

Dexmedetomidine, a selective α_2-receptor agonist is another agent that has shown to be effective in the treatment of AWS. The decreased autonomic hyperactivity and lack of respiratory compromise associated with dexmedetomidine makes it an attractive alternative in non-intubated and at-risk patients. Recent retrospective studies, have shown that dexmedetomidine demonstrates a BZD-sparing effect in the treatment of AWS; however, its use is associated with cardiovascular side effects such as bradycardia and hypotension [8, 9]. Use of dexmedetomidine by itself for treatment of AWS in critically ill patients can decrease the need for mechanical ventilation, ICU length of stay, and hospital length of stay [10]. Patients were also found to have a decrease in the incidence in delirium, an independent marker of morbidity and mortality in the ICU. Overall, the use of dexmedetomidine decreases total use of BZDs; however, due to the lack of anti-epileptic effects, it is primarily used as an adjunct rather than a primary mode of treatment.

An often overlooked component of AWS is severe malnutrition associated with electrolyte and vitamin deficiencies. Critical illness in the setting of thiamine, folate, and magnesium deficiencies, further precipitates AWS and can lead to irreparable damage. The most concerning of which is Wernicke's encephalopathy and Korsakoff syndrome which can be avoided with early thiamine administration. Folate and magnesium deficiency can also lead to confusion, psychosis, seizures, and QT prolongation. Hence, an aggressive approach towards vitamin and electrolyte replacement should be followed in all patients with AWS [11].

ANNOTATED REFERENCES FOR ALCOHOL WITHDRAWAL

1. Sarff M, Gold JA. Alcohol withdrawal syndromes in the intensive care unit. *Crit Care Med.* 2010;38(9):S494–S501.

   This is a comprehensive review of the pathophysiology, diagnostic tests, and treatment options for patients with AWS in the ICU.

2. Mirijello A, D'Angelo C, Ferrulli A, et al. Identification and management of alcohol withdrawal syndrome. *Drugs.* 2015;75(4):353–365.

   This is a "Therapy in Practice" paper with the intent to educate the reader on AWS presentation, diagnosis, and treatment algorithms.

3. Sullivan JT, Sykora K, Schneiderman J, Naranjo CA, Sellers EM. Assessment of alcohol withdrawal: the revised clinical institute withdrawal assessment for alcohol scale (CIWA-Ar). *Br J Addict.* 1989;84(11):1353–1357.

   This is a landmark 1989 study which revised the CIWA-A scale and provided a shortened 10-item scale for clinical quantification of the severity of AWS, the CIWA-Ar scale. This scale offers an increase in efficiency while at the same time retaining clinical usefulness, validity, and reliability, and is widely used in clinical practice.

4. Saitz R, Mayo-Smith MF, Roberts MS, Redmond HA, Bernard DR, Calkins DR. Individualized treatment for alcohol withdrawal. A randomized double-blind controlled trial. *JAMA*. 1994;272(7):519–523.

This randomized double-blind controlled trial assessed the difference between symptom-based or individualized treatment versus standing treatment on the intensity and duration of medication therapy in patients with alcohol withdrawal syndrome. The authors reported that prophylactic medication administration prolonged treatment and increased benzodiazepine administration in comparison to symptom-based treatment. Thus, establishing symptom-triggered therapy as a gold standard for managing alcohol withdrawal syndrome.

5. Hendey GW, Dery RA, Barnes RL, Snowden B, Mentler P. A prospective, randomized, trial of phenobarbital versus benzodiazepines for acute alcohol withdrawal. *Am J Emerg Med*. 2011;29(4):382–385.

This was a prospective study published in 2011 comparing the use of phenobarbital versus benzodiazepine in patients with alcohol withdrawal presenting to the emergency department. Forty-four patients were randomized into the study, 25 received phenobarbital and 17 received lorazepam. The researchers monitored patient's initial CIWA score, emergency room length of stay, admission rate, and 48 hour follow up CIWA score in both arms of the study. Patients in the lorazepam arm were sent home on a 5-day taper versus those in phenobarbital arm were given a 5-day placebo. The results concluded that both phenobarbital and lorazepam were similarly effective for mild to moderate alcohol withdrawal. There was no statistical difference in baseline CIWA scores, discharge scores, ED length of stay, admission, or 48-hour follow-up CIWA scores. Both medications reduced CIWA scores from baseline. With many few prospective studies on this topic, this allowed more evidence for the use of phenobarbital in alcohol withdrawal patient especially in the emergency room as an initial treatment. With the benefit of a long acting agent on board for mild or moderate alcohol withdrawal, there is a significant decrease in the amount of benzodiazepines required for treatment and eliminates the need for tapers. For more severe alcohol withdrawal patients, they may still require higher doses of phenobarbital and benzodiazepines with a taper and closer monitoring with ICU admission.

6. Tidwell WP, Thomas TL, Pouliot JD, Canonico AE, Webber AJ. Treatment of alcohol withdrawal syndrome: phenobarbital vs. CIWA-Ar protocol. *Am J Crit Care*. 2018;27(6):454–460.

This retrospective cohort study comparing the use of phenobarbital protocol versus CIWA-Ar-guided benzodiazepine protocol found that use of phenobarbital protocol decreased ICU length of stay, hospital length of stay, incidence of invasive mechanical ventilation, and use of adjunct medications. The authors concluded that phenobarbital protocol for the treatment of alcohol withdrawal was an effective alternative to the standard-of-care protocol of symptom-triggered benzodiazepine therapy.

7. Gold JA, Rimal B, Nolan A, Nelson LS. A strategy of escalating doses of benzodiazepines and phenobarbital administration reduces the need for mechanical ventilation in delirium tremens. *Crit Care Med*. 2007;35(3):724–730.

A retrospective cohort study which studied the effects of escalating doses of BZD in combination with phenobarbital in severe AWS. The results found that increasing doses in comparison to standing doses decrease the need for mechanical ventilation and ICU length of stay.

8. Crispo AL, Daley MJ, Pepin JL, Harford PH, Brown CV. Comparison of clinical outcomes in nonintubated patients with severe alcohol withdrawal syndrome treated with continuous-infusion sedatives: dexmedetomidine versus benzodiazepines. *Pharmacotherapy.* 2014;34(9):910–917.

A retrospective cohort study including non-intubated patients with severe alcohol withdrawal who were administered either a continuous dexmedetomidine infusion or a continuous benzodiazepine infusion. Primary outcome was comparing the rates of severe respiratory distress requiring mechanical ventilation or occurrence of alcohol withdrawal seizures. The study found no difference in primary outcomes, however, dexmedetomidine was associated with more adverse drug events including hypotension and bradycardia. The authors observed a benzodiazepine sparing effect with the use of dexmedetomidine and recommended the use of dexmedetomidine as an adjunct.

9. VanderWeide LA, Foster CJ, MacLaren R, Kiser TH, Fish DN, Mueller SW. Evaluation of early dexmedetomidine addition to the standard of care for severe alcohol withdrawal in the ICU: A retrospective controlled cohort study. *J Int Care Med.* 2016;31(3):198–204.

A retrospective cohort study comparing benzodiazepine requirements in critically ill patients with alcohol withdrawal syndrome who received dexmedetomidine. The study found that the use of dexmedetomidine was associated with a significant decrease in the overall use of benzodiazepines in this patient cohort. The authors concluded that use of dexmedetomidine was associated with a reduction in BZD requirement when utilized as adjunctive therapy for AWS.

10. Ludtke KA, Stanley KS, Yount NL, Gerkin RD. Retrospective review of critically ill patients experiencing alcohol withdrawal: Dexmedetomidine versus propofol and/or lorazepam continuous infusions. *Hosp Pharm.* 2015;50(3):208–213.

This retrospective chart review was conducted on ICU patients with alcohol withdrawal syndrome who received treatment with a continuous infusion of dexmedetomidine, propofol, and/or lorazepam. The study compared the incidence of mechanical ventilation, length of mechanical ventilation, and ICU as well as hospital length of stay. The authors reported a decrease in endotracheal intubation, ICU stay, and hospital length of stay with the use of dexmedetomidine infusion. Small sample size and retrospective nature of the study are the biggest limitations in recommending dexmedetomidine as a sole agent for managing AWS.

11. Flannery AH, Adkins, AD, Cook AM. Unpeeling the evidence for the banana bag: Evidence-based recommendations for the management of alcohol-associated vitamin and electrolyte deficiencies in the ICU. *Crit Care Med.* 2016;44(8):1545–1552.

The authors provide an evidence based review of the electrolyte and vitamin abnormalities associated with patients with chronic alcohol use that are admitted to the ICU. The article also discusses the pathophysiology of the metabolic derangements associated with chronic alcohol use as well as the various evidence based treatment modalities. The authors suggest abandoning the banana bag and provide recommendations on appropriate replacement dosing of various vitamins and mineral in such patients.

Landmark Article of the 21st Century

PHENOBARBITAL FOR ACUTE ALCOHOL WITHDRAWAL: A PROSPECTIVE RANDOMIZED DOUBLE-BLIND PLACEBO-CONTROLLED STUDY

Rosenson J et al., *J Emerg Med.* 2013;44(3):592–598

Commentary by Vasiliy Sim

This was a relatively small study but it is one of the largest randomized, placebo-controlled, double-blinded single institution studies performed in an urban emergency department (ED) on this subject. The study population were patients with a primary admission diagnosis of acute alcohol withdrawal syndrome. All patients were treated using a lorazepam-based modified clinical institute withdrawal assessment (CIWA) protocol. They were then randomized to either one dose of IV phenobarbital 10mg/kg in 100 mL of saline or 100 mL of normal saline. ICU admission rate (8% vs. 25%), total lorazepam used (26 mg vs. 49 mg), and the need for continuous lorazepam infusion (4% vs. 31%) was lower in phenobarbital group. There was no difference in ICU/hospital length of stay, administration of other medications, or adverse outcomes such as intubation, seizure, or restraints.

Limitations: Like many studies preceding this one, the number of randomized subjects was low. Once the patients were randomized there was no defined criteria for ICU admission and was left up to ED providers. Even though it was a blinded study, most ED clinicians would be able to tell patients who received phenobarbital simply by patient's behavior after medication was administered. This knowledge could have affected their decision for ICU admission especially since the administered dose of the phenobarbital was relatively high (twice as high as a loading dose in my institution). Phenobarbital at a high dose can lead to over sedation which will limit its application to patients whose main diagnosis is not alcohol withdrawal and in whom the neurological exam is important (neurotrauma, stroke, etc. ...). A protocolized approach to phenobarbital administration over a longer period of time will allow for lower doses administered, might achieve less over sedation, and may be more generalizable.

Conclusions: In spite of the limitations, I do not want to take away from the importance of this work. This study showed that even a single dose of phenobarbital decreased ICU admissions and total/continuous lorazepam use without an increased rate of adverse events. Phenobarbital should be considered as part of the regimen for management of acute withdrawal syndrome.Hendey GW, Dery RA, Barnes RL, Snowden B, Mentler P. A prospective, randomized, trial of phenobarbital versus benzodiazepines for acute alcohol withdrawal. *Am J Emerg Med.* 2011;29(4):382–385

CHAPTER 49

Nutrition

Review by Ulises Torres Cordero

Specialized nutrition is one of the underestimated areas in critical care. Most intensivists do not possess the armamentarium to define, diagnose, or treat the different malnutrition syndromes effectively. Realizing the presence and the severity of malnutrition changes outcomes. For these reasons, the Academy of Nutrition and Dietetics (AND) and the American Society for Parental and Enteral Nutrition (ASPEN) published a guideline to standardize the diagnostic criteria for malnutrition in 2012. There are six diagnostic criteria used in conjunction with the history and physical examination: 1) energy intake; 2) history of weight loss; 3) loss of muscle mass; 4) loss of fat; 5) edema; and 6) diminished handgrip strength. Using this tool in conjunction with a nutritional support team will assist in identifying malnutrition and possibly improving outcomes. Malnutrition in the ICU varies from 15% to 60%.

A large body of evidence has accumulated over the past decade regarding the assessment of malnutrition and the provision of nutritional support in the critical care patient. Much of these data have been summarized in the *Guidelines for the Provision and Assessment of Nutrition Support Therapy in the Adult Critically Ill Patient* published by the Society of Critical Care Medicine (SCCM) and ASPEN. There are multiple tools available for evaluating nutritional support needs, one of which is the NUTRIC score. It can be calculated using quantitative variables: age, APACHE score, SOFA score, co-morbidities, IL-6 levels, and days from hospital admission to ICU admission. Furthermore, there is a clear association between the score and mortality. In an observational study using the NUTRIC score, patients who met their caloric targets had attenuated mortality and more ventilator-free days.

The options for treatment of malnutrition are enteral nutrition (EN) and parental nutrition (PN). Evidence shows that the initiation of enteral nutrition within 24 to 48 hours of admission results in better outcomes when compared to no nutritional intake and surpasses the early initiation of PN. EN delivery is better performed through a small-bore tube into the duodenum or even jejunum, although it is acceptable to initiate in the stomach. The type of specialized nutrition should start with trophic feeds while awaiting a nutrition evaluation or full nutrition if the dietician has already made recommendations. If there is no relevant gastrointestinal pathology, then they can be increased rapidly while monitoring tolerance. It is not recommended to use gastric residual volume (GRV) measurement as part of routine care to monitor ICU patients receiving EN.

DOI: 10.1201/9781003042136-49

The type of EN formula is based on the characteristics of the patient and the dietitian recommendations. It is essential to consider the need for a combination of antioxidant vitamins, trace minerals, and other supplements as immune nutrients (arginine, glutamine, omega-3 polyunsaturated fatty acids, and RNA nucleotides) that can be very helpful for special populations. Glutamine is contraindicated in patients with acute sepsis and septic shock. Most of the studies published on immunomodulators have been successful in patients undergoing major surgery; these results have not been observed in the medical ICU population.

If the patient cannot tolerate EN and is severely malnourished, PN should be considered early; this first approach is just in the presence of severe malnutrition without any possibility of starting EN in the first 5–7 days of care. There is strong evidence to suggest that late initiation of PN has better outcomes. Casaer et al. studied two large groups in the ICU comparing early initiation to late initiation of PN. They found no difference in mortality, but the late initiation group had shorter ICU stays, fewer infections, shorter duration of mechanical ventilation, and of renal replacement therapy. PN is the second option most of the time. It can induce multiple complications such as hyperglycemia, catheter-related infection, pancreatitis, electrolyte imbalances, fluid overload, and hyperlipidemia. For PN to be effective, it has to be administered for a minimum of 5–7 days. Therefore, a short period of PN/EN combination might be the best option until the patient can tolerate 80% of the protein and caloric needs via EN.

One of the essential macronutrients is protein; unfortunately, the literature has been changing regarding the recommended amount thereby creating confusion on the correct dose and target population. Currently, the recommendation from the AND/ASPEN guidelines is to utilize high protein (2–2.5 g/kg/d). Nevertheless, a new body of evidence shows that those high doses are just beneficial for specific populations like the elderly, obese, severe traumatic injuries, severe burns, or patients undergoing renal replacement therapy (RRT). Other than these populations, the current suggested dose is no more than 1.5 g/kg/d to start the anabolic response or at least stop the catabolic effect of the underlying condition.

The COVID-19 pandemic has forced intensivists to consider new ways to approach critical care nutrition. A new set of recommendations has been published and focuses on bundled care (nutrition, skin care, medicine administration, etc.) to limit provider exposure while preserving the same quality of care. EN should be initiated within the first 24–36 hours utilizing a gastric tube inserted at the time of intubation. EN should be delivered continuously instead of boluses to avoid frequent exposure. For formula selection, it is recommended to use a standard high protein polymeric iso-osmotic formula. If PN has to be utilized, pure soy-based lipid emulsions should be limited during the first week of the acute inflammatory phase of COVID-19. Prone positioning is one of the techniques to increase oxygenation during severe viral pneumonia with COVID-19; it is recommended to deliver early EN into the stomach while elevating the head of the bed 10°–25° and not checking gastric residual volumes.

ANNOTATED REFERENCES FOR NUTRITION

Behrens S, Kozeniecki M, Knapp N, Martindale RG. Nutrition support during prone positioning: An old technique reawakened by COVID-19. *Nutr Clin Pract.* 2020;36(1):105–109.

This is a review of the recommendations and challenges while providing nutrition on a patient with COVID-19 during prone positioning. Recommendations are based on including small frequent meals of high protein, calorically dense foods and beverages for the patient who can have an oral diet, and coincide the feedings with supine positioning. For patients who need specialized nutrition, EN is preferred over PN if the gastrointestinal tract is functional; placement should be performed before turning, it is recommended having the head of the bed elevation at 25°; there is no indication for gastric residual volume checks, but if there are signs of intolerance, using prophylactic prokinetic might be helpful in addition to head elevation in preventing broncho-aspiration. Parental nutrition should be delayed until hospital stay is 5 to 7 days for low-risk patients, but early PN should be considered for patients who are at high nutrition risk. The authors emphasize on focusing care in clusters and strict PPE restrictions.

Casaer MP, Mesotten D, Hermans G, et al. Early versus late parenteral nutrition in critically ill adults. *N Engl J Med.* 2011;365(6):506–517.

This is a prospective, randomized, controlled, parallel-group, multicenter trial, randomized one to one ratio to early or late initiation of parenteral nutrition with a total of 4640 patients. The early initiation group received 20% glucose solution on the first and second day; and on the third-day parental nutrition, with those targeted to 100% of the caloric, go through combine enteral and parenteral nutrition. The late initiation group received a 5% glucose solution, and parental nutrition was initiated on the eighth to reach the calorie goal. The primary endpoint was the duration of dependency on ICU care in the secondary endpoints where new infections duration of antibiotic therapy, inflammation, weaning from mechanical ventilation, kidney injury. There were similar rates of death in both groups; however, the proportion of patients who were discharged alive from the ICU within 8 days was higher in the late initiation group; this group also had one day shorter in the ICU, shorter time in mechanical ventilation and renal replacement therapy. Also, they presented with less new infections. However, the acute inflammatory response was more pronounced than in the early initiation group.

Heyland DK, Dhaliwal R, Jiang X, Day AG. Identifying critically ill patients who benefit the most from nutrition therapy: the development and initial validation of a novel risk assessment tool. *Crit Care.* 2011;15(6):R268.

In this secondary analysis of a prospective observational study in three tertiary care surgical- medical ICU, the authors developed a score using the variables that linked starvation, inflammation, nutritional status, and clinical outcome. Using recent decreased oral intake, pre-ICU stay in the hospital as candidate variables for acute starvation in history of recent weight loss and a low BMI as measures for chronic starvation; to represent inflammatory markers they chose PCT, IL-6, and CRP. The association between risk score and mortality is attenuated in patients who meet their caloric targets. That increased nutritional risk is associated with reduced mortality in high-risk patients only. They demonstrated a statistically significant relation with 28-day mortality and ventilator 3 days except for BMI.

Leyderman I, Yaroshetskiy A, Klek S. Protein requirements in critical illness: Do we really know why to give so much? *J Parenter Enter Nutr.* 2020;44(4):589–598.

In this comprehensive review, the authors address the question of utilizing high doses of protein (2.0–2.5 g/kg/d) for critical care patients in general. They analyze the importance of anabolic resistance, where the elderly are the only demonstrated population to benefit from higher doses of protein. Utilizing nitrogen balance as a marker or protein requirements also showed that the selected population (renal replacement therapy) benefited from high protein doses. Using isotope-labeled studies also demonstrated that doses of 1.5 g/kg/d showed the lowest levels of catabolism in most patients and just a selective population (elderly and obese) benefited from higher doses. The authors also describe possible problems in the liver and during sepsis while using high dose protein. There is enough evidence to suggest that doses of 1.5 g/kg/d are adequate for most critical care patients. There are specific populations that might need higher doses (elderly, obese, trauma, burn, RRT), yet more evidence is needed to refute or confirm this approach to the latter populations.

Martindale R, Patel JJ, Taylor B, et al. Nutrition therapy in critically ill patients with coronavirus disease (COVID-19). *J Parenter Enter Nutr.* 2020;44(7):1174–1184.

This paper summarizes the first attempt to standardize recommendations for critical care nutrition support in patients with COVID-19 infection. The recommendations are based on three main principles: 1) "cluster care," 2), adherence to the Centers for Disease Control and Prevention guidelines on minimizing aerosol droplet exposure, and 3) preservation of PPE use. It is recommended initiating early EN within 24 to 36 hours of admission through an orogastric or nasogastric feeding tube, starting with a low dose hypocaloric or trophic in advancing slowly over the first week to meet the energy goal of 15 to 20 kcal per kilo of actual body weight of a standard high protein polymeric iso-osmotic enter a formula. Recommendations are given about monitoring prone positioning therapy and renal replacement therapy.

McCarthy MS, Martindale RG. Immunonutrition in critical illness: what is the role? *Nutr Clin Pract.* 2018;33(3):348–358.

This publication attempts to define what immunonutrition (IMN) is, review the essential nutrients, the role in clinical illnesses, and their proposed mechanism of action. There is enough evidence to show that immunonutrition is favorable to modulate the inflammatory response to injury and infection and improve clinical outcomes. These immunonutrients include amino acids, nucleotides, and fats, specifically glutamine, arginine, omega-3 PUFA, and RNA nucleotides. The three primary targets for these metabolic-modulating nutrients are mucosal barrier function, cellular defense function, and local or systemic inflammation prevention. Multiple benefits have been mentioned in the literature, but the only robust data showing IMN's significant benefit is in patients undergoing major surgery.

McClave SA, Taylor BE, Martindale R, et al. Guidelines for the provision and assessment of nutrition support therapy in the adult critically ill patient: Society of Critical Care Medicine (SCCM) and American Society for Parenteral and Enteral Nutrition (ASPEN). *J Parenter Enter Nutr.* 2016;40(2):159–211.

These clinical guidelines are the most comprehensive nutrition guidelines presented by the ASPEN and SCCM after reviewing the evidence of each recommendation classified from high-quality grade in randomized controlled trials, and low-quality grade for observational studies, cohort, case series, and case studies. Over most of the recommendations are based on expert consensus. It is recommended to review all the aspects of nutrition assessment, how to initiate EN, dosing, monitoring tolerance and adequacy of EN, parental nutrition indications, and specific examples for different pathologies like nutrition and pulmonary failure, renal failure, hepatic failure, acupuncture Titus, and a particular subset of populations in the surgical arena obesity, chronic illness, and sepsis.

Patel JJ, Kozeniecki M, Peppard WJ, et al. Phase 3 pilot randomized controlled trial comparing early trophic enteral nutrition with "no enteral nutrition" in mechanically ventilated patients with septic shock. *J Parenter Enteral Nutr.* 2020;44(5):866–873.

This is a phase 3 single center pilot parallel-group randomized controlled study, aimed to compare early traffic EN with no EN in mechanically ventilated medical ICU patients with septic shock; the study was not powered to give definitive conclusions on the outcomes. Nevertheless, the early end group reached 1.2 kcal/mL formula within 16 hours while on vasopressor. The no EN group was withheld until the vasopressor support was discontinued for at least 3 hours averaging 48 hours to start. Complications in the EN group were vomiting in 20% of the cases compared to 56% and then no EN group. There was no occlusive mesenteric ischemia (NOMI) or ileus in either group; this differs from the REDOX, CALORIES, and TARGET trials, large contemporary RCTs where NOMI occurred in 0.3%, 0.9%, and 0.05%, respectively.

Landmark Article of the 21st Century

EARLY VERSUS LATE PARENTERAL NUTRITION IN CRITICALLY ILL ADULTS

Casaer MP et al., *N Engl J Med.* 2011;365:506–517

Commentary by Michael P Casaer and Greet Van den Berghe

For decades, nutrition therapy in intensive care units (ICUs) strived at attenuating the dramatic acute catabolism. For this purpose, early administration of preferentially enteral nutrition (EN) was advocated. If EN couldn't cover the estimated needs, the guidelines recommended to complement EN with parenteral nutrition (PN), but they disagreed on when to initiate PN.

This question was addressed by the EPaNIC-trial, the first large nutrition randomized, controlled trial (RCT) in the ICU and adhering to new standards of trial-registration and conduct. Patients were randomized to receive either PN, targeting nutritional target, if EN was insufficient on ICU-day-2 (Early-PN) or to receive no PN before day 8 (Late-PN).

Late-PN, despite the resulting nutritional deficit, resulted in faster recovery, fewer infections and complications, better muscle force and a shorter ICU and hospital stay. In 517 patients admitted after complicated abdominal or esophageal surgery, Late-PN resulted in 1 week of near-starvation, yet its beneficial effects were even more pronounced.

Thereafter, we conducted a similar RCT (PEPaNIC) in pediatric ICUs in Belgium, the Netherlands, and Canada. Despite their limited reserves and higher presumed metabolic needs, children, particularly neonates, benefitted even more from Late-PN.

The deleterious effect of Early-PN on muscle force was explained by inhibition of autophagy, an intracellular mechanism for damage clearing. These data and detailed analyses of the relation between macronutrient intake and outcome in EPaNIC and PEPaNIC revealed that not the parenteral route per se, but the early high dose of amino acids may have hampered recovery.

EPaNIC showed that is possible, ethical, and crucial to evaluate established therapies in adequately powered RCTs.

CHAPTER 50

Telemedicine in the ICU

Review by Craig M. Lilly and Jason Kovacevic

The penetration of personal electronics into daily living has created a greater appreciation for key convenience and functional advantages that electronic devices have over their analog antecedents. The ways that video feeds can enhance our appreciation of music or short video clips can enhance task-based learning have guided the application of audio-video technologies to critical care medicine. It is not surprising in this era with dramatic growth of interactions by social media that an increasing number of patients and providers prefer the option of telemedicine assisted care delivery [1–3]. The recent growth in the use of telemedicine tools for the critically ill has been driven by the wide realization that providers can deliver high-quality evaluation and management services at lower costs and infection risk than they can provide using geography restricted rounding models [4]. The article highlighted here established that implementation of an ICU telemedicine program can simultaneously improve outcomes and reduce costs at an academic medical center.

The implementation of hub and spoke model tele-ICUs rapidly expanded in the early 2000s with the number of tele-ICU programs increasing from less than 20 to over 200 in the intervening 10 years. Similarly, the number of ICU beds covered by tele-ICU grew over this time period to more than 5000 beds covered by formal tele-ICU services [4]. During the pre-pandemic period of formal ICU telemedicine program growth there was wide recognition that access to high quality specialty medical care was particularly limited among the geographically isolated people served by the Health Resources and Services Administration (HRSA) and that the ability of ICU telemedicine programs to improve access to specialty care in these settings was worthy of fiscal support [5].

The practical ability of ICU telemedicine programs to improve the efficiency of critical care at urban tertiary medical centers where access to specialty care was not as limited as for rural patients, was far more controversial. Equipoise with regard to the ability of ICU telemedicine programs to standardize adult critical care delivery practices and observe clinically important changes in outcomes was driven in no small part by early reports from tertiary centers that failed both to replicate the model [6].

A more carefully implemented and better controlled study was needed to address whether, and explore how, hub and spoke model ICU telemedicine programs can impact care delivery and cost structure at academic medical centers. A 2011 study published in the *Journal of the American Medical Association* measured the association of a homogeneously applied hub and spoke model ICU telemedicine intervention at a large academic medical center [7]. The primary outcome of the study was severity and case mix adjusted hospital mortality with secondary outcomes of ICU mortality and hospital and ICU length of stay. The hospital mortality rate was 13.6% (95% confidence interval [CI], 11–15.4%) during the preintervention period compared with 11.8% (95% CI, 10.9–12.8%) during the tele-ICU intervention period (adjusted odds ratio [OR], 0.40 [95% CI, 0.31–0.52]). The ICU mortality rate was 10.7% for the preintervention group and 8.6% for the tele-ICU group and yielded an OR of 0.37 (95% CI, 0.28–0.49; $p = 0.003$) after adjustment for acuity, locus of care, physiological parameters, laboratory values, and time trends. The intervention was associated with shorter hospital length of stay (9.8 vs. 13.3 days, respectively; hazard ratio for discharge, 1.44 [95% CI, 1.33–1.56]). The mean length of ICU stay was 6.4 days in the preintervention group and 4.5 days in the tele-ICU group. HR was 1.26 (95% CI, 1.17–1.36; $p < 0.001$) after adjustment. The results for medical, surgical, and cardiovascular ICU patients were similar. Significantly, outcomes from step-wedge and before and after analyses yielded equivalent results.

In order to define the association of ICU telemedicine program implementation with improved outcomes, the study included internal validity analyses that measured the association of the intervention with adherence to the critical care best practices that the ICU leadership team had targeted, calculated the effects of differences in adherence with the rates of the preventable complications they were designed to reduce, and calculated their contributions to the changes in mortality and length of stay outcomes. These analyses revealed that 25–30% of the association of the ICU telemedicine intervention with lower mortality and shorter length of stay was accounted for by increased rates of adherence to ICU best practices. ICU telemedicine critical care best practice review, communication, and remediation achieved significantly higher rates of adherence than daily ICU bedside team review of a reminder list alone.

The step-wedge analysis also provided evidence of internal validity and evidence that the association of the intervention with better outcomes could not be fully accounted for by secular trends toward better critical care alone. Because patients were assigned to a specific ICU bed based on availability some patients were assigned to a same type ICU in which the ICU telemedicine hardware was installed while their counterparts were assigned to an ICU where the intervention was not yet available. Comparison of concurrent patients revealed that patients who were assigned to units that had the intervention had outcomes that were similar to those of the ICU telemedicine intervention group, and those assigned to units where the intervention was not yet available had outcomes similar to the those of the preintervention control group.

This study [7] advanced the field of telemedicine because it demonstrated that the addition of ICU telemedicine support to well-staffed academic medical center that aggressively used the best available non-electronic tools could improve mortality and length of stay outcomes. Its publication was followed by multicenter trials that demonstrated its generalizability by showing that its main findings were also evident among a group of diverse and geographically dispersed [8] health care systems [9, 10], studies that addressed cost concerns by finding significant direct and logistical support-related financial benefits to adopting "hub" institutions [11], as well as clinical and financial benefits to "spoke" institutions who leveraged off-hours access to ICU specialists to retain their critically ill adults [12].

In addition to the ability for ICU telemedicine programs to standardize ICU care delivery and prevent, better recognize, and deliver earlier interventions for episodes of physiological instability, the COVID-19 pandemic has created new use case scenarios for ICU telemedicine tools. The pandemic has witnessed a broadening of use [1] to eliminate unnecessary room entry events, reduce the number of provider aerosol exposure events, and to reduce the associated waste of personal protective equipment [2]. Hospital mortality, length of stay, and preventable complications among critically ill patients before and after tele-ICU reengineering of critical care processes was the gateway to new dimensions of ICU care [7].

ANNOTATED REFERENCES FOR TELEMEDICINE IN THE ICU

1. Kichloo A, Albosta M, Dettloff K, et al. Telemedicine, the current COVID-19 pandemic and the future: A narrative review and perspectives moving forward in the USA. *Fam Med Community Health.* 2020;8(3).
2. Moazzami B, Razavi-Khorasani N, Dooghaie Moghadam A, Farokhi E, Rezaei N. COVID-19 and telemedicine: Immediate action required for maintaining healthcare providers well-being. *J Clin Virol.* 2020;126:104345.

   These references detail patient and provider perspectives on the role of telemedicine during the COVID-19 pandemic.

3. Welch BM, Harvey J, O'Connell NS, McElligott JT. Patient preferences for direct-to-consumer telemedicine services: a nationwide survey. *BMC Health Serv Res.* 2017;17(1):784.

   This study documents current patient preferences for the convenience and safety of telemedicine- based encounters.

4. Lilly CM, Zubrow MT, Kempner KM, et al. Critical care telemedicine: evolution and state of the art. *Crit Care Med.* 2014;42(11):2429–2436.

   This review documents the pre-pandemic adoption of ICU telemedicine hub and spoke model tele-ICUs.

5. Ward MM, Carter KD, Ullrich F, et al. Averted transfers in rural emergency departments using telemedicine: rates and costs across six networks. *Telemed J E Health.* 2020.

   Fiscal support from the federal government was an important driver of the increased access to critical care specialist services for rural Americans provided by tele-ICUs.

6. Thomas EJ, Lucke JF, Wueste L, Weavind L, Patel B. Association of telemedicine for remote monitoring of intensive care patients with mortality, complications, and length of stay. *JAMA.* 2009;302(24):2671–2678.

   This academic medical center study demonstrated that when telemedicine programs were implemented by administrative fiat without bedside intensivist support that improvements of outcomes were not significant.

7. Lilly CM, Cody S, Zhao H, et al. Hospital mortality, length of stay, and preventable complications among critically ill patients before and after tele-ICU reengineering of critical care processes. *JAMA*. 2011;305(21):2175–2183.

    This landmark study found that collaborative interprofessional ICU telemedicine-supported reengineering of critical care delivery processes was associated with improved mortality and length of stay that could be accounted for by care standardization metrics.

8. Lilly CM, Fisher KA, Ries M, et al. A national ICU telemedicine survey: validation and results. *Chest*. 2012;142(1):40–47.

    This study which was sponsored by the ACCP created a validated tool for assessing adult critical care processes. This made it possible to distinguish tele-ICU implementations where processes of care were changed from those with processes of care that did not change.

9. Lilly CM, McLaughlin JM, Zhao H, et al. A multicenter study of ICU telemedicine reengineering of adult critical care. *Chest*. 2014;145(3):500–507.

    This multicenter study of a geographically dispersed and nationally representative cohort of institutions that implemented hub and spoke ICU telemedicine programs found the main findings of the landmark study were also present among this sample of United States ICUs. It used the validated process of care tool (reference 8) to associate larger improvements with greater changes in the targeted processes of care. This allowed identification of the process factors that may mediate ICU telemedicine-associated improvement in length of stay and mortality. It also identified substantial variation among adopting institutions with regard to factors that were amenable to modification after tele-ICU implementation.

10. Kahn JM, Le TQ, Barnato AE, et al. ICU telemedicine and critical care mortality: A national effectiveness study. *Med Care*. 2016;54(3):319–325.

    This study confirmed that mortality benefits of tele-ICU programs were evident in large administrative datasets. It is particularly convincing because these effects were evident using methods that allowed admixture of patients who did not receive tele-ICU supported care to be included in the telemedicine intervention group.

11. Lilly CM, Motzkus CA. ICU telemedicine: Financial analyses of a complex intervention. *Crit Care Med*. 2017;45(9):1558–1561.

    The financial benefits of ICU telemedicine programs and the benefits of leveraging them to provide logistical support are detailed over a time period that is long enough to identify durable effects. It provides insights into the macroeconomics of adult ICU care that many intensivists are not familiar with. The study quantifies the effects of increasing access to ICU care using real-time methods that reduce length of stay and increase volume. Its main finding is that the financial benefits of ICU telemedicine program implementation to the United States hub institutions greatly exceeded its costs.

12. Fifer S, Everett W, Adams M, Vincequere J. Critical care, critical choices the case for tele-ICUs in intensive care. New England Healthcare Institute; Massachusetts Technology Collaborative; 2010.
    http://www.masstech.org/teleICU.pdf.

    This study, funded by the New England Healthcare Institute, documents increased access to critical care specialty care for the patients of spoke hospitals. In addition, it documents the financial benefits. This finding was by supported independent PriceWaterhouse Cooper audits of this and the financial outcomes paper (reference 11) and acuity adjustment methods.

Landmark Article of the 21st Century

HOSPITAL MORTALITY, LENGTH OF STAY, AND PREVENTABLE COMPLICATIONS AMONG CRITICALLY ILL PATIENTS BEFORE AND AFTER TELE-ICU REENGINEERING OF CRITICAL CARE PROCESSES

Lilly C et al., *JAMA.* 2011;305(21):2175–2183

Commentary by Craig M. Lilly

In my role as the medical director of an ICU at a 600-bed, major Harvard teaching hospital, I became aware that we were limited by a lack of timely, accurate, and actionable data about our processes of critical care delivery. Telemedicine solutions that allowed real-time action based on accurate data became commercially available around 2003. While the patient safety advantages of a tele-ICU implementation were clear, provider concerns about chain of command and regarding the ability of faculty to effectively communicate care plans to a colleague prevented adoption. While this provider versus patient centered debate was being vetted, I was invited to lead an implementation at UMass Memorial Heath Care (UMMHC) as a member of the University of Massachusetts Medical School faculty.

This was a golden opportunity to test the hypothesis that using cameras, microphones, accurate data, and timely reports, could significantly and positively impact both cost and quality metrics. Moreover, I would be able to apply telemedicine support to an ICU delivery system that had already been optimized, to the extent this was possible, without electronic tools. It was necessary to install an operational electronic medical record system, integrate audio and video components, and get buy-in for not changing the agreed upon evidence-based practice standards, ICU schedules, and organizational structure during the study. Accomplishing these tasks would not have been possible without the extraordinary support and wisdom of Shawn Cody, PhD, our ICU nurse leader, and Richard S. Irwin, MD, the chair of the UMMMC Critical Care Operations Committee.

Index

Printed in the United States
by Baker & Taylor Publisher Services